Mood Disorders: Diagnosis and Treatment

Mood Disorders: Diagnosis and Treatment

Edited by Sean Gunner

hayle medical

New York

Hayle Medical,
750 Third Avenue, 9th Floor,
New York, NY 10017, USA

Visit us on the World Wide Web at:
www.haylemedical.com

ISBN: 978-1-63241-590-5

The publisher's policy is to use permanent paper from mills that operate a sustainable forestry policy. Furthermore, the publisher ensures that the text paper and cover boards used have met acceptable environmental accreditation standards.

Printed in China.

Cataloging-in-Publication Data

Mood disorders : diagnosis and treatment / edited by Sean Gunner.
p. cm.
Includes bibliographical references and index.
ISBN 978-1-63241-590-5
1. Affective disorders. 2. Affective disorders--Diagnosis. 3. Affective disorders--Treatment.
I. Gunner, Sean.
RC537 .M66 2019
616.852 7--dc23

Table of Contents

Preface

Mood disorders refer to a group of elevated and depressed mood conditions. These are classified as depressive disorders, bipolar disorders, substance-induced disorders or triggered by other medical conditions. Major depressive disorder or depression is a disorder that is characterized by low mood present across all situations and accompanied by a loss of interest in normally enjoyable activities, low self-esteem, low energy and pain caused by an unidentifiable cause. Antidepressants are generally recommended for people with depression. Bipolar disorder is another mental disorder, which causes periods of abnormally elevated mood and depression. During the elevated phase, an individual feels abnormally energetic, happy or irritable, while during depressive periods, there may be a general negative outlook towards life, crying and poor eye contact with people. Antipsychotics, mood stabilizers and melatonin may be prescribed for the treatment of bipolar disorders. This book is a compilation of chapters that discuss the most vital concepts and emerging trends in the diagnosis and treatment of mood disorders. It aims to give a general view of the different types of mood disorders and their implications in the psychological health of individuals. Students, researchers, experts and all associated with psychiatry, psychology and neurology will benefit alike from this book.

This book has been the outcome of endless efforts put in by authors and researchers on various issues and topics within the field. The book is a comprehensive collection of significant researches that are addressed in a variety of chapters. It will surely enhance the knowledge of the field among readers across the globe.

It gives us an immense pleasure to thank our researchers and authors for their efforts to submit their piece of writing before the deadlines. Finally in the end, I would like to thank my family and colleagues who have been a great source of inspiration and support.

Editor

1

Depression in Working Adults: Comparing the Costs and Health Outcomes of Working When Ill

Fiona Cocker[1,4*], Jan M. Nicholson[2], Nicholas Graves[3], Brian Oldenburg[1], Andrew J. Palmer[4], Angela Martin[5], Jenn Scott[6], Alison Venn[4], Kristy Sanderson[4]

1 School of Population and Global Health, University of Melbourne, Melbourne, Australia, **2** Judith Lumley Centre, La Trobe University, Melbourne, Australia, **3** School of Public Health, Queensland University of Technology, Queensland, Australia, **4** Menzies Research Institute Tasmania, University of Tasmania, Hobart, Australia, **5** Tasmanian School of Business and Economics, University of Tasmania, Hobart, Australia, **6** School of Psychology, University of Tasmania, Hobart, Tasmania, Australia

Abstract

Objective: Working through a depressive illness can improve mental health but also carries risks and costs from reduced concentration, fatigue, and poor on-the-job performance. However, evidence-based recommendations for managing work attendance decisions, which benefit individuals and employers, are lacking. Therefore, this study has compared the costs and health outcomes of short-term absenteeism versus working while ill ("presenteeism") amongst employed Australians reporting lifetime major depression.

Methods: Cohort simulation using state-transition Markov models simulated movement of a hypothetical cohort of workers, reporting lifetime major depression, between health states over one- and five-years according to probabilities derived from a quality epidemiological data source and existing clinical literature. Model outcomes were health service and employment-related costs, and quality-adjusted-life-years (QALYs), captured for absenteeism relative to presenteeism, and stratified by occupation (blue versus white-collar).

Results: Per employee with depression, absenteeism produced higher mean costs than presenteeism over one- and five-years ($42,573/5-years for absenteeism, $37,791/5-years for presenteeism). However, overlapping confidence intervals rendered differences non-significant. Employment-related costs (lost productive time, job turnover), and antidepressant medication and service use costs of absenteeism and presenteeism were significantly higher for white-collar workers. Health outcomes differed for absenteeism versus presenteeism amongst white-collar workers only.

Conclusions: Costs and health outcomes for absenteeism and presenteeism were not significantly different; service use costs excepted. Significant variation by occupation type was identified. These findings provide the first occupation-specific cost evidence which can be used by clinicians, employees, and employers to review their management of depression-related work attendance, and may suggest encouraging employees to continue working is warranted.

Editor: Leona Hakkaart, institute of Health Policy and Management, Netherlands

Funding: Dr. Cocker completed this work whilst in receipt of a Pro Vice Chancellor (Research) Australian Research Council Strategic Research Scholarship (ARC Linkage Project LP0990010). This work was funded by a National Health and Medical Research Council (NHMRC) Project Grant (ID490018) awarded to Associate Professor Sanderson who was funded by an Australian Research Council Future Fellowship (FT991524). Professor Palmer has received advisory board payments in the area of diabetes from Jansen, Johnson and Johnson, sanofi Aventis, and Novo Nordisk. The listed funders had no role in study design, data collection and analysis, decision to publish, or preparation of the manuscript.

Competing Interests: Prof. Palmer has received advisory board payments in the area of diabetes from Jansen, Johnson and Johnson, sanofi Aventis, and Novo Nordisk.

* Email: fiona.cocker@unimelb.edu.au

Introduction

The economic cost of depression is largely due to related work impairment, disability [1], and lost productivity from sickness absenteeism and presenteeism (continuing to work when ill) [2]. Presenteeism is common [3], more costly than absenteeism [3,4], and may account for up to 80% of depression-related lost productive time [2]. Internationally, this equates to an estimated 35.7 billion USD [2], 15.1 billion UK pounds [5] and 12.6 billion Australian dollars [6] annually. However, the health outcomes of presenteeism are less established [7]. Although presenteeism has been shown to increase the incidence of serious coronary events [8], and predict poor self-rated health [9] and future sickness absence [10], it may also confer health benefits via supervisor or colleague support and a maintained daily routine [11]. In fact, its potential health benefits may outweigh any negative health outcomes and economic costs.

Evidence regarding the economic costs and health benefits of absenteeism *and* presenteeism is essential to inform the design of workplace depression management strategies [12], particularly those focused on promotion and prevention. At present, the right balance between absenteeism and presenteeism for employees with depression is unknown. Therefore, current clinical practice guidelines for employers or employees seeking informed advice about when continued work attendance is optimal are lacking.

Further, despite awareness that work characteristics and demands can influence employee attitudes to work attendance or render them either unable or reluctant to take time off when sick [13], evidence of whether the costs and health consequences of absenteeism and presenteeism differ by occupation is scarce. Therefore, it is unclear whether work attendance recommendations should be tailored to different job types.

This study used population level data and a Markov cohort simulation approach to compare the costs and health outcomes of working while ill versus work absence over time amongst employed Australians reporting lifetime major depression. The model was amended to quantify variations across occupation (blue vs. white collar). With the information provided this study aimed to: i) determine whether continuing to work when ill or taking a planned, short-term sickness absence is the more cost-effective decision for employees reporting depression; and ii) determine whether subsequent recommendations should be altered by occupation type.

Method

Definition of scenarios and type of Analysis

We conducted an epidemiologic-based, analytic modelling study, using cohort simulation and a state-transition Markov model, to compare the costs and health outcomes of working while experiencing depression versus taking a sickness absence. The decision analysis approach used in this study requires presenteeism and absenteeism to be defined as mutually exclusive scenarios. Presenteeism, was therefore defined as the absence of absenteeism, consistent with previous approaches [8]. In other words, no reported depression-specific, work- and role-functioning disability days in response to the NSMHWB depression module item "About how many days out of 365 in the past 12 months were you totally unable to work or carry out your normal activities because of your (sadness/or/discouragement/or/lack of interest)?". Absenteeism, was the converse. Therefore, this analysis is based on two assumptions; a) all employed individuals with 12-month depression will experience impairment relevant to their work; and b) the categories of 12-month absenteeism and presenteeism are mutually exclusive. This method was selected as it provides a measure of depression-specific disability days and therefore removes the possible influence of co-morbid disorders of work attendance decisions.

Two subsequent models determined whether outcomes differed for blue- versus white-collar workers. All models were identically structured and generated using Data TreeAge Pro software (Williamstown, Mass.). Cohort simulation was deemed appropriate as it synthesises best available evidence to address difficult-to-answer questions, and is ideal when experimental trials are not ethical or feasible. Cohort simulation is commonly used in health economics, and related clinical and epidemiological research, to model future costs and outcomes of patients, groups or populations under alternative scenarios such as different treatment options [25] and is unique in that it is able to predict cross-sectional data and simulate life courses of people, providing longitudinal outcomes. A wide range of evidence is usually included, such as epidemiologic surveys, meta-analyses, and high-quality single studies in order to determine the benefits and costs beyond time horizon of existing data [26][37].

Analytic Structure and Time Horizon

A hypothetical cohort of employees (N = 1000) occupied and moved between seven health states over time according to probabilities (Figure 1) [14]. A 3-month cycle length was chosen to reflect the natural history of depression, and the selected health states are clinically relevant and informed by related research [14]. Where relevant, health states were assigned lost productive time, job turnover, and health service use costs, and a utility value consistent with a depression diagnosis (depressed/not depressed) and treatment status (in treatment/not in treatment). The number of people and the amount of time they spent in each health state determined the aggregate costs and health outcomes at the conclusion of the model. Costs and health outcomes were considered from the societal perspective over 1-year, and extended to a 5-year time horizon to produce results relevant to employers' decision-making time frames i.e. those interested in improving outcomes for their current employees.

Data Sources

Probabilities and costs were derived from our primary epidemiological data source, the National Survey of Mental Health and Wellbeing (2007) (NSMHWB) [15], or published literature. The NSMHWB is a stratified, random household survey conducted by the Australian Bureau of Statistics (ABS) to determine lifetime and 12-month prevalence estimates of affective and other common psychiatric disorders within the Australian population. To estimate the prevalence of specific mental disorders, the NSMHWB used the World Mental Health Survey Initiative version of the World Health Organization's Composite International Diagnostic Interview, version 3.0 (WMH-CIDI 3.0). This is a comprehensive interview used to assess the lifetime, 12-month, and 30-day prevalence of selected mental disorders by measuring symptoms and their impact on day-to-day activities. It provides an assessment of mental disorders based on the definitions and criteria of two classification systems: the Diagnostic and Statistical Manual of Mental Disorders, Fourth Edition (DSM-IV); and the WHO International Classification of Diseases, Tenth Revision (ICD-10). Both the DSM-IV and the ICD-10 have sets of criteria, necessary for diagnosis, which specify the nature and number of symptoms required, the level of distress or impairment required, and the exclusion of cases where symptoms can be attributed to general medical conditions, such as a physical injury, or to substances, including alcohol. The WMH-CIDI 3.0 was also used to collect information on the course, onset, recency and persistence of symptoms of mental disorders, the impact of mental disorders on home, work, relationship and social functioning, and treatment seeking and access to adequate treatment.

The NSMHWB received a response rate of 60% (N = 8841) and data were weighted to represent the projected Australian adult population (N = 16 015 300) thus ensuring the data and findings derived from this survey are generalisable to the total in scope population. More specifically, weighting adjusts results from a sample survey to infer results for the total in-scope population by allocating a 'weight' to each sample unit corresponding to the level at which population statistics are produced, e.g. household or person level. This weight is considered an indication of how many population units are represented by the sample unit. ABS household surveys are calibrated to population benchmarks by state, part of state, age and sex. Initial person weights were simultaneously calibrated to population benchmarks for state by part of state, age, sex, state by household composition, state by educational attainment, and state by labour force status. Household weights were derived by separately calibrating initial household selection weights to the projected household composition population counts of households containing persons aged 16–85 years, who were living in private dwellings in each state and territory of Australia, at 31 October 2007.

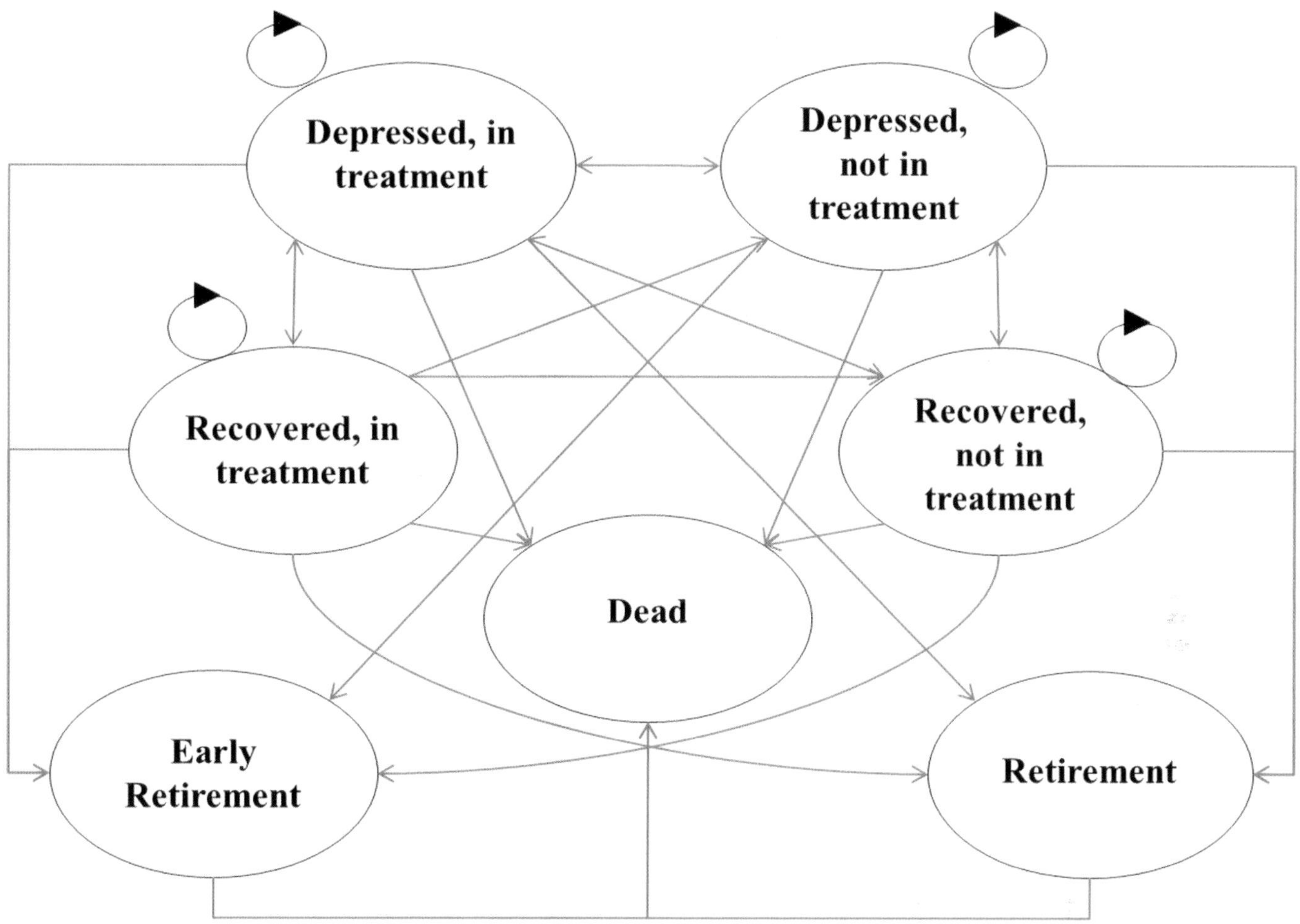

Figure 1. State transition Markov model diagram.

Occupation type was derived from the employment component of the NSMHWB, which was summarised according to the Australian and New Zealand Standard Classification of Occupation (ANZSCO) [16]. Data from published studies determined the probability [17] and cost [18] of depression-related job turnover, mean presenteeism days [19], and absenteeism and presenteeism-related lost productive time costs [2,20].

Initial Probabilities

The NSMHWB provided the major depression diagnosis used to distribute the cohort among health states (Figure 1), and the reported depression-specific disability days used to determine distribution between absenteeism and presenteeism scenarios. The probability of being in each of the health states for a hypothetical white or blue collar worker reporting absenteeism are presented in Table S2, initial probabilities for white and blue collar workers reporting presenteeism are presented in Table S3. (see Tables S1, S2, S3) [21]. Models only included individuals with depression, as determined by current 12-month symptoms or any lifetime experience. Individuals were defined as 'depressed' if they reported 12-month depression symptoms, or 'recovered' if they reported lifetime depression without 12-month symptoms. 'In treatment' referred to self-reported contact with a health professional for a mental health problem any time in the last 12-months [15]. Individuals started the simulation process in a 'depressed' or a 'recovered' state (Figure 1).

Transition Probabilities

Transition probabilities were derived from relevant secondary sources (see Table S1, S2, S3), applied in each successive 3-month cycle, and governed the cohort's movement between health states over time (see Table S1, S2, S3). Tables S1, S2 and S3 demonstrate how they differed according to occupation type (Table S1, S2, S3). Remission (with and without treatment) determined movement from a 'depressed' to a 'recovered' state, and relapse (with and without treatment) was the converse. The transition probabilities were derived from published findings from a national survey of the US population [2,4], (see Table S1) in which diagnoses were made using the Primary Care Evaluation of Mental Disorders (PRIME-MD) instrument. The PRIME-MD has been shown to have excellent agreement with clinical diagnoses made using the lengthier diagnostic interviews such as the CIDI [35,36]. Treatment initiation probabilities determined movement from a 'not in treatment' to an 'in treatment' state. Age- and sex-specific mortality/survival rates determined movement to the 'deceased' state. All depression states had an increased mortality rate due to risk of suicide, and an increased risk of early retirement (before the age of 50). The deceased and retirement health states were absorbing states, which individuals could not leave once entered.

Costs

Lost productive time, job turnover, depression-related service use and antidepressant medication costs were assigned to each health state (see Table S1, S2, S3). They were based on the probability of various cost-incurring events being experienced, the number of times that event occurred, and the unit cost assigned to that event. All costs were in 2007 Australian dollars (AUD), to reflect the reference year of the NSMHWB. Lost productive time costs involved multiplying the number of depression-specific absenteeism and presenteeism days, adjusted to a 3-month estimate, by the average daily wage. Daily wage, weekly wage and annual salary were calculated using the Australian Bureau of Statistics estimates of employee earnings and hours averaged across all occupations, and blue collar and white collar occupations separately, as defined by ANZSCO [16]. Depression-related job turnover costs included the recruitment, hiring and training costs of replacing an employee who is terminated or voluntarily leaves. The job turnover probability estimate, although deemed the best available [22], was from a sample considered unrepresentative of the general population. Therefore, probabilities were restricted to 'depressed in treatment' states [17]. The NSMHWB provided depression-specific service use and antidepressant medication costs. Number of contacts in the past year with general practitioners, psychologists, psychiatrists, mental health nurses and alternative therapists were costed using Australia's national health insurance scheme information (the Medicare Benefits Schedule). Reported 2-week antidepressant medication use was converted to 3-month probability estimates. As the type/s of antidepressant used, and duration and dosage were unknown, prescriptions were costed for 3-months using the medication type (Selective Serotonin Reuptake Inhibitors) and dosage recommended under optimal care [23].

Health Outcomes

Quality-adjusted life years (QALYs), a combination of quality (measured using utilities) and duration of life, were the primary measure of health outcome (see Table S1, S2, S3). Utilities are a global measure of the value attached to each health state and ideal to capture the broad effects on health and wellbeing possible from presenteeism and absenteeism [7,8]. The applicability of utility-weighted, population health outcomes to depression has been demonstrated [24]. The NSMHWB [15] provided utilities derived from the Assessment of Quality of Life-4D (AQoL-4D) [25], a validated measure, able to detect subtle quality-of-life differences in areas including mental health [26].

Sensitivity Analysis

Probabilistic sensitivity analysis using Monte Carlo simulation determined the total costs and health outcomes of all models. Values for all model parameters were sampled from specified distributions. These were beta distributions for probabilities, gamma distributions for costs and uniform distributions when true functional form was unknown as recommended by published guidelines for decision modelling in health economic evaluation [27]. Expected costs and health outcomes were calculated for a hypothetical cohort of 1000 workers. Re-sampling from each distribution and recalculating the costs and health outcomes from the model generated a distribution of the estimated values. 95% credible intervals were estimated from the simulated data. Costs and QALYs were both discounted at 3% [14,28].

Univariate sensitivity analysis was performed by varying single-parameter values according to credible ranges, informed by existing literature, and re-running the model. Parameters selected for further investigation were those most likely to influence differences in cost; probability and cost of job turnover, daily wage and annual salary. Daily wage, weekly wage, and annual salary were replaced with identical values for blue- and white-collar workers to explore whether observed differences between the groups were due to white-collar workers' higher mean wage. Job turnover cost, represented in both models by a large range of 0.75–1.5 times a worker's annual salary, was widened further to represent the full range of estimates reported in the literature; 0.5–10 times a worker's annual salary. Job turnover probability for workers experiencing depression was increased from 10.5% to 25% and 50%, a realistic probability according to current estimates.

Results

Base Case Model

Table 1 presents mean costs and health outcomes for absenteeism and presenteeism over one-year with 95% credible intervals. Outcomes are presented for the base case, and blue- and white-collar models. The 1-year total mean cost of absenteeism per employee with depression was $9626, presenteeism costs were $7864. While total costs and all cost contributors (job turnover costs, lost productive time, antidepressant medication and service use) were higher for absenteeism reporters than presenteeism, the only significant difference was for service use costs (Table 2). One-year health outcomes did not significantly differ for absenteeism reporters relative to presenteeism reporters, based on overlapping 95% credible intervals (Table 1).

Five-year total simulated costs per worker for absenteeism were $42 573 (95% CI: $19 269–$69 348), presenteeism costs ($37 791, 95% CI $17 475–$66 781) were not significantly different. Further, 5-year health outcomes did not significantly differ for absenteeism (2.70 QALYS; 95% CI 2.16–3.57) compared to presenteeism reporters (3.14 QALYs; 95% CI 2.34–3.75).

Blue- and White-collar Models

One-year total simulated cost of absenteeism was $6223 per blue-collar worker and $12 938 per white-collar worker (Table 1). Over 1-year, presenteeism cost an estimated $5370 per blue-collar worker and $11 178 per white-collar worker. Job turnover, lost productive time, antidepressant medication and depression-related service use costs were all significantly higher for white-collar workers (Table 2).

While not significantly different, blue-collar workers reporting absenteeism showed a trend towards better 1-year health outcomes (0.57 QALYs; 95% CI 0.51–0.60) compared to white-collar absenteeism reporters (0.54 QALYs; 95% CI 0.49–0.56). Similarly, blue-collar presenteeism reporters had slightly better health outcomes (0.65 QALYs; 95% CI 0.58–0.66) when compared to white-collar presenteeism reporters (0.66 QALYs; 95% CI 0.60–0.71) (Table 1). Within the white collar workforce, presenteeism reporters had significantly better quality of life (0.66 QALYs) compared to white collar workers who reported absenteeism (0.54 QALYs). There were no differences in health outcomes for blue collar workers reporting absenteeism versus presenteeism.

The simulated costs and health outcomes of absenteeism and presenteeism over 5-years differed for blue- versus white-collar workers. Five-year total simulated cost of absenteeism was $26 401 per blue-collar worker and $63 771 per white-collar worker. Presenteeism costs were estimated at $23 711 per blue-collar and $54 709 per white-collar worker. Five-year health outcomes did not significantly differ for blue-collar workers reporting absenteeism (2.74 QALYs) compared to white-collar absenteeism reporters

Table 1. One-year cost and health outcomes of absenteeism and presenteeism.

	Absenteeism		Presenteeism	
	Estimate	**95% Credible Interval**	**Estimate**	**95% Credible Interval**
Blue Collar				
Cost ($ AUD)	6223	4722–5997	5370	5589–6833
QALYs	0.57	0.51–0.60	0.65	0.58–0.66
White Collar				
Cost ($ AUD)	12 938	11 442–14 416	11 178	9662–12 764
QALYs	0.54	0.49–0.56	0.66	0.60–0.71
Base Case				
Cost ($ AUD)	9626	6224–11 384	7864	4452–9565
QALYs	0.60	0.40–0.84	0.68	0.48–0.89

(2.64 QALYs). Nor did they differ for blue-collar presenteeism reporters (3.12 QALYs) when compared to white-collar presenteeism reporters (3.20 QALYs).

Sensitivity Analysis

Probabilistic sensitivity analysis revealed wide 95% credible intervals around the cost of job turnover for blue-collar and white-collar workers, by absenteeism and presenteeism, for both time frames (Table 2). This highlights the importance of job turnover in terms of its contribution to the overall cost of the models and the need for a more robust estimate.

Base case results revealed 1-year absenteeism costs ranged from $7376–$46 273 per worker (Table 3). In the occupation-specific models 1-year absenteeism costs of ranged from $5075–$22 186 per blue-collar worker, and $9783–$57 740 per white-collar worker (Table 3). Over 1-year, base case presenteeism costs varied from $5500–$46 377. Further, presenteeism costs ranged from $4349–$19 864 per blue-collar worker, and $9783–$55 672 per white-collar worker (Table 3). Using a uniform daily wage and annual salary estimates revealed differences in cost outcomes between blue- and white-collar workers remained i.e. total cost was higher for white-collar workers. Varying cost of job turnover estimates for workers with and without depression symptoms had the most substantial impact on total cost outcomes (Table 4).

Table 2. One year costs of absenteeism and presenteeism.

	Absenteeism		Presenteeism	
	Cost ($ AUD)	**95% CIs**	**Cost ($ AUD)**	**95% CIs**
Blue Collar				
Lost Productive Time	2738	2693–2741	1762	1731–1764
Job Turnover	3456	2899–4055	3586	2964–4173
Service Use	2	1–4	0.16	0.06–0.24
Antidepressants	36	7–46	20	6–45
Total	6223	6326–8048	5370	4522–5952
White Collar				
Lost Productive Time	4070	3995–4075	2198	2158–2201
Job Turnover	8745	7225–10138	8880	7330–10 431
Service Use	16	6–32	4	2–5
Antidepressants	106	104–106	87	85–88
Total	12 938	11 442–14 416	11 178	9662–12764
Base Case				
Lost Productive Time	3095	1945–4457	2032	1308–2680
Job Turnover	6305	3633–7783	5692	2518–7358
Service Use	45	20–62	11	8–14
Antidepressants	179	124–172	128	112–153
Total	9626	6224–11 384	7864	4452–9565

Table 3. Absenteeism and presenteeism cost outcomes of selected one-way sensitivity analysis over one-year.

		Base Case	
		Presenteeism	Absenteeism
		$/QALY	$/QALY
	Alternative Parameters	7864	9626
Probability of Job Turnover			
Not Depressed	0.025		
	0.05	11 899	13 464
	0.075	12 627	13 530
Depressed	0.105		
	0.25	9886	12 796
	0.50	13 351	18 230
Cost of Job Turnover			
Not Depressed	512	5500	7376
	1154		
	11 615	46 377	46 271
Depressed	2080	7061	8634
	4685		
	47 318	20 997	25 674

Table 4. Absenteeism and presenteeism cost outcomes of selected one-way sensitivity analysis over one-year.

		Blue Collar			White Collar	
		Presenteeism	Absenteeism		Presenteeism	Absenteeism
		$/QALY	$/QALY		$/QALY	$/QALY
	Alternative Parameters	5370	6223	Alternative Parameters	11 178	12 938
Probability of Job Turnover						
Not Depressed	0.01			0.025		
	0.02	7 170	8036	0.05	16 533	18 331
	0.05	12 627	13 530	0.06	18 733	20 545
Depressed	0.105			0.105		
	0.25	7823	8474	0.25	15 728	17 235
	0.50	12 019	12 332	0.50	23 527	24 598
Cost of Job Turnover						
Not Depressed	223	4349	5195	717	8044	9783
	502			1614		
	4470	19 864	20 818	14 348	55 672	57 740
Depressed	2303	4395	5075	2912	9373	10 843
	5183			6553		
	46 079	19 167	22 186	38 254	26 889	31 478
Income						
Mean Annual Salary	44 252			55 595		
	72 517	7660	8431	72 517	13 811	15 529
Daily Wage	170			215		
	279	6506	7988	279	11 839	14 162

Discussion

The purpose of this analysis was to estimate the costs and health outcomes of absenteeism versus presenteeism for employed Australians experiencing major depression, and quantify variations across occupation. Within blue and white-collar groups, absenteeism reporters incurred significantly higher lost productive time, service use, and antidepressant medication costs than presenteeism reporters. Differences in lost productive time costs may be attributable to absenteeism reporters taking time off work due to more severe symptoms, which may also account for their greater antidepressant medication and service use, and the related costs. These findings suggest to employers and health professionals that absenteeism reporters should be the more immediate focus of any health promotion strategies implemented in the workplace.

However, whilst presenteeism costs were often lower than absenteeism costs, they were also substantial, thus indicating the need to better manage this behavior to prevent depression-related productivity loss. Although, not significant, the higher QALYs of employees reporting presenteeism suggests they may be milder depression cases, and their work capacity is reduced but not eliminated. Therefore, employers and health professionals could collaborate to rearrange job tasks to suit employees' abilities [1], and/or provide flexible work attendance arrangements to make the most of employees' work capacity whilst allowing time off when productivity contributions are more severely affected.

Graded sickness absence, which allows employees to work part-time, work full-time hours but perform modified tasks, or perform regular tasks with reduced input whilst receiving a partial sick leave pay and partial salary [29], has been proven effective at keeping people with reduced work ability in working life [30,31]. Such an approach may have positive effects on health and well-being through the maintenance of their daily routines, and by providing a sense of purpose and opportunities for social support from co-workers. Recognition of reduced capacity may also alleviate stress on the affected worker and improve relationships with co-workers by enabling better planning of how tasks may need to be allocated. To ensure the efficacy of such programs, complementary efforts to reduce stigma associated with mental health issues are required as modifying duties or work-time arrangements may expose employees to the negative effects of stigma and exacerbate their condition [32].

As lost productive time was valued on the basis of mean wage, wage differences between blue- and white- collar workers partly account for the differences by occupational type in overall costs. When a white-collar worker reports depression-related absenteeism or presenteeism the ensuing productivity loss is greater as their time is valued more highly within the labour market. Whilst sensitivity analyses revealed a higher mean wage does not entirely explain the observed differences, it explains the work-related variation, and demonstrates to managers and policy makers the importance of tailoring workplace intervention and promotion strategies to specific occupation types. In particular, employers of white-collar workers, particularly those with paid sick leave entitlements, for whom reducing depression-related absenteeism and presenteeism within this group would have significant cost-saving potential. However, as wages fully explain the aforementioned differences in work-related costs, from a workplace perspective, strategies designed to ameliorate depression-related absenteeism and presenteeism amongst blue-collar workers are equally important.

Higher service use and antidepressant medication costs for white-collar workers may be partly explained by the sex distribution between occupation types in our sample. That is, the combination of women being more likely to disclose depression symptoms and seek treatment [33], and the fact that 85% of females in our sample were white-collar workers, may have increased service-related costs within the white-collar group. This is relevant for managers and employers with a large proportion of female staff, such as those operating in the retail, education, or health sectors. However, these are societal costs and workplace mental health support could have broader benefits beyond specific organisations or work settings. Therefore, investment in the mental health and wellbeing of the workforce should be seen as priority for society in general as well employers.

Disparate health outcomes between occupation groups, suggest depression and related work attendance decisions affect blue and white-collar workers differently. White-collar absenteeism reporters experienced poorer QALYs than their blue-collar counterparts and depression-related absenteeism *and* presenteeism costs were higher for white collar workers. This may help to identify areas of priority in regards to mental health promotion and prevention. In particular, the costs associated with absenteeism for white-collar workers, borne by employers via lost productive time and by employees via service use and antidepressant medication costs, suggest they are an important focus of future workplace health promotion strategies with the potential to deliver individual and societal benefits.

Limitations

Lower QALYs amongst absenteeism compared to presenteeism reporters may be due to absenteeism reporters experiencing more severe symptoms which restrict their work ability and impact quality-of-life. However, whether presenteeism reporters have higher QALYs due to benefits of continued work attendance, or whether continuing to work is due to higher quality-of-life, remains unclear. Analysis of absenteeism versus presenteeism costs and health outcomes stratified by severity of depression may allow recommendations as to whether presenteeism is advisable, and whether absenteeism reporters should be encouraged to return to work promptly. The inability to source each model input stratified by depression severity status precluded such an analysis being conducted and was one of this study's major limitations.

Further, job turnover was the largest contributor to overall cost, but sensitivity analysis revealed the probability and cost estimates for job turnover used had substantial uncertainty around them; 95% credible intervals were wide. Additionally, potentially relevant costs, including those attributable to depression-related workplace accidents, were excluded due to inability to find a reliable estimate which met established quality of evidence criteria [22]. Exploratory sensitivity analysis revealed workplace accidents costs contributed substantially to total cost and future effort should be directed at understanding the magnitude of this problem.

Presenteeism behaviour was defined in the initial scenarios as the absence of depression-related absenteeism in the 12-months prior to the NSMHWB interview. This initial classification assumes that the categories of 12-month absenteeism and presenteeism were mutually exclusive, which is not always correct. Recent research has identified that episodes of absenteeism are often preceded and followed by episodes of presenteeism [38]. This highlights that employed individuals reporting depression can experience both absenteeism and presenteeism within a given period of time. Therefore there may be some error in classification at baseline based on this definition. However, while there was a NSMHWB item which asked respondents to report the number disability, or presenteeism, days they experienced in the past year, separate to an item which asked individuals to report their number of absence days, it was not depression specific. Therefore, although the method we employed to define presenteeism may be considered a limitation, it was depression-specific and removed the possible influence of co-morbid disorders on work attendance decisions. Further, as we modelled what happened to our hypothetical cohort in 3-month cycles, individuals were assigned probabilities of lost productive time based on both absenteeism and presenteeism as we know they move in and out of these states over time.

Absenteeism reporters had lower QALYs, albeit not significantly, compared to presenteeism reporters. This may be due to individuals reporting absenteeism experiencing more severe symptoms which restrict their work ability and by extension their quality-of-life. However, what remains unclear is whether individuals reporting presenteeism have higher quality-adjusted life years due to benefits of continued work attendance such as social support, structured routine and income or whether continuing to work is due to higher quality-of-life. This highlights the need for longitudinal data examining the impact of continued work attendance not only on Quality of Life amongst employed individuals reporting depression, but also whether any observed changes are as a result of their changes in the severity of their depression. Such data would enable further exploration s of absenteeism versus presenteeism costs and health outcomes stratified by severity of depression, and may allow recommendations as to whether continuing to work is advisable and whether absenteeism reporters should be encouraged to return to work as soon as possible. The inability to source individual model inputs stratified by depression severity status precluded such an analysis being conducted in the present study.

Strengths

This study's most notable strength was the use of a quality epidemiological data source providing representative estimates of the Australian working population [15]. This allows generalizability of our findings and facilitates their translation to all employed Australians. Another strong point is the major depression diagnoses provided by the NSMHWB, determined using the modified version of the World Mental Health Survey Initiative version of the Composite International Diagnostic Interview (WMH-CIDI). This instrument has undergone extensive methodological testing and development which ensures the international comparability of our results. Additionally, occupation type is an objectively measured variable which eliminates the potential for answers regarding working characteristics to be influenced by response style (acquiescence, social desirability), personality characteristics and negative affect [34]; an important consideration within a sample of individuals experiencing depression.

Conclusion

These findings could inform workplace health promotion strategies aimed at improving the management of depression and related work attendance behaviour, and benefit employees, employers and broader society via investment in a healthy and productive workforce. Informing employers and health care professionals of the health *and* economic benefits of presenteeism for employees experiencing depression could encourage them to adapt work environments, allow employees to perform modified tasks, and offer flexible work time arrangements to promote continued work attendance [29]. Such action may decrease productivity loss, as employers use their employees' remaining work ability more effectively, and reduce turnover and employee replacement costs as employees with depression continue to be productive members of the workforce [30]. Secondly, and of interest to health professionals, such workplace modifications may have positive, long-term effects on health and well-being via maintained daily routine and co-worker support. Finally, the exploration of these outcomes by occupation type allows work attendance recommendations to be tailored to specific occupation types. Such information may be of particular importance for specific occupations or sectors with strong attendance demands such as small businesses, who lack the human capital to compensate for the lost productivity associated with absenteeism, or health care professionals with difficult to substitute skills.

Supporting Information

Table S1 Data inputs and assumptions in base case model.

Table S2 Data inputs and assumptions in absenteeism model.

Table S3 Data inputs and assumptions in presenteeism model, where estimates differ from absenteeism model.

Table S4 Absenteeism and presenteeism days and associated lost productive time by occupation type.

Acknowledgments

This work was completed as part of Dr Fiona Cocker's doctoral thesis at the Menzies Research Institute Tasmania, University of Tasmania.

Author Contributions

Conceived and designed the experiments: FC JN NG BO JS KS. Performed the experiments: FC KS. Analyzed the data: FC KS. Contributed reagents/materials/analysis tools: FC NG AP KS. Wrote the paper: FC JN NG BO AP AM AV JS KS.

References

1. Sanderson K, Tilse E, Nicholson J, Oldenburg B, Graves N (2007) Which presenteeism measures are more sensitive to depression and anxiety? Journal of Affective Disorders 101: 65–74.
2. Stewart WF, Ricci JA, Chee E, Hahn SH, Morganstein D (2003) Cost of lost productive work time among US workers with depression. Journal of the American Medical Association 289: 3135–3144.
3. Sanderson K, Andrews G (2006) Common mental disorders in the workforce: recent findings from descriptive and social epidemiology. Canadian Journal of Psychiatry 51: 63–75.
4. Stewart WF, Ricci JA, Chee E, Hahn SR, Morganstein D (2003) Cost of lost productive work time among US workers with Depression. JAMA 289: 3135–3144.
5. Cox A, Ness K, Carlson R (2010) International perspectives on depression in the workplace.
6. LaMontagne A, Sanderson K, Cocker F (2010) Estimating the economic benefits of eliminating job strain as a risk factor for depression. Melbourne, Australia: Victorian Health Promotion Foundation (VicHealth).
7. Aronsson G, Gustafsson K (2005) Sickness presenteeism: Prevalence, attendance-pressure factors, and an outline of a model for research. JOEM 47: 958–966.
8. Kivimaki M, Head J, Ferrie JE, Hemingway H, Shipley MJ, et al. (2005) Working while ill as a risk factor for serious coronary events: The Whitehall II Study. American Journal of Public Health 95: 98–100.

9. Bergstrom G, Bodin L, Hagberg J, Lindh T, Aronsson G, et al. (2009) Does sickness presenteeism have an impact of future general health? Int Arch Occup Environ Health 82: 1179–1190.
10. Bergstrom G, Bodin L, Hagberg J, Aronsson G, Josephson M (2009) Sickness presenteeism today, sickness absenteeism tomorrow? A prospective study in sickness presenteeism and future sickness absenteeism. JOEM 51: 629–638.
11. Väänänen A, Toppinen-Tannera S, Kalimoa R, Mutanene P, Vahterad J, et al. (2003) Job characteristics, physical and psychological symptoms, and social support as antecedents of sickness absence among men and women in the private industrial sector. Social Science & Medicine 57: 807–824.
12. Aronsson G, Gustafsson K, Dallner M (2000) Sick but yet at work. An empirical study of sickness presenteeism. J Epidemiol Community Health 54: 502–509.
13. Hilton MF, Scuffham P, Sheridan JS, Cleary CM, Whiteford HA (2008) Mental ill-health and the differential effect of employee type on absenteeism and presenteeism. Journal of Occupational and Environmental Medicine 50: 1228–1243.
14. Wang PS, Patrick A, Avorn J, Azocar F, Ludman E, et al. (2006) The costs and benefits of enhanced depression care to employers. Archives of General Psychiatry 63: 1345–1353.
15. Australian Bureau of Statistics (2007) National Survey of Mental Health and Wellbeing (Cat. No. 4326.0), Basic CURF. Canberra, ACT: Australian Bureau of Statistics.
16. Australian Bureau of Statistics (2006) The Australian and New Zealand Standard Classification of Occupations (ANZSCO) First Edition (cat. no. 1220.0). Canberra, ACT: ABS.
17. Lerner D, Adler DA, Chang H, Lapitsky L, Hood MY, et al. (2004) Unemployment, job retention, and productivity loss among employees with depression. Psychiatric Services 55: 1371–1378.
18. Australian Federal Department of Education Employment and Workplace Relations (2008) Evaluating work and family strategies in your workplace. In: Relations AFDoEEaW, editor. Canberra:ACT: Commonwealth of Australia.
19. Simon GE, Revicki D, Heiligenstein J, Grothaus L, VanKorff M, et al. (2000) Recovery from depression, work productivity, and health care costs among primary care patients. General Hospital Psychiatry 22: 153–162.
20. Rost K, Smith JL, Dickinson M (2004) The effect of improving primary care depression management on employee absenteeism and productivity: A randomised trial. Medical Care 42: 1202–1210.
21. Teesson M, Slade T, Mills K (2009) Comorbidity in Australia: findings of the 2007 National Survey of Mental Health and Wellbeing. Australian and New Zealand Journal of Psychiatry 43: 606–614.
22. Braithwaite S, Roberts MS, Justice AC (2007) Incorporating quality of evidence into decision analytic modelling. Ann Int Med 146: 133–141.
23. Therapeutic Guidelines Limited. Psychotropic Writing Group (2008) Therapeutic Guidelines: psychotropic; Dowden J, editor. Melbourne: Therapeutic Guidelines Limited.
24. Sanderson K, Andrews G, Corry J, Lapsley H (2004) Modelling change in preference values from descriptive health status using the effect size. Quality of Life Research 13: 1255–1264.
25. Hawthorne G, Richardson J, Osborne R (1999) The Assessment of Quality of Life (AQoL) instrument: a psychometric measure of health-related quality of life. Quality of Life Research 8: 209–224.
26. Hawthorne G, Osborne R (2005) Population norms and meaningful differences for the Assessment of Quality of Life (AQoL) measure. Blackwell Publishing Ltd. pp. 136–142.
27. Briggs AH (2000) Handling uncertainty in cost-effectiveness models. Pharmacoecon 17: 479–500.
28. Gold M, Siegel J, Russell L, Weinstein MC, editors (1996) Cost effectiveness in Health and Medicine. New York, NY: Oxford University Press.
29. Kausto J, Miranda H, Martimo KP, Viikari-Juntura E (2008) Partial sick leave - review of its use, effects and feasibility in the Nordic countries. Scand J Work Environ Health 34: 239–249.
30. Kausto J, Virta L, Luukkonen R, Viikari-Juntura E (2010) Associations between partial sickness benefit and disability pensions: initial findings of a Finnish nationwide register study. BMC Public Health 10: 1–11.
31. Markussen S, Mykletun A, Røed K (2010) The Case for Presenteeism. Oslo, Norway: Ragnar Frisch Centre for Economic Research and IZA Norwegian Institute of Public Health.
32. Martin A (2010) Individual and contextual correlates of managers' attitudes toward depressed employees. Human Resource Management 49: 647–668.
33. Burgess PM, Pirkis JE, Slade TN, Johnston AK, Meadows GN, et al. (2009) Service use for mental health problems: findings from the 2007 National Survey of Mental Health and Wellbeing. Aust NZ J of Psychiatry 43: 615–623.
34. Birnbaum HG, Leong SA, Greenberg PE (2003) The economics of women and depression: an employer's perspective. J Affect Disorders 74: 15–22.
35. Spitzer RL, Williams JW, Kroenke K (1994). Utility of a new procedure for diagnosing mental disorders in primary care: The prime-md 1000 study. JAMA 272: 1749–56.
36. Loerch B, Szegedi A, Kohnen R, Benkert O (2000). The primary care evaluation of mental disorders (PRIME-MD), German version: a comparison with the CIDI. J Psych Res 34: 211–20.
37. Kruijshaar ME, Barendregt J, Vos T, de Graaf R, Spijker J (2005).Lifetime prevalence estimates of major depression: An indirect estimation method and a quantification of recall bias. Euro J Epi 20: 103–11.
38. Leineweber C, Westerlund H, Hagberg J, Svedberg P, Alexanderson K (2012). Sickness presenteeism is more than an alternative to sickness absence: results from the population-based SLOSH study. Int Arch Occup Env Health 85: 905–14.

The Association of Depression and Anxiety with Pain: A Study from NESDA

Eric W. de Heer[1,2*], Marloes M. J. G. Gerrits[3], Aartjan T. F. Beekman[3,4], Jack Dekker[5,6], Harm W. J. van Marwijk[7], Margot W. M. de Waal[8], Philip Spinhoven[9,10], Brenda W. J. H. Penninx[3], Christina M. van der Feltz-Cornelis[1,2,11]

1 TopClinical Center for Body, Mind, and Health, GGz Breburg Tilburg, Tilburg, The Netherlands, **2** Tilburg School of Behavioral and Social Sciences, Tranzo Department, University of Tilburg, Tilburg, The Netherlands, **3** Department of Psychiatry, EMGO Institute for Health and Care research, VU University Medical Centre, Amsterdam, The Netherlands, **4** GGZ inGeest, Mental Health Institute, Amsterdam, The Netherlands, **5** Arkin, Mental Health Institute, Amsterdam, The Netherlands, **6** Department of Clinical Psychology, VU University, Amsterdam, The Netherlands, **7** Department of General Practice, EMGO Institute for Health and Care Research, VU University Medical Centre, Amsterdam, The Netherlands, **8** Department of Public Health and Primary Care, Leiden university Medical Centre, Leiden, The Netherlands, **9** Institute of Psychology, Leiden University, Leiden, The Netherlands, **10** Department of Psychiatry, Leiden University Medical Centre, Leiden, The Netherlands, **11** Trimbos Institute, Utrecht, the Netherlands

Abstract

Chronic pain is commonly co-morbid with a depressive or anxiety disorder. Objective of this study is to examine the influence of depression, along with anxiety, on pain-related disability, pain intensity, and pain location in a large sample of adults with and without a depressive and/or anxiety disorder. The study population consisted of 2981 participants with a depressive, anxiety, co-morbid depressive and anxiety disorder, remitted disorder or no current disorder (controls). Severity of depressive and anxiety symptoms was also assessed. In separate multinomial regression analyses, the association of presence of depressive or anxiety disorders and symptom severity with the Chronic Pain Grade and location of pain was explored. Presence of a depressive (OR = 6.67; P<.001), anxiety (OR = 4.84; P<.001), or co-morbid depressive and anxiety disorder (OR = 30.26; P<.001) was associated with the Chronic Pain Grade. Moreover, symptom severity was associated with more disabling and severely limiting pain. Also, a remitted depressive or anxiety disorder showed more disabling and severely limiting pain (OR = 3.53; P<.001) as compared to controls. A current anxiety disorder (OR = 2.96; p<.001) and a co-morbid depressive and anxiety disorder (OR = 5.15; P<.001) were more strongly associated with cardio-respiratory pain, than gastro-intestinal or musculoskeletal pain. These findings remain after adjustment for chronic cardio respiratory illness. Patients with a current and remitted depressive and/or anxiety disorder and those with more severe symptoms have more disabling pain and pain of cardio-respiratory nature, than persons without a depressive or anxiety disorder. This warrants further research.

Editor: H. Sunny Sun, National Cheng Kung University Medical College, Taiwan

Funding: The infrastructure for the NESDA study is funded through the Geestkracht program of the Netherlands Organisation for Health Research and Development (Zon-MW, grant number 10-000-1002) and is supported by participating universities and mental health care organisations (VU University Medical Center, GGZ inGeest, Arkin, Leiden University Medical Center, GGZ Rivierduinen, University Medical Center Groningen, Lentis, GGZ Friesland, GGZ Drenthe, IQ Healthcare, Netherlands Institute for Health Services Research [NIVEL], and the Netherlands Institute of Mental Health and Addiction [Trimbos]. The funders had no role in study design, data collection and analysis, decision to publish, or preparation of the manuscript.

Competing Interests: The authors of this manuscript have read the journal's policy and have the following competing interests: ATFB reports grants from Eli Lilly, grants from Astra Zeneca, grants from Jansen, grants from Shire, personal fees (as a speaker) from Eli Lilly, and personal fees (as a speaker) from Lundbeck, outside the submitted work. JD and CMFC report grants from Eli Lilly, outside the submitted work. BWJHP reports grants from Dutch government, ministry o f Health (ZonMw), during the conduct of the study.

* Email: e.deheer@ggzbreburg.nl

Introduction

Chronic pain is common in up to 70% of patients with depressive and anxiety disorders [1–9]. Chronic pain and depression most likely have a bidirectional association: depression is a predictor of persistent pain and pain is a predictor of the persistence of depression [1,3,10]. A possible explanation is that impaired functioning caused by pain can lead to social isolation, which in turn can lead to a negative effect on depressive symptoms, and vice versa [11,12]. Furthermore, different brain areas, such as the amygdala and hypothalamus, play a role in both depression and pain [13,14]. Also, when depression and chronic pain are co-morbid, recognition and treatment of depression are less effective, as patients mostly only present their physical complaints and receive treatment accordingly [1].

Most studies up to now have only considered the relationship of pain with depression, whereas its association with anxiety disorders has been less examined. It is likely that the association of pain and anxiety is equally important, as depression and anxiety commonly appear together. Pain may cause feelings of anxiety, which in turn can make one more sensitive to pain, with persistence of the pain experience as a consequence [15]. Furthermore, anxiety disorders and chronic pain share underlying cognitive and behavioural processes, such as increased attention towards threat and anxious avoidance of physical exertion [16,17]. Fear avoidance can play a role in chronic pain, with the (acute) pain experience leading to pain catastrophising and pain-related fear which in turn will lead to greater disability and persistent pain experience [15]. Therefore, we need more comprehensive insight by studying both depression and anxiety in concert (separately and as co-morbid problems) with pain [18–20]. Another reason to study the cross-sectional relationship between depressive and anxiety disorders and pain is that pain also has a negative impact on the prognosis of psychopathology and psychiatric treatment outcome, with pain leading to more treatment resistance [2,21–23]. Pain may be a marker of a more difficult-to-treat disorder, and lead to a longer time before remission [24].

Pain is a common presenting symptom in depression and anxiety and several studies have explored this association for specific pain symptoms, such as back pain [25–27] or neck pain [27,28]. However, pain symptoms often occur in more than one location and thus may be clustered; clustering of (medically unexplained) physical symptoms was examined by Wessely et al. [29], Nimnuan et al. [30], and Fink et al. [31]. These studies found different clusters of pain symptoms, the most prominent being musculoskeletal, gastro-intestinal, and cardio-respiratory pain. Associations were found between depressive, but mostly anxiety symptoms and cardio-respiratory pain, musculoskeletal pain and gastro-intestinal pain. However, the strength of these associations and the correlation with pain-related disability has not yet been explored [32–34]. Therefore, this study will explore the association of clustered locations of pain (musculoskeletal, gastro-intestinal, and cardio-respiratory) with depression and anxiety, while taking severity of pain and pain-related disability into account.

We aim to examine and compare the impact of current and remitted depressive, anxiety and co-morbid disorders on different pain-variables in a large sample of individuals with depressive and/or anxiety disorders versus normal controls. We will explore if severity of depressive or anxiety symptoms is associated with severity of pain and pain-related disability, and whether these associations are stronger for certain clustered pain locations. We expect that not only a depressive disorder will have a strong association with abovementioned pain-variables, but that an anxiety disorder will show a comparably strong association, with comorbid depression and anxiety showing the strongest association.

Methods

Sample

The present study used data from the Netherlands Study of Depression and Anxiety (NESDA): an ongoing longitudinal cohort study in which 2981 participants, recruited from the community, general practice and secondary mental health care, are monitored to investigate the long-term course and consequences of depressive and anxiety disorders. Penninx et al. [35] provide a detailed description of the NESDA study design and sampling procedures. NESDA was designed to include patients with depressive and anxiety disorders at different stages of development of their disorder. In order to achieve this, participants were recruited from the community, in primary care and in specialised mental health care [35]. At baseline, healthy controls, persons with a prior history, and persons with a current depressive and/or anxiety disorder, between 18 and 65 years old, were included. The sample was stratified for setting (community, primary care, and specialised mental health). Furthermore, the sample includes a range of psychopathology: from those without a depressive or anxiety disorder (controls) to those with a current, first or recurrent (in the past 6 months) depressive or anxiety disorder and those with a remitted disorder (at baseline, a depressive and/or anxiety disorder was diagnosed in the past, but no diagnoses were present at 6 months before baseline). The disorders included dysthymia, major depressive disorder, general anxiety disorder, panic disorder, social phobia, and agoraphobia. Exclusion criteria were not being fluent in Dutch and a primary diagnosis of psychotic, obsessive compulsive, bipolar or severe addiction disorder. The research protocol was approved by the Ethical Committee of participating universities and written informed consent was obtained from all participants. Interviews were conducted by specially trained research staff.

The sample consists of 2329 persons with a current diagnosis of depression (n = 396) or anxiety disorder (n = 543), a remitted disorder (n = 628) and 652 persons without a history of depressive and/or anxiety disorder and no current diagnosis of depression or anxiety disorder. All 2981 participants were interviewed, by specially trained clinical research staff, for depression and/or anxiety in the baseline interview using the DSM IV based Composite International Diagnostic Interview (CIDI, version 2.1), a reliable and valid instrument for assessing depressive and anxiety disorders [36].

The baseline measurement of NESDA, collected between September 2004 and February 2007, was used for this study. Next to the structured interview to assess mental health, self-report questionnaires were used to assess physical health (such as chronic disease, pain, and severity of mental health).

Measures

Pain assessment. Pain was assessed using the 7-item Chronic Pain Grade (CPG) Scale by von Korff [37]. The CPG is a reliable and valid instrument for chronic pain populations and the general population [37,38]. The CPG is a good instrument for measuring pain-related variables and for making a hierarchical classification of pain intensity and pain-related disability. It has good internal consistency (with a Cronbach's alpha of 0.91) and the item-total correlations are all high, ranging from .69 to .83.

The CPG grades (chronic) pain using pain intensity and pain-related disability. Pain intensity is based on the mean of the average, worst, and present pain on a scale of 0–100. Pain-related disability is based on the mean of interference with usual activities, work/household activities, and family/social activities on a scale of 0–100, and the number of days (0–180) one is unable to carry out usual activities due to pain in the previous 6 months. To create 5 grades for chronic pain, the following calculations were used: pain intensity was divided into low intensity (score <50) and high intensity (score ≥50). To calculate the score of pain-related disability, an overall score of 0–6 was created by assigning 0–3 points for disability score (0–29 = 0; 30–49 = 1; 50–69 = 2; 70–100 = 3) and adding 0–3 points for number of disability days (0–6 days = 0; 7–14 days = 1; 15–30 days = 2; >30 days = 3). With these scores, 5 grades of chronic pain can be calculated:

grade 0 (no pain symptoms);

grade 1 (low pain intensity (<50) – low disability (<3 points));

grade 2 (high intensity (≥50) – low disability (<3 points));

Table 1. Baseline characteristics of total NESDA sample (N = 2981).

		N (%)	Mean (SD)
Demographics			
Female gender		1979 (66.4)	
Age in years			41.9 (13.1)
Level of education	Basic	199 (6.7)	
	Intermediate	1736 (58.2)	
	High	1046 (35.1)	
Partner or married		2066 (69.3)	
Psychopathology characteristics			
No psychopathology		652 (21.9)	
Remitted disorder		628 (21.0)	
	# of depressive episodes		1.73 (5.9)
Current depressive disorder		396 (13.3)	
	# of depressive episodes		10.29 (71.3)
Current anxiety disorder		543 (18.2)	
Current depressive and anxiety disorder		762 (25.6)	
	# of depressive episodes		9.88 (72.6)
Severity of depression (QIDS)*	None	1121 (37.6)	
	Mild	820 (27.5)	
	Moderate	627 (21.0)	
	(Very) Severe	374 (12.5)	
Severity of anxiety (BAI)**	Normal	1477 (49.5)	
	Mild	758 (25.4)	
	Moderate	493 (16.5)	
	Severe	218 (7.3)	
Other characteristics			
Musculoskeletal chronic disease		648 (21.7)	
Gastro-intestinal chronic disease		335 (11.2)	
Cardio respiratory chronic disease		775 (26.0)	
Antidepressant use		785 (26.4)	
Use of other psychotropic drugs		700 (23.5)	

*39 missing.
**35 missing.

grade 3 (high disability – moderately limiting (3–4 disability points, regardless of intensity));

grade 4 (high disability – severely limiting (5–6 disability points, regardless of intensity)).

Along with the CPG, we also assessed the specific pain location. To locate the specific pain location, an inventory was made, with a self-report questionnaire, of pain symptoms in the back, neck, head, stomach, joints, chest, and face. Participants could report one or more of these pain locations, and were asked which of these pain locations bothered them the most in the last six months. We then categorised these pain locations as musculoskeletal (back, neck, head, joints, face), gastro-intestinal (stomach), and cardio respiratory (chest) pain symptoms. Participants could report multiple pain symptoms across the categories.

Depression and anxiety. The presence of a depressive or anxiety disorder was established using the CIDI. In this study, psychopathology profiles were made for each participant. A participant either had no psychopathology (n = 652), a remitted disorder (depression and/or anxiety) (n = 628), a current depressive disorder (n = 396), a current anxiety disorder (n = 543) or a current co-morbid depressive and anxiety disorder (n = 762) (in the past 6 months).

In addition to this categorical approach of disorders (yes/no), we also assessed severity of depressive and anxiety symptoms. Severity of depressive symptoms was assessed with the Quick Inventory of Depressive Symptomatology-Self-Report (QIDS-SR) [39], in which no pain items are included. The QIDS-SR is the shortened version of the self-rated Inventory of Depressive Symptomatology (IDS-SR) [40] and is a 16-item questionnaire with a range of 0 to 27 with high internal consistency (Cronbach's $\alpha = 0.86$). A score of 0–5 refers to none to mild depressive symptoms, a score of 6–10 refers to mild severity, a score of 11–15 refers to moderate severity, and a score of 16 or higher refers to (very) severe depressive symptoms. Severity of anxiety symptoms was assessed with the Beck Anxiety Inventory (BAI) [41], which also does not include any pain items. The BAI is a 27-item questionnaire ranging from 0 to 63 also with high internal

Table 2. Baseline pain characteristics divided by psychopathology.

		Total	No psychopathology	Remitted disorder	Current depressive disorder	Current anxiety disorder	Current depressive and anxiety disorder
		N = 2981	N = 652	N = 627	N = 396	N = 543	N = 762
CPG*	Grade 0, N (%)	170 (5.7)	82 (12.6)	33 (5.3)	19 (4.8)	23 (4.2)	13 (1.7)
	Grade 1, N (%)	1635 (54.8)	441 (67.6)	379 (60.4)	194 (49.0)	315 (58.0)	306 (40.2)
	Grade 2, N (%)	605 (20.3)	81 (12.4)	134 (21.4)	86 (21.7)	118 (21.7)	186 (24.4)
	Grade 3, N (%)	311 (10.4)	29 (4.4)	48 (7.7)	60 (15.2)	52 (9.6)	122 (16.0)
	Grade 4, N (%)	259 (8.7)	19 (2.9)	33 (5.3)	37 (9.3)	35 (6.4)	135 (17.7)
Pain location	No pain, N (%)	170 (5.7)	82 (12.6)	33 (5.3)	19 (4.8)	23 (4.2)	13 (1.7)
	Musculoskeletal, N (%)	2753 (92.4)	552 (84.7)	586 (93.3)	374 (94.4)	507 (93.4)	734 (96.3)
	Gastro-intestinal, N (%)	1432 (48.0)	207 (31.7)	250 (39.8)	216 (54.5)	278 (51.2)	481 (63.1)
	Cardio respiratory, N (%)	764 (25.6)	77 (11.8)	117 (18.6)	101 (25.5)	156 (28.7)	313 (41.1)

*1 missing.

consistency (Cronbach's $\alpha = 0.92$). A score of 0–9 refers to normal severity, whereas a score of 10–18 refers to mild severity, a score of 18–29 refers to moderate severity, and a score higher than 29 refers to severe anxiety symptoms [42].

Covariates. Covariates were selected a priori based on previous research on the association of depression and anxiety with pain. Socio-demographic factors included gender, age, level of education, and partner status. Furthermore, the presence of chronic diseases was taken into account as a covariate. Based on self-report during the initial interview, the presence of a chronic disease was assessed. These chronic diseases were then categorised, by a physician, into cardio respiratory disease (coronary heart disease, angina pectoris, heart failure, chronic nonspecific lung disease, stroke, hypertension), gastro-intestinal disease (diabetes, (gastro-intestinal) ulcer, ulcerative colitis or Crohn's disease, liver cirrhosis, hepatitis) and musculoskeletal disease (arthritis, osteoarthritis, rheumatism). Because medication can have an analgesic influence on pain, the use of antidepressants and other psychotropic drugs were also selected as covariates. Also, the number of depressive episodes was taken into account as a covariate.

Statistical Analyses. All statistical analyses were performed in SPSS 19 for Windows. Descriptive analyses were used to assess baseline characteristics across the total sample. To assess the associations of type of disorder with the CPG, we used multinomial logistic regression analyses. For the pain outcome variable (the CPG) we used the group with no pain (CPG0) as a reference category. For type of disorder, the healthy control group without depression or anxiety was selected as a reference category. In this analysis we controlled for all the covariates.

We used adjusted multinomial analyses to assess the association of severity of depressive and anxiety symptoms with the outcome variable CPG, with the lowest severity category as the reference category.

Furthermore, we used four separate logistic regression analyses to examine the association of depression and/or anxiety with the outcome variable of location of pain (1. no pain, 2. musculoskeletal pain (controlling for the presence of musculoskeletal disease), 3. gastro-intestinal pain (controlling for the presence of gastro-intestinal disease), and 4. cardio respiratory pain (controlling for the presence of cardio respiratory disease)). Here also, having no depressive or anxiety disorder was used as a reference category.

Results

Table 1 presents the baseline characteristics of the total population. Of the total sample, 652 participants reported no psychopathology, and slightly less participants (628) reported a remitted depressive and/or anxiety disorder (with a mean of 1.73 depressive episodes). The least participants had a current depressive disorder (with a mean of 10.29 depressive episodes), followed by a current anxiety disorder. Most participants reported a current comorbid depressive and anxiety disorder, with a mean of almost 10 depressive episodes. 26.4% of the total sample used antidepressant medication. Of the 2981 participants, 170 (5.7%) reported no pain symptoms. Most participants (92.4%) reported having musculoskeletal pain, followed by gastro-intestinal pain (1432 participants), and cardio respiratory pain (764 participants). Table 2 shows the pain characteristics, separated in no psychopathology, remitted disorder, current depressive disorder, current anxiety disorder, and current depressive and anxiety disorder. Of the total sample and of each of the abovementioned groups, most participants had low intensity and low pain-related disability (CPG1), and pain of musculoskeletal origin. Especially when a depressive disorder is comorbid with an anxiety disorder, more

Table 3. Associations of presence of current depressive disorder, current anxiety disorder, current co-morbid depression and anxiety and remitted depression or anxiety with the Chronic Pain Grade, with no depression and/or anxiety disorder as a reference category.

	CPG1[a,b]	CPG2[a,b]	CPG3[a,b]	CPG4[a,b]
	OR (95% CI)	*OR (95% CI)*	*OR (95% CI)*	*OR (95% CI)*
No psychopathology	reference	reference	reference	reference
Remitted depression/anxiety	1.87 (1.17–2.97)*	3.45 (2.02–5.87)**	3.49 (1.81–6.73)**	3.53 (1.67–7.43)*
Depression current	1.35 (0.72–2.55)	3.53 (1.76–7.08)**	7.14 (3.28–15.54)**	6.67 (2.81–15.88)**
Anxiety current	2.10 (1.25–3.54)*	4.06 (2.26–7.30)**	5.15 (2.57–10.31)**	4.84 (2.22–10.57)**
Co-morbid depression and anxiety current	3.13 (1.56–6.25)*	10.18 (4.87–21.26)**	19.72 (8.77–44.35)**	30.26 (12.68–72.23)**

*p<.05;
**p<.001.
[a]reference category is no pain.
[b]adjusted for age, gender, level of education, partner status, antidepressant use, use of other psychotropic drugs, chronic diseases, and number of depressive episodes.

participants report highly disabling and severely limiting pain (CPG4).

Association of depression and/or anxiety with the CPG

Table 3 shows results from the adjusted multinomial logistic regression analysis assessing the association of depression and/or anxiety with the CPG. The results show a significant association and the odds ratios (ORs) rise per CPG level. For all CPG levels, the ORs were significantly elevated compared to the reference group. Having a co-morbid depressive and anxiety disorder, as compared to having no disorder, showed the strongest association (OR = 30.26; 95% CI = 12.68–72.23). Also, when compared to having no depression or anxiety, there is still a high odds of having disabling pain symptoms when the depressive or anxiety disorder is remitted (CPG1: OR = 1.87; 95% CI = 1.17–2.97; CPG4: OR = 3.53; 95% CI = 1.67–7.43). However, the confidence intervals do overlap. Therefore, four sensitivity analyses were performed, each with an other psychopathology group (remitted disorder, current depressive disorder, current anxiety disorder, comorbid depression and anxiety) as a reference category, in order to examine the possible differences in associations between pain and various depressive and anxiety disorder categories (Tables 4–7). With a current depressive disorder or anxiety disorder as reference group, the results show no significant differences between these disorders on the CPG. A current anxiety disorder and a current depressive disorder also show no significant difference with a remitted disorder. Only a co-morbid depressive and anxiety disorder had a significantly higher association with the CPG compared to a remitted, current depressive, and current anxiety disorder. These findings were similar to those in the analysis with the reference group of healthy controls. The unadjusted results did not differ from the adjusted results.

Because the reference group for pain (CPG0) was small (N = 170), another sensitivity analysis was conducted where CPG0 and CPG1 were combined to form the reference category (Table 8). This analysis showed that the association between type of disorder and CPG mostly remains: as can be seen in table 8, all associations became less strong after combining CPG0 and CPG1 as a reference category, but remained significant.

Association of severity of depressive and anxiety symptoms with the CPG

Table 9 shows the association of the severity of depressive symptoms (as measured with the QIDS) and anxiety symptoms (as measured with the BAI) with the CPG. Similar to the main finding, as the severity of the depressive symptoms increases, the odds of having highly disabling and severely limiting pain increases as well. The same accounts for the association between severity of anxiety symptoms and the CPG. The unadjusted results did not differ from the adjusted results.

Table 4. Associations of presence of current depressive disorder, current anxiety disorder, current co-morbid depression and anxiety and remitted depression or anxiety with the Chronic Pain Grade, with remitted disorder as a reference category.

	CPG1[a,b]	CPG2[a,b]	CPG3[a,b]	CPG4[a,b]
	OR (95% CI)	*OR (95% CI)*	*OR (95% CI)*	*OR (95% CI)*
Remitted depression/anxiety	reference	reference	reference	reference
No psychopathology	.54 (.34–.85)*	.29 (.17–.50)**	.29 (.15–.55)**	.28 (.14–.60)*
Depression current	.72 (.39–1.36)	1.03 (.52–2.01)	2.04 (.98–4.25)	1.89 (.85–4.20)
Anxiety current	1.13 (.64–2.00)	1.18 (.64–2.18)	1.47 (.74–2.94)	1.37 (.65–2.91)
Co-morbid depression and anxiety current	1.68 (.84–3.36)	2.95 (1.43–6.09)*	5.65 (2.61–12.22)**	8.58 (3.84–19.21)**

*p<.05;
**p<.001.
[a]reference category is no pain.
[b]adjusted for age, gender, level of education, partner status, antidepressant use, use of other psychotropic drugs, chronic diseases, and number of depressive episodes.

Table 5. Associations of presence of current depressive disorder, current anxiety disorder, current co-morbid depression and anxiety and remitted depression or anxiety with the Chronic Pain Grade, with current depressive disorder as a reference category.

	CPG1[a,b]	CPG2[a,b]	CPG3[a,b]	CPG4[a,b]
	OR (95% CI)	*OR (95% CI)*	*OR (95% CI)*	*OR (95% CI)*
Depression current	reference	reference	reference	reference
No psychopathology	.74 (.39–1.40)	.28 (.14–.57)**	.14 (.0–31)**	.15 (.06–.36)**
Remitted depression/anxiety	1.38 (.74–2.59)	.98 (.50–1.91)	.49 (.24–1.02)	.53 (.24–1.17)
Anxiety current	1.56 (.79–3.05)	1.15 (.56–2.35)	.72 (.34–1.54)	.73 (.32–1.65)
Comorbid depression and anxiety current	2.31 (1.10–4.85)*	2.88 (1.34–6.21)*	2.76 (1.25–6.09)*	4.53 (2.00–10.30)**

*p<.05;
**p<.001.
[a]reference category is no pain.
[b]adjusted for age, gender, level of education, partner status, antidepressant use, use of other psychotropic drugs, chronic diseases, and number of depressive episodes.

Because the reference group for pain (CPG0) was small (N = 170), a sensitivity analysis was conducted where CPG0 and CPG1 were combined to form the reference category (table 10). This analysis showed that the association found between severity of depressive and anxiety symptoms and CPG mostly remains, with more severe depressive or anxiety symptoms being more strongly associated with more disabling and limiting pain, when CPG0 and CPG1 were combined to have a larger reference group. Here also, all associations were less strong, with some associations (especially the association of severe anxiety symptoms with the CPG2 and CPG4) remaining statistically significant, while other associations (e.g. the association of mild and moderate anxiety symptoms with CPG3) becoming non-significant.

Association of depression and/or anxiety with musculoskeletal, gastro-intestinal, and cardio respiratory pain symptoms

Table 11 shows the multinomial logistic regression analyses assessing the association of depression and/or anxiety with three clustered pain locations. For those with pain, the highest ORs are seen in co-morbid depression and anxiety. The ORs for musculoskeletal pain range from 2.28 (95% CI = 1.53–3.42) for a depressive or anxiety disorder in remission to 3.88 (95% CI = 2.33–6.47) for a co-morbid depressive and anxiety disorder. For gastro-intestinal pain, the ORs range from 1.40 (95% CI = 1.10–1.78) for a depressive or anxiety disorder in remission to 3.31 (95% CI = 2.57–4.27) for a co-morbid depressive and anxiety disorder. Cardio respiratory pain shows a range in ORs from 1.74 (95% CI = 1.27–2.40) for a depressive or anxiety disorder in remission to 5.15 (95% CI = 3.80–6.98) for co-morbid depressive and anxiety disorder. The unadjusted results did not differ from the adjusted results.

Discussion

The high proportion of participants with anxiety and depressive disorders in this study reflects the sampling strategy for including sufficient numbers of respondents to examine individuals at different stages of development and severity of depression and anxiety. This study demonstrates considerable associations between presence of depressive and anxiety disorders (current and remitted) and symptom severity with different pain dimensions, namely pain-related disability, pain intensity, and the location of pain symptoms (musculoskeletal, gastro-intestinal, and cardio respiratory).

Presence and severity of depressive or anxiety disorder

Our results show that having a mood or anxiety disorder increases the odds of highly disabling and severely limiting pain. Also, the severity of the depressive and anxiety symptoms are significantly associated with pain-related disability and limiting

Table 6. Associations of presence of current depressive disorder, current anxiety disorder, current co-morbid depression and anxiety and remitted depression or anxiety with the Chronic Pain Grade, with current anxiety disorder as a reference category.

	CPG1[a,b]	CPG2[a,b]	CPG3[a,b]	CPG4[a,b]
	OR (95% CI)	*OR (95% CI)*	*OR (95% CI)*	*OR (95% CI)*
Anxiety current	reference	reference	reference	reference
No psychopathology	.48 (.28–.80)*	.25 (.14–.44)**	.19 (.10–.39)**	.21 (.10–.45)**
Remitted depression/anxiety	.89 (.450–1.57)	.85 (.46–1.57)	.68 (.34–1.35)	.73 (.34–1.54)
Depression current	.64 (.33–1.26)	.87 (.43–1.78)	1.39 (.65–2.97)	1.38 (.61–3.13)
Comorbid depression and anxiety current	1.49 (.72–3.06)	2.51 (1.18–5.30)*	3.83 (1.74–8.42)*	6.25 (2.76–14.15)**

*p<.05;
**p<.001.
[a]reference category is no pain.
[b]adjusted for age, gender, level of education, partner status, antidepressant use, use of other psychotropic drugs, chronic diseases, and number of depressive episodes.

Table 7. Associations of presence of current depressive disorder, current anxiety disorder, current co-morbid depression and anxiety and remitted depression or anxiety with the Chronic Pain Grade, with comorbid depressive- and anxiety disorder as a reference category.

	CPG1[a,b]	CPG2[a,b]	CPG3[a,b]	CPG4[a,b]
	OR (95% CI)	*OR (95% CI)*	*OR (95% CI)*	*OR (95% CI)*
Comorbid depression and anxiety current	reference	reference	reference	reference
No psychopathology	.32 (.16–.64)*	.10 (.05–.21)**	.05 (.02–.11)**	.03 (.01–.08)**
Remitted depression/anxiety	.60 (.30–1.20)	.34 (.16–.70)*	.18 (.08–.38)**	.12 (.05–.26)**
Depression current	.43 (.21–.91)*	.35 (.16–.75)*	.36 (.16-.80)*	.22 (.10–.50)**
Anxiety current	.67 (.33–1.39)	.40 (.19–.85)*	.26 (.12–.57)*	.16 (.07–.36)**

*p<.05;
**p<.001.
[a]reference category is no pain.
[b]adjusted for age, gender, level of education, partner status, antidepressant use, use of other psychotropic drugs, chronic diseases, and number of depressive episodes.

pain, with more severe symptoms having higher odds for highly disabling and severely limiting pain.

Depressive and anxiety disorders may add to pain as they increase the likelihood of social isolation, increased attention towards threat and avoidance of physical exertion [11,12,16,17]. Depression and anxiety disorders also share the same pathophysiological pathways as pain [43–45]. They facilitate the central modulation of the pain response, in the periaqueductal gray, amygdala, and hypothalamus [1,13,14], and when deficits occur in these areas, modulation of signals from the body are disturbed, leading to a more severe experience of pain. Although these brain areas all play a role in depression, anxiety, and pain, not every individual responds the same to pain stimuli [46–48]. Some individuals are more sensitive to pain than others. The use of EEG may help in identifying neuronal markers for sensitivity to pain [46], and whether there are differences between depressive and anxious individuals. Furthermore, depression and anxiety induce stress and increases the production of pro-inflammatory cytokines [49–51], which may increase pain [52,53]. The finding showing higher pain-related disability in co-morbid depression and anxiety in our study is similar to findings from the STAR*D studies [54–56].

Depressive or anxiety disorder in remission

Regarding the association of a remitted disorder and pain, we expected persons with remitted depression or anxiety to have similar pain symptoms as controls without depression or anxiety. However, this is not the case. Persons with a remitted depressive or anxiety disorder still showed high odds on the pain outcomes when compared to those that have no such disorder. This is remarkable, because this means that having a remitted disorder is not the same as having no disorder with regards to pain. This raises several questions.

First, pain symptoms may be residual symptoms in depressive and anxiety disorder. This finding may suggest that pain in patients with remitted depressive or anxiety disorder might be indicative of a risk for recurrence, as disability in life (e.g. disability to fulfil his or her role at home) is an important risk factor for the recurrence of anxiety disorders [57], and our results show that those with a remitted diagnosis still have high odds of having pain symptoms and pain-related disability.

Another explanation for the high odds of pain symptoms in remitted depression or anxiety might be that treatment, if it was provided, for the depressive or anxiety disorder is not effective for pain symptoms, or treatment should be different when pain is co-morbid with the depressive or anxiety disorder. For example, it has been suggested that patients with depression and pain are a

Table 8. (Results from sensitivity analysis, with CPG0 and CPG1 combined) Associations of presence of current depressive disorder, current anxiety disorder, current co-morbid depression and anxiety and remitted depression or anxiety with the Chronic Pain Grade, with no depression and/or anxiety disorder as a reference category.

	CPG2[a,b]	CPG3[a,b]	CPG4[a,b]
	OR (95% CI)	*OR (95% CI)*	*OR (95% CI)*
No psychopathology	reference	reference	reference
Remitted depression/anxiety	1.99 (1.45–2.73)**	2.01 (1.22–3.30)*	2.03 (1.10–3.73)*
Depression current	2.78 (1.93–4.01)**	5.61 (3.39–9.29)**	5.23 (2.77–9.85)**
Anxiety current	2.09 (1.50–2.92)**	2.65 (1.61–4.35)**	2.48 (1.34–4.59)*
Comorbid depression and anxiety current	3.63 (2.61–5.04)**	7.01 (4.38–11.23)**	10.72 (6.07–18.96)**

*p<.05;
**p<.001.
[a]reference category is no pain.
[b]adjusted for age, gender, level of education, partner status, antidepressant use, use of other psychotropic drugs, chronic diseases, and number of depressive episodes.

Table 9. Association of severity of depressive symptoms and anxiety symptoms with the Chronic Pain Grade.

		CPG1[a,b]	CPG2[a,b]	CPG3[a,b]	CPG4[a,b]
		OR (95% CI)	*OR (95% CI)*	*OR (95% CI)*	*OR (95% CI)*
QIDS[b]	None	reference	reference	reference	reference
	Mild	2.59 (1.55–4.34)**	3.72 (2.13–6.49)**	3.99 (2.13–7.49)**	4.05 (1.99–8.23)**
	Moderate	1.10 (0.59–2.02)	1.56 (.91–3.40)	3.32 (1.62–6.80)*	2.91 (1.31–6.48)*
	(Very) Severe	1.11 (.43–2.87)	2.18 (.81–5.87)	4.66 (1.65–13.16)*	7.93 (2.70–23.35)**
BAI[c]	Normal	reference	reference	reference	reference
	Mild	1.76 (.59–12.51)	2.41 (1.36–4.29)*	2.66 (1.42–4.97)*	3.07 (1.54–6.12)*
	Moderate	2.23 (.99–5.03)	4.22 (1.82–9.79)*	3.89 (1.60–9.45)*	6.69 (2.66–16.84)**
	Severe	2.73 (1.02–3.02)*	6.70 (1.44–31.20)*	8.29 (1.73–39.59)*	13.32 (2.73–64.97)*

*p<.05;
**p<.001.
[a]reference category is no pain.
[b]adjusted for age, gender, level of education, partner status, chronic diseases, antidepressant use, use of other psychotropic drugs, number of depressive episodes, and severity of anxiety symptoms.
[c]adjusted for age, gender, level of education, partner status, chronic diseases, antidepressant use, use of other psychotropic drugs, number of depressive episodes, and severity of depressive symptoms.

distinctively other group of patients than those with depression without pain, with the former having a focus on health and the latter having a focus on a negative view of the self [58,59]. If that is the case, the treatment should be different for depressive disorder with pain and depressive disorder without pain. The same could possibly apply to patients with an anxiety disorder with or without pain. This finding warrants further research, to examine if having a depressive or anxiety disorder in remission may be a possible risk factor for subsequent long lasting chronic pain.

Pain location

Of the total sample, 92.4% reported pain symptoms of musculoskeletal nature, followed by 48% reporting gastro-intestinal pain and 25.6% of cardio respiratory pain. Because musculoskeletal pain has by far the highest prevalence in this study, we expected that this pain location would have the highest association with depression and anxiety. However, this expectation was not confirmed. Our findings show that those with a current depressive disorder or a remitted depressive or anxiety disorder have high odds for having musculoskeletal pain, but the odds for having pain of cardio respiratory origin are also large when compared to having no depressive or anxiety disorder. Furthermore, persons having a current anxiety or co-morbid depressive and anxiety disorder show high odds for having cardio respiratory pain. These findings remain after adjustment for chronic cardio respiratory illness.

In a review by Celano & Huffman [60], depressive disorder was associated with cardiac disease, such as coronary artery disease. This also applies to anxiety which appears to be a risk factor for coronary heart disease and cardiac mortality [61]. The finding

Table 10. (Results of sensitivity analysis, with CPG0 and CPG1 combined) Association of severity of depressive symptoms and anxiety symptoms with the Chronic Pain Grade.

		CPG2[a,b]	CPG3[a,b]	CPG4[a,b]
		OR (95% CI)	*OR (95% CI)*	*OR (95% CI)*
QIDS[b]	None	reference	reference	reference
	Mild	1.55 (1.18–2.02)*	1.65 (1.11–2.46)*	1.67 (1.00–2.80)*
	Moderate	1.67 (1.21–2.33)*	3.14 (2.04–4.83)**	2.75 (1.58–4.78)**
	(Very) Severe	2.05 (1.36–3.09)*	4.37 (2.61–7.33)**	7.42 (4.08–13.649)**
BAI[c]	Normal	reference	reference	reference
	Mild	1.42 (1.09–1.85)*	1.57 (1.09–2.24)*	1.81 (1.14–2.87)*
	Moderate	1.99 (1.44–2.75)**	1.83 (1.19–2.81)*	3.15 (1.91–5.19)**
	Severe	2.59 (1.63–4.13)**	3.12 (1.86–5.53)**	5.16 (2.83–9.41)**

*p<.05;
**p<.001.
[a]reference category is no pain.
[b]adjusted for age, gender, level of education, partner status, chronic diseases, antidepressant use, use of other psychotropic drugs, number of depressive episodes, and severity of anxiety symptoms.
[c]adjusted for age, gender, level of education, partner status, chronic diseases, antidepressant use, use of other psychotropic drugs, number of depressive episodes, and severity of depressive symptoms.

Table 11. Associations of remitted psychopathology, current depressive disorder, current anxiety disorder, and current co-morbid depression and anxiety with pain location, with no depression and/or anxiety as reference category.

	No pain[a]	Musculoskeletal[a]	Gastro-intestinal[a]	Cardio respiratory[a]
	OR (95% CI)	*OR (95% CI)*	*OR (95% CI)*	*OR (95% CI)*
No psychopathology	reference	reference	reference	reference
Remitted depression/anxiety	.47 (.30–.75)*	2.28 (1.53–3.42)**	1.40 (1.10–1.78)*	1.74 (1.27–2.40)*
Depression current	.52 (.28–.97)*	2.64 (1.53–4.56)**	2.43 (1.84–3.22)**	2.63 (1.86–3.70)**
Anxiety current	.39 (.24–.66)**	2.29 (1.49–3.51)**	2.08 (1.61–2.68)**	2.96 (2.16–4.04)**
Co-morbid depression and anxiety current	.19 (.10–.38)**	3.88 (2.33–6.47)**	3.31 (2.57–4.27)**	5.15 (3.80–6.98)**

*p<.05;
**p<.001.
a = adjusted for age, gender, level of education, partner status, antidepressant use, use of other psychotropic drugs, number of depressive episodes, and chronic disease.

that anxiety shows such high odds for cardio respiratory pain symptoms, even when we controlled for cardio respiratory disease, could be due to the fact that anxious patients with chest pain are more sensitive to bodily sensations [62]; in that case, the experience of pain would be centrally modulated in such a way as to elevate the odds for experiencing pain. However, another explanation might be possible as well; stress induced anxiety has an elevating effect on cytokines [49], and elevated cytokines lead to pain symptoms. This might explain our findings.

In the STAR*D study, depressed patients (with less sleep quality and sympathetic arousal) showed an association with higher cardiac risk, which may be similar to our findings [63] whereby having a depressive disorder had higher odds for having cardio respiratory pain when compared to having no depressive or anxiety disorder. Even when we controlled for having a chronic disease of cardio respiratory origin, the association remained strong and significant. Previous research showed that having a mental illness is a possible risk factor for cardiovascular disease [64,65]. Our finding that a depression/anxiety, whether or not in remission, shows a strong association with cardiac pain is worth exploring in further longitudinal research to explore a possible causal relation of depression and/or anxiety (current or in remission) with cardiac disease, of which cardio respiratory pain might be an early indicator.

Strengths of the study

A strength of this study is the large sample size. Also, because patients with a depressive or anxiety disorder often report pain in multiple locations, the categorisation of pain locations makes these results clinically relevant and widely applicable. Moreover, this study not only examines the association of pain with depressive or anxiety disorder, but also with co-morbid depression and anxiety, as well as with remitted disorders. Additionally, in the analyses of the pain symptoms, the no pain group was the reference category which is new compared to earlier studies that compared low pain with high pain – which is subject to interpretation bias as pain is a subjective experience. In our study, we had a healthy control group with no pain in which better contrasts could be made with those who had pain.

Limitations

This study also has some limitations. First, it is not possible to make inferences about causality because this was a cross-sectional observational study. Second, some of the subgroups of our sample were smaller than the other groups, such as those with no pain symptoms (CPG0, N = 170). However, a sensitivity analysis revealed that the association between severity of depressive and anxiety symptoms and CPG mostly remains, with more severe depressive or anxiety symptoms being more strongly associated with more disabling and limiting pain when CPG0 and CPG1 were combined to have a larger reference group. Therefore, these associations can be considered valid and of clinical relevance as they indicate a clear difference in association with depression or anxiety between patients with and without pain. Another possible limitation is the self-reporting of physical illness, which might lead to overreporting or underreporting of chronic physical illness; however, a study by Kriegsman et al. [66] shows that patients report their physical illness fairly accurately when compared to the reports of their general practitioner, even when taking depressive symptomatology into account. Furthermore, no information was available whether a physical illness was organic or functional, which may have its effect on pain. For example, individuals with an organic disease describe their pain as consistent, whereas those without an organic disease describe their pain as variable and diffuse [67]. Also, PTSD has been linked to increased risk for pain [68,69]. Therefore, future research that examines the association of anxiety disorders with pain should also include PTSD.

Conclusion

This study shows that depressive and anxiety disorders have a similar and very strong association with the CPG (which includes pain-related disability and pain intensity) and musculoskeletal pain, cardio respiratory pain, and gastro-intestinal pain compared to a control group without depressive or anxiety disorder. Depression and anxiety share the same pathophysiological pathways as pain and can have a reciprocal effect on each other, which could explain these associations. Moreover, even a remitted disorder has a strong association with pain. This might mean that patients with depression or anxiety and pain are a different group and need different treatment than patients that do not have pain accompanying their depression or anxiety. Depression and anxiety also have a strong association with cardio respiratory pain, and this association remained after correction for cardiovascular or respiratory illness. This strong association between depression/anxiety (current or in remission) with cardio respiratory pain is an interesting finding, which warrants further longitudinal research to examine a possible causal relation of cardiac pain and a mental disorder (current or in remission) with cardiac disease.

Author Contributions

Conceived and designed the experiments: BWJHP ATFB PS HWJM. Performed the experiments: BWJHP ATFB PS HWJM. Analyzed the data: EH MMJGG BWJHP HWJM MWMW PS. Contributed reagents/materials/analysis tools: BWJHP ATFB PS HWJM. Contributed to the writing of the manuscript: EH MMJGG ATFB JD BWJHP HWJM MWMW PS CMFC.

References

1. Bair MJ, Robinson RL, Katon W, Kroenke K (2003) Depression and pain comorbidity: a literature review. Arch Intern Med 163: 2433–2445.
2. Demyttenaere K, Bruffaerts R, Lee S, Posada-Villa J, Kovess V, et al. (2007) Mental disorders among persons with chronic back or neck pain: results from the World Mental Health Surveys. Pain 129: 332–342.
3. Gureje O, Von Korff M, Kola L, Demyttenaere K, He Y, et al. (2008) The relation between multiple pains and mental disorders: results from the World Mental Health Surveys. Pain 135: 82–91.
4. Gureje O, Von Korff M, Simon GE, Gater R (1998) Persistent pain and well-being: a World Health Organization Study in Primary Care. JAMA 280: 147–151.
5. Means-Christensen AJ, Roy-Byrne PP, Sherbourne CD, Craske MG, Stein MB (2008) Relationships among pain, anxiety, and depression in primary care. Depress Anxiety 25: 593–600.
6. Stahl S, Briley M (2004) Understanding pain in depression. Hum Psychopharmacol 19: S9–S13.
7. Wise TN, Fishbain DA, Holder-Perkins V (2007) Painful physical symptoms in depression: a clinical challenge. Pain Med 8: S75–82.
8. Burloux G, Forestier P, Dalery J, Guyotat J (1989) Chronic pain and posttraumatic stress disorders. Psychother Psychosom 52: 119–124.
9. Ayuso Mateos JL, Bayon Perez C, Santo-Domingo Carrasco J, Olivares D (1989) Atypical chest pain and panic disorder. Psychother Psychosom 52: 92–95.
10. Ohayon MM, Schatzberg AF (2003) Using chronic pain to predict depressive morbidity in the general population. Arch Gen Psychiatry 60: 39–47.
11. Saito T, Kai I, Takizawa A (2012) Effects of a program to prevent social isolation on loneliness, depression, and subjective well-being of older adults: a randomized trial among older migrants in Japan. Arch Gerontol Geriatr 55: 539–547.
12. Jang Y, Haley WE, Small BJ, Mortimer JA (2002) The role of mastery and social resources in the associations between disability and depression in later life. Gerontologist 42: 807–813.
13. Ossipov MH, Dussor GO, Porreca F (2010) Central modulation of pain. J Clin Invest 120: 3779–3787.
14. Millan MJ (2002) Descending control of pain. Prog Neurobiol 66: 355–474.
15. Vlaeyen JW, Linton SJ (2000) Fear-avoidance and its consequences in chronic musculoskeletal pain: a state of the art. Pain 85: 317–332.
16. Asmundson GJ, Katz J (2009) Understanding the co-occurrence of anxiety disorders and chronic pain: state-of-the-art. Depress Anxiety 26: 888–901.
17. Sareen J, Cox BJ, Clara I, Asmundson GJ (2005) The relationship between anxiety disorders and physical disorders in the U.S. National Comorbidity Survey. Depress Anxiety 21: 193–202.
18. McWilliams LA, Cox BJ, Enns MW (2003) Mood and anxiety disorders associated with chronic pain: an examination in a nationally representative sample. Pain 106: 127–133.
19. Beesdo K, Jacobi F, Hoyer J, Low NC, Hofler M, et al. (2010) Pain associated with specific anxiety and depressive disorders in a nationally representative population sample. Soc Psychiatry Psychiatr Epidemiol 45: 89–104.
20. Gerhardt A, Hartmann M, Schuller-Roma B, Blumenstiel K, Bieber C, et al. (2011) The prevalence and type of Axis-I and Axis-II mental disorders in subjects with non-specific chronic back pain: results from a population-based study. Pain Med 12: 1231–1240.
21. Gerrits MM, Vogelzangs N, van Oppen P, van Marwijk HW, van der Horst H, et al. (2012) Impact of pain on the course of depressive and anxiety disorders. Pain 153: 429–436.
22. Papakostas GI, Petersen T, Denninger J, Sonawalla SB, Mahal Y, et al. (2003) Somatic symptoms in treatment-resistant depression. Psychiatry Res 118: 39–45.
23. Teh CF, Morone NE, Karp JF, Belnap BH, Zhu F, et al. (2009) Pain interference impacts response to treatment for anxiety disorders. Depress Anxiety 26: 222–228.
24. Karp JF, Scott J, Houck P, Reynolds CF 3rd, Kupfer DJ, et al. (2005) Pain predicts longer time to remission during treatment of recurrent depression. J Clin Psychiatry 66: 591–597.
25. Gilkey DP, Keefe TJ, Peel JL, Kassab OM, Kennedy CA (2010) Risk factors associated with back pain: a cross-sectional study of 963 college students. J Manipulative Physiol Ther 33: 88–95.
26. Janwantanakul P, Sitthipornvorakul E, Paksaichol A (2012) Risk factors for the onset of nonspecific low back pain in office workers: a systematic review of prospective cohort studies. J Manipulative Physiol Ther 35: 568–577.
27. Kindler LL, Jones KD, Perrin N, Bennett RM (2010) Risk factors predicting the development of widespread pain from chronic back or neck pain. J Pain 11: 1320–1328.
28. Croft PR, Lewis M, Papageorgiou AC, Thomas E, Jayson MI, et al. (2001) Risk factors for neck pain: a longitudinal study in the general population. Pain 93: 317–325.
29. Wessely S, Nimnuan C, Sharpe M (1999) Functional somatic syndromes: one or many? Lancet 354: 936–939.
30. Nimnuan C, Hotopf M, Wessely S (2001) Medically unexplained symptoms: an epidemiological study in seven specialities. J Psychosom Res 51: 361–367.
31. Fink P, Toft T, Hansen MS, Ornbol E, Olesen F (2007) Symptoms and syndromes of bodily distress: an exploratory study of 978 internal medical, neurological, and primary care patients. Psychosom Med 69: 30–39.
32. Lucchetti G, Oliveira AB, Mercante JP, Peres MF (2012) Anxiety and fear-avoidance in musculoskeletal pain. Curr Pain Headache Rep 16: 399–406.
33. Walter SA, Jones MP, Talley NJ, Kjellstrom L, Nyhlin H, et al. (2013) Abdominal pain is associated with anxiety and depression scores in a sample of the general adult population with no signs of organic gastrointestinal disease. Neurogastroenterol Motil 25: 741–e576.
34. Shahid M, Rehmani R, Khan MM (2004) Anxiety and depression among young adults with chest pain. J Coll Physicians Surg Pak 14: 700.
35. Penninx BW, Beekman AT, Smit JH, Zitman FG, Nolen WA, et al. (2008) The Netherlands Study of Depression and Anxiety (NESDA): rationale, objectives and methods. Int J Methods Psychiatr Res 17: 121–140.
36. Wittchen HU (1994) Reliability and validity studies of the WHO–Composite International Diagnostic Interview (CIDI): a critical review. J Psychiatr Res 28: 57–84.
37. Von Korff M, Ormel J, Keefe FJ, Dworkin SF (1992) Grading the severity of chronic pain. Pain 50: 133–149.
38. Smith BH, Penny KI, Purves AM, Munro C, Wilson B, et al. (1997) The Chronic Pain Grade questionnaire: validation and reliability in postal research. Pain 71: 141–147.
39. Rush AJ, Trivedi MH, Ibrahim HM, Carmody TJ, Arnow B, et al. (2003) The 16-Item Quick Inventory of Depressive Symptomatology (QIDS), clinician rating (QIDS-C), and self-report (QIDS-SR): a psychometric evaluation in patients with chronic major depression. Biol Psychiatry 54: 573–583.
40. Rush AJ, Gullion CM, Basco MR, Jarrett RB, Trivedi MH (1996) The Inventory of Depressive Symptomatology (IDS): psychometric properties. Psychol Med 26: 477–486.
41. Beck AT, Epstein N, Brown G, Steer RA (1988) An inventory for measuring clinical anxiety: psychometric properties. J Consult Clin Psychol 56: 893–897.
42. Kabacoff RI, Segal DL, Hersen M, Van Hasselt VB (1997) Psychometric properties and diagnostic utility of the Beck Anxiety Inventory and the State-Trait Anxiety Inventory with older adult psychiatric outpatients. J Anxiety Disord 11: 33–47.
43. Bair MJ, Robinson RL, Eckert GJ, Stang PE, Croghan TW, et al. (2004) Impact of pain on depression treatment response in primary care. Psychosom Med 66: 17–22.
44. Campbell LC, Clauw DJ, Keefe FJ (2003) Persistent pain and depression: a biopsychosocial perspective. Biol Psychiatry 54: 399–409.
45. Maes M, Yirmyia R, Noraberg J, Brene S, Hibbeln J, et al. (2009) The inflammatory & neurodegenerative (I&ND) hypothesis of depression: leads for future research and new drug developments in depression. Metab Brain Dis 24: 27–53.
46. Schulz E, Zherdin A, Tiemann L, Plant C, Ploner M (2012) Decoding an individual's sensitivity to pain from the multivariate analysis of EEG data. Cereb Cortex 22: 1118–1123.
47. Mogil JS (1999) The genetic mediation of individual differences in sensitivity to pain and its inhibition. Proc Natl Acad Sci U S A 96: 7744–7751.
48. Ziv M, Tomer R, Defrin R, Hendler T (2010) Individual sensitivity to pain expectancy is related to differential activation of the hippocampus and amygdala. Hum Brain Mapp 31: 326–338.
49. Maes M, Song C, Lin A, De Jongh R, Van Gastel A, et al. (1998) The effects of psychological stress on humans: increased production of pro-inflammatory cytokines and a Th1-like response in stress-induced anxiety. Cytokine 10: 313–318.
50. Felger JC, Lotrich FE (2013) Inflammatory cytokines in depression: neurobiological mechanisms and therapeutic implications. Neuroscience 246: 199–229.
51. Sharpley CF, Agnew LL (2011) Cytokines and depression: findings, issues, and treatment implications. Rev Neurosci 22: 295–302.
52. de Oliveira CM, Sakata RK, Issy AM, Gerola LR, Salomao R (2011) Cytokines and pain. Rev Bras Anestesiol 61: 255–259, 260–255, 137–242.
53. Shubayev VI, Kato K, Myers RR (2010) Cytokines in Pain. In: Kruger L, Light AR, editors. Translational Pain Research: From Mouse to Man. Boca Raton, FL: Llc.
54. Fava M, Alpert JE, Carmin CN, Wisniewski SR, Trivedi MH, et al. (2004) Clinical correlates and symptom patterns of anxious depression among patients with major depressive disorder in STAR*D. Psychol Med 34: 1299–1308.
55. Fava M, Rush AJ, Alpert JE, Carmin CN, Balasubramani GK, et al. (2006) What clinical and symptom features and comorbid disorders characterize outpatients with anxious major depressive disorder: a replication and extension. Can J Psychiatry 51: 823–835.

56. Fava M, Rush AJ, Alpert JE, Balasubramani GK, Wisniewski SR, et al. (2008) Difference in treatment outcome in outpatients with anxious versus nonanxious depression: a STAR*D report. Am J Psychiatry 165: 342–351.
57. Scholten WD, Batelaan NM, van Balkom AJ, Wjh Penninx B, Smit JH, et al. (2013) Recurrence of anxiety disorders and its predictors. J Affect Disord 147: 180–185.
58. Pincus T, Williams A (1999) Models and measurements of depression in chronic pain. J Psychosom Res 47: 211–219.
59. Tossani E (2013) The concept of mental pain. Psychother Psychosom 82: 67–73.
60. Celano CM, Huffman JC (2011) Depression and cardiac disease: a review. Cardiol Rev 19: 130–142.
61. Roest AM, Martens EJ, de Jonge P, Denollet J (2010) Anxiety and risk of incident coronary heart disease: a meta-analysis. J Am Coll Cardiol 56: 38–46.
62. Cheng C, Wong WM, Lai KC, Wong BC, Hu WH, et al. (2003) Psychosocial factors in patients with noncardiac chest pain. Psychosom Med 65: 443–449.
63. Fraguas R Jr, Iosifescu DV, Alpert J, Wisniewski SR, Barkin JL, et al. (2007) Major depressive disorder and comorbid cardiac disease: is there a depressive subtype with greater cardiovascular morbidity? Results from the STAR*D study. Psychosomatics 48: 418–425.
64. Gladigau EL, Fazio TN, Hannam JP, Dawson LM, Jones SG (2014) Increased cardiovascular risk in patients with severe mental illness. Intern Med J 44: 65–69.
65. Nielsen TJ, Vestergaard M, Christensen B, Christensen KS, Larsen KK (2013) Mental health status and risk of new cardiovascular events or death in patients with myocardial infarction: a population-based cohort study. BMJ Open 3.
66. Kriegsman DM, Penninx BW, van Eijk JT, Boeke AJ, Deeg DJ (1996) Self-reports and general practitioner information on the presence of chronic diseases in community dwelling elderly. A study on the accuracy of patients' self-reports and on determinants of inaccuracy. J Clin Epidemiol 49: 1407–1417.
67. Leavitt F, Garron DC, D'Angelo CM, McNeill TW (1979) Low back pain in patients with and without demonstrable organic disease. Pain 6: 191–200.
68. Beck JG, Clapp JD (2011) A different kind of co-morbidity: Understanding posttraumatic stress disorder and chronic pain. Psychol Trauma 3: 101–108.
69. Roth RS, Geisser ME, Bates R (2008) The relation of post-traumatic stress symptoms to depression and pain in patients with accident-related chronic pain. J Pain 9: 588–596.

3

Successful Application of Adaptive Emotion Regulation Skills Predicts the Subsequent Reduction of Depressive Symptom Severity but neither the Reduction of Anxiety nor the Reduction of General Distress during the Treatment of Major Depressive Disorder

Carolin M. Wirtz[1,2]*, Anna Radkovsky[1], David D. Ebert[1,3], Matthias Berking[2]

1 Department of Clinical Psychology and Psychotherapy, University of Marburg, Marburg, Hesse, Germany, **2** Department of Clinical Psychology and Psychotherapy, University of Erlangen- Nuremberg, Erlangen, Baveria, Germany, **3** Division for Clinical Psychology and Psychotherapy, Department for Psychology, Leuphana University Lueneburg, Lueneburg, Lower Saxony, Germany

Abstract

Objective: Deficits in general emotion regulation (ER) skills have been linked to symptoms of depression and are thus considered a promising target in the treatment of Major depressive disorder (MDD). However, at this point, the extent to which such skills are relevant for coping with depression and whether they should instead be considered a transdiagnostic factor remain unclear. Therefore, the present study aimed to investigate whether successful ER skills application is associated with changes in depressive symptom severity (DSS), anxiety symptom severity (ASS), and general distress severity (GDS) over the course of treatment for MDD.

Methods: Successful ER skills application, DSS, ASS, and GDS were assessed four times during the first three weeks of treatment in 175 inpatients who met the criteria for MDD. We computed Pearson correlations to test whether successful ER skills application and the three indicators of psychopathology are cross-sectionally associated. We then performed latent growth curve modelling to test whether changes in successful ER skills application are negatively associated with a reduction of DSS, ASS, or GDS. Finally, we utilized latent change score models to examine whether successful ER skills application predicts subsequent reduction of DSS, ASS, or GDS.

Results: Successful ER skills application was cross-sectionally associated with lower levels of DSS, ASS, and GDS at all points of assessment. An increase in successful skills application during treatment was associated with a decrease in DSS and GDS but not ASS. Finally, successful ER skills application predicted changes in subsequent DSS but neither changes in ASS nor changes in GDS.

Conclusions: Although general ER skills might be relevant for a broad range of psychopathological symptoms, they might be particularly important for the maintenance and treatment of depressive symptoms.

Editor: Antonio Verdejo García, University of Granada, Spain

Funding: The authors have no support or funding to report.

Competing Interests: The authors have declared that no competing interests exist.

* Email: carolin.wirtz@staff.uni-marburg.de

Introduction

Major depressive disorder (MDD) is one of the most common mental disorders [1] and is considered to be a leading cause of disease burden worldwide [2]. Despite the availability of effective pharmacological and psychological treatments [3], outcome research also indicates that even when treated with evidence-based interventions, MDD remains a highly prevalent [1], usually recurrent [4], and potentially chronic problem [5,6]. In patients suffering from MDD, anxiety, nervousness, and their somatic correlates are common comorbid symptoms. For example, Melartin and colleagues [7] found that nearly 60% of patients with an episode of MDD suffered from at least one comorbid anxiety disorder. The most frequent comorbid anxiety disorder in patients with MDD is social phobia, followed by generalized anxiety disorder, and panic disorder [8,9]. MDD with high levels of anxiety symptoms has been found to be associated with an even greater functional impairment, chronicity [10], delayed response to treatment [11], more severe depression, and an increased risk of suicidality [12]. Moreover, the presence of a comorbid anxiety disorder predicts a poorer long-term outcome and a greater familial prevalence of MDD [11,13]. These findings indicate that more research is needed to improve the efficacy and sustainability of psychotherapeutic treatments for MDD especially when co-occurring anxiety disorders have to be taken into account. Such research should include studies aiming to identify mechanisms that facilitate change in evidence-based treatments for depression and anxiety symptoms [14,15]. Potentially relevant mechanisms include transdiagnostic factors, which can be hypothesized to be relevant for either common symptoms co-occurring in depressive and anxiety disorders or common causes of these two forms of psychopathology disorders. With regard to common symptoms, several studies have shown that depression and anxiety disorders share a general distress factor [16–18].

Recent research has focused on general deficits in emotion regulation (ER) as a putative factor in the maintenance of various forms of psychopathology [19–23]. ER refers to the set of processes whereby people seek to monitor, evaluate, and redirect the spontaneous flow of their emotions to accomplish their needs and goals [24–26]. Deficits in general ER skills may contribute to the development of both MDD and anxiety disorders in several ways. First, the inability to down-regulate undesired affective states may lead to an escalation or perpetuation of each of these states and may thus enhance an individual's likelihood of meeting the diagnostic criteria for anxiety disorders or depression [27,28]. Second, deficits in ER skills may lead to increased aversive emotional experiences in general and may thus increase an individual's vulnerability to developing mental disorders in general [21,23]. More specifically, the absence of effective ER skills likely amplifies the risk that an individual's evaluates the current situation as aversive and beyond one's control, which is a relevant antecedent of anxiogenic and depressogenic information processing [29,30]. Finally, in the absence of effective ER skills, the interaction of subthreshold symptoms of anxiety and depression may significantly impede an individual's attempt to cope with both anxiety and depression. For example, (subthreshold) anxiety may interfere with the individual's attempt to engage in positive activities when working to overcome depression; similarly, feelings of dysphoria, helplessness, and hopelessness may interfere with the individual's attempt to confront feared stimuli in order to overcome anxiety [31,32].

Based on the assumption that deficits in ER contribute to the development and maintenance of various mental disorders, Berking [33–35] proposed a skill-based model of adaptive coping with emotions (ACE) that facilitates the use of the notoriously broad and abstract concept of ER for clinical purposes. The ACE model conceptualizes adaptive ER as a situation-dependent interaction between the following ER skills: (1) the ability to be consciously aware of emotions, (2) the ability to identify emotions, (3) the ability to correctly label emotions, (4) the ability to identify what has caused and what maintains one's present emotions, (5) the ability to actively modify emotions in an adaptive manner, (6) the ability to accept undesired emotions when they cannot be changed, (7) the ability to tolerate undesired emotions when they cannot be changed, (8) the ability to approach and confront situations that are likely to trigger negative emotions if this is necessary to attain personally relevant goals, and (9) the ability to provide compassionate self-support when working to cope with challenging emotions. The model additionally includes the hypothesis that only the acceptance/tolerance and modification of undesired emotions are ultimately relevant for mental health. All other skills are only necessary to the extent that they facilitate an individual's ability to successfully accept/tolerate or modify undesired emotions.

Numerous studies have provided empirical evidence on the relevance of skills included in the ACE model for both depression and anxiety disorders. For example, cross-sectional studies suggest that symptom severity in both MDD and anxiety disorders are associated with difficulties in identifying and labeling emotions [36–39], accepting and tolerating negative emotions [40–47], compassionately supporting oneself when facing challenging emotions [48–50], and adaptively modifying emotions [51–53]. Moreover, in both disorders, patients report experiencing high levels of shame and hopelessness [54,55] and using dysfunctional ER strategies when working to cope with challenging experiences such as rumination or avoidance [19,56].

Longitudinal studies suggest that deficits in ER predict the subsequent severity of depression and anxiety symptoms in clinical and nonclinical samples. For example, in nonclinical samples, deficits in ER skills application negatively predicted subsequent anxiety symptom severity over a 2-week period [33] and the level of both depression and anxiety over a 5-year interval [57,58]. Additional longitudinal evidence is provided by studies showing that rumination in response to undesired emotions prospectively predicted the level of depressive symptoms as well as the prevalence of anxiety disorders in clinical and nonclinical samples as well as adults, adolescents, and children [59–61]. Studies that have failed to find evidence for the importance of general ER skills for both depression and anxiety include a study by McLaughlin and colleagues [32], in which ER also predicted subsequent increases in anxiety symptoms but did not predict the level of depressive symptoms in a large sample of adolescents over a 7-month period. Similarly, in the aforementioned study by Berking [33], ER skills significantly predicted anxiety symptoms and negative affect, but a nonsignificant trend was found for the ability of ER skills to predict subsequent depression. However, in another study, ER skills negatively predicted the level of depressive symptoms over a 5-year interval in a nonclinical sample [58]. Therefore, Berking and colleagues argued that general ER skills are relevant first for preventing the onset of anxiety and negative affect and subsequently for preventing the onset of depressive symptoms. However, at this point, this hypothesis has not yet been systematically investigated.

In addition to clarifying moderators explaining the partly inconsistent findings regarding the transdiagnostic relevance of ER skills, the present study investigates the reciprocal associations between general ER skills and symptoms of depression, anxiety, and general distress over the course of treatment, as studies on these associations are lacking in the literature to this point. In particular, a general distress factor has been included in the analyses in the present study because it has frequently been associated with depressive and anxiety disorders. Distress may simply be a symptom occurring in both forms of psychopathology, or it may even be the common cause for the onset of depressive and anxiety disorders. If fostering ER skills reduces the intensity of symptoms of these three domains, adopting such a transdiagnostic approach might be more economical than compiling a number of strategies that each focus on one domain of psychopathology [20].

The present study thus aimed to clarify the reciprocal associations between the successful application of arguably adaptive general ER skills (as included in the ACE model) and depressive symptom severity (DSS), anxiety symptom severity (ASS), and general distress symptom severity (GDS) over the course of treatment for MDD. More specifically, we first tested whether the ability to successfully apply adaptive ER skills would be cross-sectionally associated with lower levels of DSS, ASS, or GDS during four stages of treatment for MDD. Second, we tested whether changes in successful ER skills application would be negatively associated with changes in DSS, ASS, or GDS during treatment for MDD. Finally, we aimed to clarify whether successful ER skills application would predict subsequent changes in DSS, ASS, and GDS during treatment for MDD.

Methods

Procedures and Participants

The study was conducted in a German mental health hospital between August 2010 and August 2012 [62]. Once a week, participants completed a set of self-report questionnaires that assessed successful ER skills application, depressive symptom severity (DSS), anxiety symptom severity (ASS), and general psychological distress severity (GDS) (see Measures). Given that the majority of patients who were treated in the hospital stayed for at least three weeks, we chose to cover this 3-week period in the analyses. The assessments took place on a weekly basis, starting in the first week of hospital admission. If participants missed an assessment, they were allowed to make up the assessment within the next two days. All participants were invited to complete the four points of assessment, which were provided through an online assessment tool. Data entry, transmission, and storage were strictly protected from unauthorized access. All study procedures followed internationally accepted human research guidelines, such as the Helsinki Protocol, and received approval by the ethics committee of Marburg University. All participants provided their written consent to participate in the study. The written consent has been approved by the ethics committee.

In order to be eligible for the study, participants were required to meet the following criteria: (a) current diagnosis of MDD according to the DSM-IV criteria, (b) pre-treatment BDI score of 11 or above, (c) 18 years of age or above, (d) sufficient German language skills to complete the questionnaires, and (e) no current alcohol or drug addiction, psychoses, bipolar disorder, brain damage, or other severe somatic disorders requiring other treatments. Based on sensitivity and specificity analyses, Riedel and colleagues [63] recently recommended 11 or above as a clinical cut-off score for the German version of the BDI, which is used in the present study. To maximize the external validity of the findings, no further exclusion criteria were considered (e.g., regarding comorbidity, antidepressant medication, or suicidal tendencies).

Within the first week of treatment, diagnostic assessments were conducted. Participants were interviewed with the Structured Clinical Interview for the DSM-IV (German version: SCID [64]). All raters who conducted the diagnostic interviews had a Bachelor's degree or higher in clinical psychology and had all received extensive training in the SCID interview (18 hours of training by a certified trainer). In addition, all raters were supervised by experienced psychotherapists (either psychologists or physicians with a Master's degree or higher in psychology or medicine).

The final sample consisted of 175 participants. The average total length of treatment was about seven weeks ($M = 7.2$; $SD = 2.35$; *range* = 2.85–22.89). The majority of the participants had at least one comorbid Axis I diagnosis (58.9%). The most common comorbidity included anxiety disorders (any anxiety disorder: 51.4%; social phobia: 26.1%; agoraphobia: 20.7%; generalized anxiety disorder: 18%; panic disorder: 14.4%; posttraumatic stress disorder: 10.8%), followed by comorbid somatoform disorders (35.1%) and dysthymia (13.5%). About one-third of the participants (36%) met the criteria for at least two comorbid Axis I disorders. About one-quarter of the participants (23.0%) met the criteria for at least one Axis II disorder. Among these disorders, the most common were avoidant personality disorder (8.6%), obsessive-compulsive personality disorder (3.9%), and borderline personality disorder (3.3%).

All of the participants were Caucasian (which is quite representative of the German population), the majority were women (57.7%), and the average age was 46.7 years ($SD = 10.8$, *range* = 18–71). The highest level of education ("Abitur") was reported by 40% of the sample, 35.4% reported to have completed the second highest level of education ("Realschulabschluss"), and 15.4% had completed the lowest level of education. Nearly half of the participants (44.6%) were married, 13.1% were divorced, and 28% had never been married; moreover, 59.4% had at least one child.

Treatment

During the treatment period under investigation, the participants received an average of 3.63 hours ($SD = 1.29$, *range* = 3.00–6.00) of individual and 23.64 hours ($SD = 1.58$, *range* = 16.00–26.00) of group psychotherapy. About half of the group-based therapy specifically focused on depression, utilizing cognitive behavioral therapy techniques developed and validated for this disorder [65]. All of the participants received group treatment for depression during the first three weeks (followed by group therapy for comorbid disorders, such as anxiety disorders, if they were present). Psychotherapeutic interventions were supplemented with sports and arts therapy as well as medical treatment when necessary. All treatments were based on a cognitive behavioral rationale and included techniques such as behavior analyses, behavioral activation, cognitive restructuring, and relaxation training [66]. Psychotherapeutic treatment was delivered by experienced therapists and therapists in training-all of whom had a Master's degree in psychology or medicine. Supplementary treatments were delivered by trained nurses, sports and art therapists, physiotherapists, and medical doctors. Treatment integrity was ensured through regular team meetings and weekly supervision by licensed senior therapists. Treatment approaches that explicitly and exclusively targeted general ER skills were not included in any of the interventions [35,67,68].

Measures

Emotion-Regulation Skills Questionnaire. To assess successful ER skills application, we used the German version of the Emotion-Regulation Skills Questionnaire (ERSQ [69]). The ERSQ is a self-report questionnaire consisting of 27 items. Each of the nine skills is assessed on a 5-point Likert-type scale (*0 = not at all* to *4 = almost always*), which are preceded by the stem *"Last week I …"*. Based on the ACE model, successful skills application is assessed through the following nine subscales: *awareness* (e.g., "I paid attention to my feelings."), *sensations* (e.g., "My physical sensations were a good indication of how I was feeling."), *clarity* (e.g., "I was clear about what emotions I was experiencing."), *understanding* (e.g., "I was aware of why I felt the way I felt."), *modification* (e.g., "I was able to influence my negative feelings."), *acceptance* (e.g., "I accepted my emotions."), *tolerance* (e.g., "I felt I could tolerate my negative feelings."), *readiness to confront distressing situations when necessary to attain personally relevant goals* (e.g., "I did what I had planned, even if it made me feel uncomfortable or anxious."), and *self-support* (e.g., "I supported myself in emotionally distressing situations."). The total score of the ERSQ is computed as the mean of all 27 items. Previous studies have provided evidence that all scales of the ERSQ have good internal consistency; at least adequate retest reliability; good convergent, discriminate, and factorial validity; and significant sensitivity to change [33,57,58,62,69–73]. As indicated in Table 1,

Table 1. Descriptive Statistics for BDI and ERSQ over Time.

Measure	Time 1				Time 2				Time 3				Time 4			
	M	*SD*	*N*	*α*	*M*	*SD*	*N*	*α*	*M*	*SD*	*N*	*α*	*M*	*SD*	*N*	*α*
$ERSQ_{Total}$	2.87	.74	171	.96	3.07	0.76	112	.97	3.20	0.77	111	.96	3.25	0.79	101	.96
$DASS_{Stress}$	8.12	4.78	172	.88	7.44	4.48	114	.90	6.94	4.57	113	.86	6.72	4.66	105	.91
$DASS_{Depression}$	8.11	5.57	172	.92	7.05	4.82	114	.92	6.31	4.76	113	.91	5.72	4.75	105	.94
$DASS_{Anxiety}$	5.06	4.65	172	.85	4.41	3.72	114	.87	4.41	4.39	113	.86	4.23	4.18	105	.87

Note. ERSQ = Emotion-Regulation Skills Questionnaire, DASS = Depression Anxiety Stress Scale, *M* = Mean, *SD* = Standard Deviation, *N* = Number of completers, Means and standard deviations are based on FIML estimation.

in the present study, the internal consistencies were very good for the ERSQ score at all four assessment points (αT1–4 = .96–.97).

Depression Anxiety Stress Scale—21-item version. To assess separate scores for DSS, ASS, and GDS, we used the Depression Anxiety Stress Scale (DASS-21 [74]). Sample items include "I couldn't seem to experience any positive feelings" (depression), "I felt scared without any good reason" (anxiety), and "I found it hard to wind down" (general distress). Participants indicate how much each item applied to them over the past week on a 4-point Likert-scale. All subscales demonstrate very good internal consistency (α ranging from.88 to.94) in a clinical sample [75] and adequate retest-reliability (coefficients ranging from.71 to.81) in a clinical sample [76]. In the current study, the DASS-21 showed good internal consistencies for all four points of assessment (αT1–4 = .85–.92).

Statistical Analyses

Cross-sectional association and associations of change. To test whether successful ER skills application is negatively correlated with DSS, ASS, and GDS (Hypothesis 1), we computed Pearson product-moment coefficients (*r*) for all four assessment points. To determine whether changes in successful ER skills application are negatively associated with changes in DSS, ASS, and GDS over the course of treatment for MDD (Hypothesis 2), we used bivariate latent growth curve (LGC) modeling, which is based on structural equation modeling (SEM) [77,78]. Statistically, SEM represents an extension of general linear modeling procedures, such as ANOVA and multiple regression analysis. However, we prefer SEM to more parsimonious approaches, as SEM 1) allows for complex hypotheses that include interactions and reciprocal relationships to be tested, 2) allows for latent variable modeling to be used and thereby the effects of random measurement error to be corrected, and 3) allows for a model to be tested as an explanation of the underlying process, which has given rise to the empirical data.

In bivariate LGC, an individual growth curve is calculated for each of the two variables, and each growth curve correlated with the other growth curve. As an example of the association between ER and DSS, Figure 1 illustrates the path diagram of the bivariate latent growth curve model that is used in this study. The means of individual slopes and intercepts describe the group trend of change in the total sample (fixed effects), and the variability of the mean slope and intercept factors (random effects) represent the extent of intraindividual change [79,80]. The correlations of intercepts indicate the strength of the association between the initial level of successful ER skills application and the initial level of DSS, ASS, and GDS, and the slopes of the correlations indicate the strength of the association between changes in successful ER skills application and changes in depression, anxiety and general distress during treatment [80,81]. Following procedures proposed by Grimm [80], we fixed loadings for the intercept to one and fixed loadings for the slope to model linear growth, starting with zero for the first assessment point and ending with three for the final measurement at T4.

Prediction of subsequent latent change. To test whether successful ER skills application predicts subsequent reduction of DSS, ASS, and GDS (Hypothesis 3), we used latent change score analyses (LCS [78,82]). LCS models have recently been introduced into treatment outcome research to help identify relevant predictors of change by clarifying reciprocal pathways between two (or more) variables over time (e.g., [83–88]). LCS modeling integrates latent growth curve models and cross-lagged regression models to examine reciprocal dynamic processes between two variables. More specifically, time-lagged associations

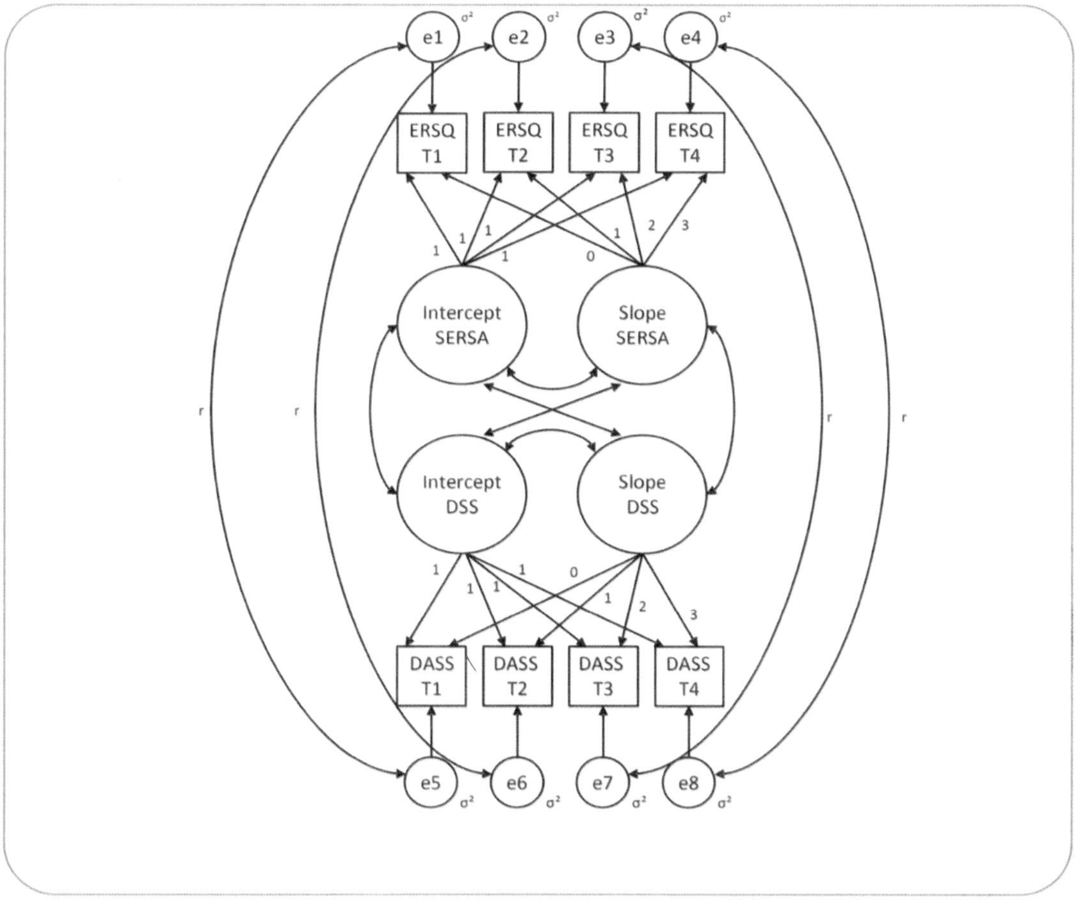

Figure 1. Path Diagram of the Bivariate Growth Curve Model. ERSQ = Emotion-Regulation Skills Questionnaire, DASS = Depression Anxiety Stress Scale, SERSA = Successful Emotion Regulation Skills Application, DSS = Depressive Symptoms Severity, e = residual error, σ^2 = variance, r = cross-construct error covariance (set equal across time); residual errors were allowed to covary across constructs within time to avoid bias due to variance related to specific assessment occasions and to increase model parsimony [80].

between Variable A and subsequent changes in Variable B and time-lagged associations between Variable B and subsequent changes in Variable A are estimated in the same model. To the extent that the influence of an unknown third variable associated with the dependent variable can be excluded (e.g., through sound theoretical assumptions or statistical procedures), significant associations between Variable A and subsequent changes in Variable B provide evidence for a causal effect of A on B (and vice versa).

Figure 2 illustrates the LCS model that we used to test Hypothesis 3 (as an example, we utilized the association between successful ER skills application (SERSA) and DSS). As indicated in the figure, the trajectory for true scores of both variables comprises an initial level of the unobserved score (intercept) and the accumulation of *true* latent changes in the unobserved variable. Latent change scores (ΔDSS and ΔSERSA in Figure 1) are computed as a function of (a) a constant change factor (slope), referring to systematic change over time; (b) a proportion parameter (β), representing the influence of the same variable at the previous measurement; and (c) a coupling parameter (γ), representing influence of the other variable at the previous time point. These coupling parameters describe dynamic aspects of the model, as they represent the impact of one variable at time *t-1* on the other variable at the next point of time *t* [80,81].

By setting different restrictions for the coupling parameters, specific hypotheses about the dynamic associations of, e.g., depression and ER skills application can be tested. Following the recommendations of Ferrer and McArdle [81] and McArdle and Grimm [89], we compared the model fit across the unrestricted model and the three nested models resulting from restricting the coupling parameters in accordance with assumptions regarding the prospective associations. In particular, we tested the following models (as an example, we again present the associations between DSS and SERSA): (a) a coupling effect exists for both parameters (bidirectional model, $\gamma SERSA \neq 0$, $\gamma DSS \neq 0$), (b) a coupling effect exists only for the SERSA to DSS association (unidirectional model, $\gamma SERSA \neq 0$, $\gamma DSS = 0$), (c) a coupling effect exists only for the DSS to SERSA association (unidirectional model, $\gamma SERSA = 0$, $\gamma DSS \neq 0$), and (d) no coupling effects exist for any of the parameters ($\gamma SERSA = 0$; $\gamma DSS = 0$). More specifically, we tested whether the bidirectional or either of the unidirectional models would show significantly better fit than the no-coupling model. The same procedure was applied for the LCS analyses for ASS and GDS. The cross-sectional associations between both variables were incorporated by a) allowing the error variance to covary between each point of assessment and b) correlating the intercept of SERSA with the intercept of DSS, ASS, or GDS.

The evaluation of the SEM model fit was based on current recommendations [90,91]. Aside from the χ^2 statistic, we used

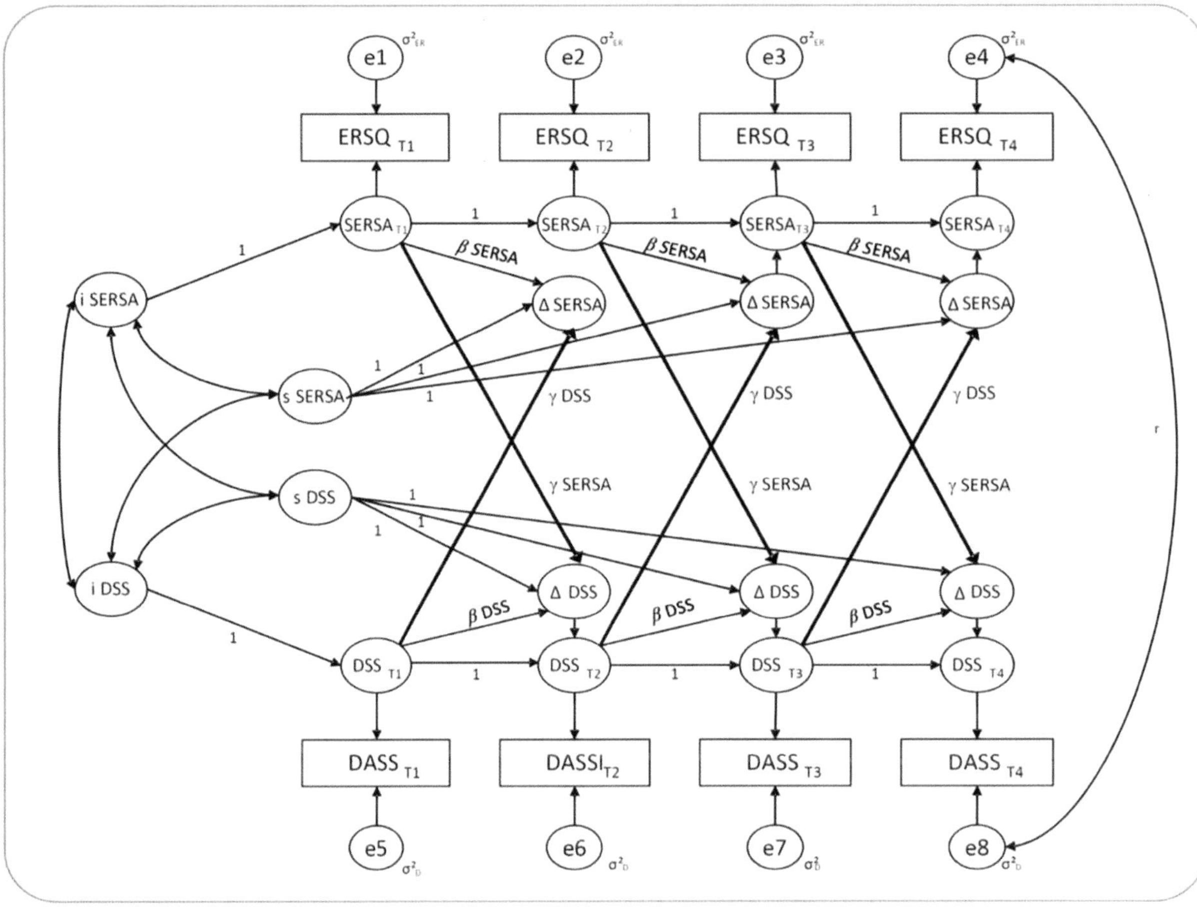

Figure 2. Path Diagram of the Bivariate Latent Change Score Model. ERSQ = Emotion-Regulation Skills Questionnaire, DASS = Depression Anxiety Stress Scale, SERSA = Successful Emotion Regulation Skills Application, DSS = Depressive Symptoms Severity, r = cross-construct error covariance, i = intercept, s = slope, γ = coupling parameter, β = proportion parameter, Δ = latent change score; for purpose of clarity, cross-construct error covariances are only shown for T4, but are also included for the other measurement points; error variances were set equal within constructs; loadings of growth factors and autoregressive proportions were set equal to one; proportion and coupling parameters were set equal across time within constructs; for model identification, means of errors and intercept of observed variables were set equal to zero [81,89].

three fit indices that were most suitable for our data characteristics (moderate sample size and missing values). Hu and Bentler [91] suggested that *good fit* is indicated by Comparative Fit Index (CFI) values greater than or equal to.95, Standardized Root Mean Square Residual (SRMR) values less than or equal to.08, and Root Mean Square Error of Approximation (RMSEA) values less than or equal to.06. We also report the RMSEA confidence interval and the p value for the null hypothesis that the RMSEA coefficient in the population is not greater than.05 (p close fit [92]).

With regard to missing values, we used the full information maximum likelihood estimation (FIML), which is recommended for use with longitudinal data models [80] and is considered to be superior to other methods, such as listwise or pairwise deletion [93]. Analyses were performed with an alpha level of 0.05, and bidirectional tests were used for all of the hypotheses. We used SPSS 19 (SPSS Inc., Chicago, IL, USA) for the preliminary analyses and MPlus 7 for SEM [94].

Results

Preliminary analyses confirmed that all the statistical assumptions (normality, linearity, collinearity, and reliability) required for using SEM with FIML were met. Indicators suggested a good (χ^2 and RMSEA statistics) to very good (SRMR and CFI values) model fit for the LGC model and a good fit for the LCS model (see Table 2).

Cross Sectional Associations and Associations of Change

As shown in Table 3, the ERSQ total score was negatively correlated with DSS, ASS, and GDS at all four assessment points. This finding supports the hypothesis that successful ER skills application is negatively associated with depressive and anxiety symptom severity as well as psychological distress. According to Cohen [95], the correlation coefficient indicates a moderate to large effect size.

Bivariate LGC modeling was conducted to examine whether changes in successful ER skills application are associated with changes in DSS, ASS, and GDS. The mean intercepts and slopes for successful ER skills application, DSS, ASS, and GDS significantly differed from zero (see Table 4), suggesting that significant intraindividual change in these variables occurred in the sample (fixed effects). Moreover, for all the variables (except for the anxiety scale of the DASS-21), the variance of the mean intercept and slope significantly differed from zero, suggesting that the intraindividual change significantly differed across individuals (random effects). For successful ER skills application, DSS, ASS,

Table 2. Fit indices of the models tested.

Model	χ^2	df	χ^2/df	SRMR	CFI	RMSEA (*p* of close-fit)	90%-CI of RMSEA
Bivariate latent growth curve model							
ERSQ & $DASS_{Stress}$	29.78	21	1.42	.04	.99	.05 (.48)	.00-.09
ERSQ & $DASS_{Depression}$	34.51*	21	1.64	.04	.98	.06 (.29)	.02-.10
ERSQ & $DASS_{Anxiety}$	31.63	21	1.51	.04	.99	.05 (.40)	.00-.09
Bivariate latent change score model							
ERSQ & $DASS_{Stress}$	25.50	23	1.11	.03	.99	.03 (.79)	.00-.07
ERSQ & $DASS_{Depression}$	24.74	23	1.08	.03	.99	.02 (.81)	.00-.07
ERSQ & $DASS_{Anxiety}$	29.36	23	1.28	.05	.99	.04 (.63)	.00-.08

Note. IFI = Incremental Fit Index; CFI = Comparative Fit Index; RMSEA = Root Mean Square Error of Approximation; CI = Confidence Interval; ERSQ = Emotion-Regulation Skills Questionnaire; BDI = Beck Depression Inventory; ** $p < .01$.

and GDS, the correlations between the intercepts and slopes were nonsignificant, indicating that a change in the variables is not associated with the pretreatment level. As also shown in Table 4, the intercept of the ERSQ was significantly (negatively) correlated with the DSS, ASS, and GDS intercepts. This finding replicates the findings from the cross-sectional correlations on a latent level; that is, higher pretreatment successful ER values indicate lower pretreatment symptom severity.

Finally, consistent with Hypothesis 2, the slopes of successful ER skills application and DSS and the slopes of successful ER skills application and GDS were significantly (negatively) correlated. This finding indicates that an increase in overall successful ER skills application is significantly associated with a decrease in DSS and GDS and vice versa. However, a significant correlation was not found for the slopes of successful ER and ASS.

Prediction of the Subsequent Latent Change

Time-lagged associations between successful ER skills application and DSS, ASS, and GDS were tested by using the LCS model illustrated in Figure 2. As shown in Table 5, the cross-lagged effect from successful ER skills application on subsequent changes in DSS (γSERSA = −2.65, $p = .035$) was significant and negative. Consistent with Hypothesis 3, this finding indicates that successful ER skills application predicts changes in the subsequent level of DSS. Patients reporting more successful ER skills application were likely to experience a greater reduction of DSS. In contrast, the other coupling effect predicting changes in successful ER skills application from previous DSS scores was nonsignificant (γDSS = -.01, $p = .95$). These findings are consistent with those of a previous study by Radkovsky and colleagues62 that assessed the cross-sectional and bivariate relationship between ER and DSS measured by the BDI. The cross-lagged effect from successful ER skills application on subsequent changes in GDS (γSERSA = −1.12, $p = .23$) and ASS (γSERSA = -.20, $p = .76$) was negative but nonsignificant. Additionally, the other coupling effects predicting changes in successful ER skills application from previous GDS (γstS = -.03, $p = .21$) and ASS (γASS = -.02, $p = .52$) scores were nonsignificant.

For each of the three LCS model, we tested whether the fit of the bidirectional model (e.g., unrestricted estimation of γSERSA and γDSS) and the two unidirectional models (γSERSA or γDSS set to zero) differed significantly from the fit of the no-coupling model (γSERSA and γDSS set to zero). For the LCS models, neither the ASS nor the GDS model resulted in a significant improvement in the model fit relative to the no-coupling model. However, we found a significant improvement for the unidirectional model relative to the no-coupling model in the DSS model (see Table 6). This finding again indicates that changes in general ER predict subsequent changes in DSS but not vice versa.

Discussion

Research suggests that deficits in emotion regulation (ER) are an important factor driving the maintenance of depression and hence a promising treatment target when working to reduce depressive symptoms. A particular advantage of enhancing individuals' *general* ER skills (i.e., skills that are effective for coping with a broad range of undesired affective states) is that these skills can also be assumed to facilitate individuals' ability to cope with symptoms that often co-occur with depressive symptoms and that arguably contribute to the maintenance of depression, such as anxiety symptoms. However, at this point, the associations between the successful application of adaptive ER skills and symptoms of depression and anxiety have not been investigated during the

Table 3. Correlations of $ERSQ_{total}$ Score and the DASS Scales for Each Assessment Point.

Measure	r Time 1	r Time 2	r Time 3	r Time 4	r Total Time
$DASS_{Stress}$	−.48**	−.55**	−.46**	−.60**	−.52
$DASS_{Depression}$	−.62**	−.62**	−.61**	−.68**	−.63
$DASS_{Anxiety}$	−.45**	−.57**	−.49*	−.53**	−.51

Note. ERSQ = Emotion-Regulation Skills Questionnaire, DASS = Depression Anxiety Stress Scale, *r* = Pearson-Correlation, *r* Total Time = correlation averaged across all assessment points; * $p<.05$, ** $p<.01$.

course of treatment in individuals who meet the criteria for MDD. Therefore, we assessed self-reports of successful ER skills application, depressive symptom severity (DSS), and anxiety symptom severity (ASS) over four assessment points in a sample of 175 inpatients receiving treatment with cognitive behavioral therapy for MDD. To assess the potentially confounding effects of general distress as a common factor of depression and anxiety, we also assessed self-reports of general distress severity (GDS). After testing whether ER is cross-sectionally associated with DSS, ASS, and/or GDS, we used latent curve modeling to test whether changes in successful ER skills application are negatively associated with changes in DSS, ASS, and/or GDS, and we used latent change score modeling to test whether successful ER skills application predicts the subsequent reduction of DSS, ASS, and/or GDS. In the results, successful ER skills application was significantly associated with (lower levels of) DSS, ASS, and GDS. Moreover, an increase in successful ER skills application was significantly associated with a decrease in DSS and GDS but not ASS. Finally, successful skills application significantly predicted the subsequent reduction of DSS. Unexpectedly, successful ER skills application significantly predicted the subsequent reduction of neither ASS nor DSS.

The finding that successful ER skills application was consistently associated with lower levels of (subsequent) DSS contributes to a body of evidence supporting the hypotheses that deficits in ER constitute an important factor driving the risk for and the maintenance of MDD [21,35,96–98]. Additionally, the findings that successful ER skills application was cross-sectionally associated with lower levels of ASS and that successful ER skills application was negatively associated with ASS provide some support for the transdiagnostic importance of general ER skills [23,28,99,100]. However, the findings that (a) the cross-sectional associations were smaller for ASS than for DSS, (b) the association between the slope for successful ER skills application and the slope for ASS was nonsignificant, and (c) successful ER skills application did not significantly predict subsequent ASS indicates that general ER skills might be more important in the context of depression than in the context of anxiety.

This hypothesis is consistent with preliminary evidence indicating that depressed individuals often struggle with a broad range of aversive affective states, including sadness, dysphoria, helplessness, hopelessness, a lack of positive emotions, stress/tension, anxiety, guilt, and shame [101,102], whereas in the context of anxiety disorders, the focus is commonly more restricted to an external threat, anxiety, or its somatic symptoms [101,103–105]. Thus, in the context of depression, general ER skills should be particularly helpful, as they help an individual to cope with a broad range of negative affective states that he or she is suffering from. In contrast, the ability to cope with anxiety-related problems might instead be facilitated by enhancing specific ER skills that are particularly effective for coping with anxiety. Moreover, deficits in ER are associated with difficulties in sustaining and/or increasing positive emotions. As anhedonia is one symptom thought to separate depression from anxiety disorders, the enhancement of general emotion regulation skills should be particularly effective for patients suffering from depression.

Another interesting finding in the present study is that successful ER skills application was not significantly associated with general distress in the LCS analyses. This finding is consistent with multiphase theories of affect generation [35,106–108]. These theories postulate that a perceived misfit between salient goals and needs and the perception of goal attainment and need satisfaction initially elicits unspecific negative affect; furthermore, individuals subsequently analyze the misfit between the perceived state and the desired state in detail and make prognoses about how the misfit will likely develop in the future. For these cognitive processes, the perceived ability to cope with one's emotions is crucial. If the individual anticipates that she/he will be able to cope with the undesired affective state, no challenging secondary affective reactions, such as anxiety or depression, will occur. However, if the individual anticipates having trouble coping with the undesired affective state, anxiety will occur. If the individual anticipates that he/she will be completely unable to control the undesired affective state and therefore assumes that this state will be stable over time, depressogenic schema will be activated [109]. The findings from the present study provide support for these theories in a clinical context, as they suggest that the ability to cope with general distress does not necessarily reduce the distress itself but may prevent the development of symptoms of a mental disorder (such as depression).

Strengths of this study include the use of a large and carefully diagnosed clinical sample, multiple assessments, a routine health care setting, and advanced statistical methods that have recently been introduced to clarify reciprocal associations in longitudinal data. A major limitation of the study includes the exclusive use of self-reports, as the process of emotion regulation notably functions in an explicit and implicit manner. Therefore, the exclusive use of self-reports may miss crucial information regarding the participants' implicit emotion regulation strategies, as the participants may not be fully aware of these strategies. Thus, future research should use multiple methods, e.g., experimental [110] and biological [111] paradigms, to assess ER in treated and untreated samples while combining latent change score analysis with multitrait-multimethod approaches [112] to diminish the occurrence of measurement errors. Moreover, the ER measure that was used in the present study assesses how participants respond to their "negative feelings" or "emotions" and hence does not discriminate between ER skills across distinct affective states. This is problematic because the measure does not help to identify which skills are particularly helpful for coping with a specific form of psychopathology. Thus, future research should assess regulation skills separately across various affective states [113] and should test

Table 4. Latent Growth Curve Model: Parameter Estimates for Intercepts, Slopes and Correlations of Slopes and Intercepts.

Measure	Intercept				Slope				Correlation of Slopes		Correlation of Intercepts	
	M	*SE*	σ^2	*SE*	*M*	*SE*	σ^2	*SE*	*Estimate*	*SE*	*Estimate*	*SE*
$DASS_{Stress}$	8.03^{***}	.35	15.25^{***}	2.38	$-.48^{***}$	.11	$.64^{*}$	.29	$-.061^{*}$	.029	-1.53^{***}	.288
$ERSQ_{total}$	2.90^{***}	.06	$.43^{***}$	.06	$.12^{**}$	.02	$.02^{**}$	.01	–	–	–	–
$DASS_{Depression}$	7.99^{***}	.40	21.67^{***}	3.15	$-.82^{***}$	.12	$.76^{***}$	.35	$-.094^{**}$	.034	-2.24^{***}	.348
$ERSQ_{total}$	2.90^{***}	.06	$.44^{***}$	.06	$.13^{**}$	.02	$.02^{*}$	.01	–	–	–	–
$DASS_{Anxiety}$	4.85^{***}	.32	13.76^{***}	2.06	$-.25^{**}$	.10	.17	.22	.005	.023	-1.31^{***}	.265
$ERSQ_{total}$	2.90^{***}	.06	$.04^{***}$	.06	$.13^{***}$	.02	$.02^{*}$	.01	–	–	–	–

Note. Unstandardized parameter estimates are presented; *M* = Mean, *SE* = Standard Error, σ^2 = Variance, ERSQ = Emotion Regulation Skills Questionnaire, DASS = Depression Anxiety Stress Scale; Residual variance set equal over time within construct; $^{*}p<.05$, $^{**}p<.01$, $^{***}p<.001$.

Table 5. Bivariate Latent Change Score Model: Estimates of Regression Coefficients.

	Coupling Parameter				Proportion Parameter			
	γ_{SERSA} (SERSA → $_{\Delta}$StS)		γ_{StS} (StS → $_{\Delta}$SERSA)		β_{SERSA} (SERSA → $_{\Delta}$SERSA)		β_{StS} (StS → $_{\Delta}$StS)	
Model	Estimate	S.E.	Estimate	S.E.	Estimate	S.E.	Estimate	S.E.
$DASS_{Stress}$	−1.13	0.93	−.03	.03	$-.55^{***}$	.13	$-.74^{***}$	.15
$DASS_{Depression}$	-2.65^{*}	1.25	−.01	.03	$-.46^{**}$	.17	$-.79^{***}$	.17
$DASS_{Anxiety}$	−0.20	0.65	−.02	.03	$-.47^{***}$	.12	$-.79^{***}$	.18

Note. Unstandardized parameter estimates are presented; coefficients β_{SERSA}, β_{SS}, γ_{SERSA} and $_{DSS}$ as denoted in Fig. 2; SE = Standard Error, SERSA = successful Emotion Regulation skills application, StS = Symptoms Severity, $_{\Delta}$ = Difference between two subsequent time points of assessment; $^{*}p<.05$, $^{**}p<.01$, $^{***}p<.001$.

Table 6. Bivariate LCS Models: Stepwise Test of Coupling Effects ($\Delta\ \chi^2/\Delta$ df for comparisons with no-coupling model).

	Bidirectional model	Unidirectional model γ_{SERSA}	Unidirectional model γ_{Sts}
	SERSA ↔ StS	SERSA $\rightarrow_{\Delta}$StS	StS $\rightarrow_{\Delta}$SERSA
	$\gamma_{SERSA} \neq 0$, $\gamma_{Sts} \neq 0$	$\gamma_{SERSA} \neq 0$, $\gamma_{Sts} = 0$	$\gamma_{SERSA} = 0$, $\gamma_{Sts} \neq 0$
$DASS_{Stress}$	4.9/2	3.3/1	3.4/1
$DASS_{Depression}$	4.7/2	4.6/1*	0.4/1
$DASS_{Anxiety}$	0.6/2	0.1/1	0.5/1

Note. Coefficients γ_{SERSA} and γ_{SS} as denoted in Fig. 2; SERSA = Successful Emotion Regulation Skills Application, StS = Symptoms Severity; $^*p<.05$.

the hypothesis that successfully utilizing arguably effective ER skills to cope with several undesired affective states is particularly important in the context of depression, whereas in the context of anxiety, the ability to effectively use anxiety regulation skills might be far more important than the ability to effectively use regulation skills related to other affective states.

Moreover, adaptive ER notably needs to be conceptualized as a dynamic process in which multiple strategies are used [19,34]. Thus, future research should assess how affective and regulatory processes interact over time and which patterns of ER strategy utilization are most effective for coping with specific mental-health problems.

An additional limitation of this study is the selection criteria, which limit the generalizability of the results, as only German-speaking inpatients with a current diagnosis of MDD and a pre-treatment BDI score of 11 or above were eligible for the study. Moreover, because of the selection criteria, the DASS-21 was merely approximately normally distributed at certain assessment points. However, nonparametric tests (e.g., Spearman's Rho) achieved comparable results. In addition, future studies 1) should prolong the interval of assessment, as the first three weeks of inpatient treatment may be too short to assess substantial effect of emotion regulation on depression, anxiety, and distress, and 2) should use a larger sample size owing to the complexity of the model.

Finally, significant associations might be driven by a third factor that affects both ER and symptoms of mental disorders. As the number of factors that can be assessed and statistically controlled for is always limited, future research should focus on experimental studies (i.e., randomized clinical trials) in which the focus on enhancing either general or specific ER skills is systemically varied. If this research assesses how the type of psychopathology moderates the effects of such interventions on psychopathology, the extent to which enhancing general ER skills can be used within transdiagnostic interventions to effectively foster patients' ability to cope with various challenges for mental health can be clarified.

Supporting Information

Demographic Data S1.

Data S1.

Author Contributions

Conceived and designed the experiments: DDE MB. Performed the experiments: CMW AR. Analyzed the data: CMW AR. Contributed reagents/materials/analysis tools: CMW AR. Wrote the paper: CMW AR MB.

References

1. Kessler RC, Berglund P, Demler O, Robert J, Koretz D, et al. (2003) The epidemiology of major depressive disorder. Results from the national comorbidity survey replication (NCS-R). JAMA 23: 3095–3105.
2. Mathers C, Fat DM, Boerma JT (2008) The global burden of disease: 2004 update. Geneva, Switzerland: World Health Organization.
3. Cuijpers P, van Straten A, van Oppen P, Andersson G (2008) Are psychological and pharmacologic interventions equally effective in the treatment of adult depressive disorders? A meta-analysis of comparative studies. J Clin Psychiatry 69: 1675–85.
4. Kupfer DJ (1991) Long-term treatment of depression. J Clin Psychiatry 52: 28–34.
5. Keller MB, Lavori PW, Mueller TI, Endicott J, Coryell W, et al. (1992) Time to recovery, chronicity, and levels of psychopathology in major depression. Arch Gen Psychiat 49: 809–816.
6. Torpey DC, Klein DN (2008) Chronic depression: Update on classification and treatment. Curr Psychiatry Rep 10: 458–464.
7. Melartin TK, Rytsala HJ, Leskela US, Lestela-Mielonen PS, Sokero TP, et al. (2002) Current comorbidity of psychiatric disorders among DSM-IV major depressive disorder patients in psychiatric care. J Clin Psychiatry 63: 126–134.
8. Gaynes BN, Magruder KM, Burns BJ, Wagner HR, Yarnall KS, et al. (1999) Does a Coexisting Anxiety Disorder Predict Persistence of Depressive Illness in Primary Care Patients With Major Depression? Gen Hosp Psychiat 21: 158–167.
9. Sanderson WC, Beck AT, Beck J (1990) Syndrome comorbidity in patients with major depression or dysthymia: prevalence and temporal relationships. Am J Psychiatry 147: 1025–1028.
10. VanValkenberg C, Akiskal H, Puzantian V, Rosenthal T (1984) Anxious depressions: clinical, family history and naturalistic outcome-comparisons with panic and major depressive disorders. J Affect Disord 6: 67–82.
11. Clayton PJ, Grove WM, Coryell W, Keller M, Hirschfeld R, et al. (1991) Follow-up and family study of anxious depression. Am J Psych 148: 1512–1517.
12. Fava M, Alpert JE, Carmin CN, Wisniewski SR, Trivedi MH, et al. (2004) Clinical correlates and symptom patterns of anxious depression among patients with major depressive disorder in STAR*D. Psychol Med 34: 1299–1308.
13. Coryell W, Endicott J, Winokur G (1992) Anxiety syndromes as epiphenomena of primary major depression: outcome and familial psychopathology. Am J Psychiatry 149: 100–107.
14. Kazdin AE, Nock MK (2003) Delineating mechanisms of change in child and adolescent therapy: Methodological issues and research recommendations. J Child Psychol Psych 44: 1116–1129.
15. Laurenceau, Hayes AM, Feldman GC (2007) Some methodological and statistical issues in the study of change processes in psychotherapy. Clin Psychol Rev 27: 682–695.
16. Veit CT, Ware JE (1983) The structure of psychological distress and well-being in general populations. J Consult Clin Psych 51: 730–742.
17. Clark LA, Watson D (1991) Tripartite model of anxiety and depression: psychometric evidence and taxonomic implications. J Abnorm Psychol 100: 316–336.
18. Henry JD, Crawford JR (2005) The short-form version of the Depression Anxiety Stress Scales (DASS-21): Construct validity and normative data in a large non-clinical sample. Brit J Clin Psychol 44: 227–239.

19. Aldao A, Nolen-Hoeksema S, Schweizer S (2010) Emotion-regulation strategies across psychopathology: A meta-analytic review. Clin Psychol Rev 30: 217–237.
20. Berking M, Wupperman P (2012) Emotion regulation and mental health: recent findings, current challenges, and future directions. Curr Opin Psychiatry 25: 128–134.
21. Mennin DS, Fresco DM (2009) Emotion regulation as an integrative framework for understanding and treating psychopathology. In: Kring AM, Sloan DM, editors. Emotion regulation and psychopathology: A transdiagnostic approach to etiology and treatment. New York, NY: Guilford Press. pp. 356–379.
22. Campbell-Sills L, Ellard KK, Barlow DH (2013) Emotion regulation in anxiety disorders. In: Gross JJ, editor. Handbook of Emotion Regulation. New York, NY: Guilford Press. pp. 230–249.
23. Hofmann SG, Sawyer AT, Fang A, Asnaani A (2012) Emotion dysregulation model of mood and anxiety disorders. Depress Anxiety 29: 409–416.
24. Gross JJ (2013) Conceptual and empirical foundations. In: Gross JJ, editor. Handbook of Emotion Regulation. New York: Guilford. pp. 13–21.
25. Koole SL (2009) The psychology of emotion regulation: An integrative review. Cogn Emot 23: 4–41.
26. Thompson RA (1994) Emotion regulation: A theme in search of definition. Monogr Soc Res Child Dev 59: 25–52.
27. American Psychiatric Association (2013) Diagnostic and statistical manual of mental health disorders: DSM-V (5th ed.). Washington, DC: American Psychiatric Publishing.
28. Barlow DH (1991) Disorders of Emotion. Psychol Inq 2: 58–71.
29. Decker ML, Turk CL, Hess B, Murray CE (2008) Emotion regulation among individuals classified with and without generalized anxiety disorder. J Anxiety Disord 22: 485–494.
30. Teasdale JD, Barnard PJ (1993) Affect, cognition, and change: Remodeling depressive thought. Hove, U.K.: Lawrence Erlbaum Associates.
31. Alloy LB, Kelly KA, Mineka S, Clements CM, Maser JD, et al. (1990) Comorbidity of anxiety and depressive disorders: A helplessness-hopelessness perspective. In: Jack M, Cloninger CR, editors. Comorbidity of mood and anxiety disorders. Arlington, VA: American Psychiatric Association. pp. 499–543.
32. McLaughlin K, Hatzenbuehler ML, Mennin DS, Nolen-Hoeksema S (2011) Emotion dysregulation and adolescent psychopathology: A prospective study. Behav Res Ther 49: 544–554.
33. Berking M, Orth U, Wupperman P, Meier LL, Casper LL (2008) Prospective effects on emotion regulation on emotional adjustment. J Couns Psychol 55: 485–494.
34. Berking M, Schwarz J (2013) The Affect regulation training. In Gross J., editor. Handbook of Emotion Regulation. New York: Guilford. pp. 350–392.
35. Berking M, Whitley B (2013) Affect regulation training. 1st ed. New York: Springer.
36. Honkalampi K, Saarinen P, Hintikka J, Virtanen V, Viinamaki H (1999) Factors associated with alexithymia in patients suffering from depression. Psychother Psychosom 68: 270–275.
37. Rude S, McCarthy C (2003) Emotional functioning in depressed and depression-vulnerable college students. Cognition Emotion 17: 799–806.
38. Baker R, Holloway J, Thomas PW, Thomas S, Owens M (2004) Emotional processing and panic. Behav Res Ther 42: 1271–1287.
39. Cox BJ, Swinson RP, Shulman ID, Bourdeau D (1995) Alexithymia in panic disorder and social phobia. Compr Psychiat 36: 195–198.
40. Brody CL, Haaga DAF, Kirk L, Solomon A (1999) Experiences of anger in people who have recovered from depression and never-depressed people. J Nerv Ment Dis 187: 400–405.
41. Campbell-Sills L, Barlow DH, Brown TA, Hofmann SG (2006) Effects of suppression and acceptance on emotional responses of individuals with anxiety and mood disorders. Behav Res Ther 44: 1251–1263.
42. Conway M, Csank PAR, Holm SL, Blake CK (2000) On individual differences in rumination on sadness. Journal Pers Assess 75: 404–425.
43. Hayes SC, Strosahl KD, Wilson KG, Bissett RT, Pistorello J, et al. (2004) Measuring experimental avoidance: A preliminary test of working model. Psychol Rec 54: 553–578.
44. Leahy RL (2002) A model of emotional schemas. Cogn Behav Prac 9: 177–191.
45. Naragon-Gainey K (2010) Meta-analysis of the relations of anxiety sensitivity to the depressive and anxiety disorders. Psychol Bull 136: 128–150.
46. Parker JD, Taylor GJ, Bagby RM, Acklin MW (1993) Alexithymia in panic disorder and simple phobia: a comparative study. Am J Psych 150: 1105–1107.
47. Kashdan TB, Steger MF (2006) Expanding the topography of social anxiety. An experience-sampling assessment of positive emotions, positive events, and emotion suppression. Psychol Sci 17: 120–128.
48. Hofmann SG, Grossman P, Hinton DE (2001) Loving-kindness and compassion meditation: Potential for psychological interventions. Clin Psychol Rev 31: 1126–1132.
49. Kuyken W, Watkins E, Holden E, White K, Taylor RS, et al. (2010) How does mindfulness-based cognitive therapy work? Behav Res Ther 48: 1105–1112.
50. Martin RC, Dahlen ER (2005) Cognitive emotion regulation in the prediction of depression, anxiety, stress, and anger. Pers Individ Dif 39: 1249–1260.
51. Catanzaro SJ, Wasch HH, Kirsch I, Mearns J (2000) Coping-related expectancies and dispositions as prospective predictors of coping responses and symptoms. J Pers 68: 757–788.
52. Kassel JD, Bornovalova M, Mehta N (2007) Generalized expectancies for negative mood regulation predict change in anxiety and depression among college students. Behav Res Ther 45: 939–950.
53. Kraaij V, Garnefski N, Van Gerwen L (2003) Cognitive coping and anxiety symptoms among people who seek help for fear of flying. Aviat Space Env Med 74: 273–277.
54. Fergus TA, Valentiner DP, McGrath PB, Jencius S (2010) Shame- and guilt-proneness: Relationships with anxiety disorder symptoms in a clinical sample. J Anxiety Disord 24: 811–815.
55. Abramson LY, Metalsky FI, Alloy LB (1989) Hopelessness depression: A theory based subtype of depression. Psychol Rev 96: 358–372.
56. Feldner MT, Zvolensky MJ, Eifert GH, Spira AP (2003) Emotional avoidance: an experimental test of individual differences and response suppression using biological challenge. Behav Res Ther 41: 403–411.
57. Wirtz CM, Hofmann SG, Riper H, Berking M (2013) Emotion Regulation Predicts Anxiety over a Five-Year Interval: A Cross-Lagged Panel Analysis. Depress Anxiety 30: 1–9.
58. Berking M, Wirtz CM, Svaldi J, Hofmann SG (2014) Successful Emotion Regulation Skills Application Negatively Predicts Depressive Symptom Severity over Five Years in Individuals Suffering from at least some Depressive Symptoms. Under review by Behav Res Ther.
59. Nolen-Hoeksema S, Morrow J (1991) A prospective study of depression and posttraumatic stress symptoms after a natural disaster: the 1989 Loma Prieta earthquake. J Pers Soc Psychol 61: 115–121.
60. Roelofs J, Rood L, Meesters C, te Dorsthorst V, Bögele S, et al. (2009) The influence of rumination and distraction on depressed and anxious mood: a prospective examination of the response styles theory in children and adolescents. Eur Child Adolesc Psychiatry 18: 635–642.
61. Calmes CA, Roberts JE (2007) Repetitive Thought and Emotional Distress: Rumination and Worry as Prospective Predictors of Depressive and Anxious Symptomatology. Cognit Ther Res 31: 343–356.
62. Radkovsky A, McArdle JJ, Bockting CLH, Berking M (2014) Successful Emotion Regulation Skills Application Predicts Subsequent Reduction of Symptom Severity During Treatment of Major Depressive Disorder. J Consult Clin: in press.
63. Riedel M, Möller, Obermeier M, Schennach-Wolff R, Bauer M, et al. (2010) Response and remission criteria in major depression: A validation of current practice. J Psychiat Res 44: 1063–1068.
64. Wittchen, Zaudig M, Fydrich T (1997) Strukturiertes Klinisches Interview für DSM-IV. Manual zum SKID-I und SKID-II. [Structured clinical interview for DSM-IV. Manual for SCID-I and SCID-II.].Göttingen: Hogrefe.
65. Beck AT, Rush AJ, Shaw BF, Emery G (2010) Kognitive Therapie der Depression [Cognitive therapy for depression]. Weinheim, Germany: Beltz.
66. Barlow DH (2008) Clinical handbook of psychological disorders: A step-by-step treatment manual. New York, NY: Guilford Press.
67. Greenberg LS (2002) Emotion-focused therapy: Coaching clients to work through their feelings. Washington, DC: American Psychological Association.
68. Linehan MM (1993) Cognitive-behavioral treatment of Borderline Personality Disorder. New York, NY: Guilford Press.
69. Berking M, Znoj H (2008) Entwicklung und Validierung eines Fragebogens zur standardisierten Selbsteinschätzung emotionaler Kompetenzen [Development and validation of the emotion-regulation skills questionnaire (ERSQ-27)]. Z Psychiatr Psychol Psychother 56: 141–152.
70. Berking M, Margraf M, Ebert D, Wuppermann P, Hofmann SG, et al. (2011) Deficits in emotion-regulation skills predict alcohol use during and after cognitive-behavioral therapy for alcohol dependence. J Consult Clin Psychol 79: 307–318.
71. Berking M, Poppe C, Luhmann M, Wuppermann P, Jaggy V, et al. (2012) Is the association between various emotion-regulation skills and mental health mediated by the ability to modify emotions? Results from two cross-sectional studies. J Behav Ther Exp Psychiatry 43: 931–937.
72. Berking M, Ebert D, Cuijpers P, Hofmann SG (2013) Emotion-regulation skills training enhances the efficacy of cognitive behavioral therapy for major depressive disorder. Psychother Psychosom 82: 234–245.
73. Berking M, Meier C, Wupperman P (2010) Enhancing emotion-regulation skills in police officers – results of a controlled study. Behav Ther 41: 329–339.
74. Lovibond PF, Lovibond SH (1995) The structure of negative emotional states: Comparison of the Depression Anxiety Stress Scales (DASS) with the Beck Depression and Anxiety Inventories. Behav Res Ther 33: 335–342.
75. Antony MM, Bieling PJ, Cox BJ, Enns MW, Swinson RP (1998) Psychometric properties of the 42-item and 21-itemversions of the depression anxiety stress scales in clinical groups and a community sample. Psychol Assess 10: 176–181.
76. Brown TA, Chorpita BF, Korotitsch W, Barlow DH (1997) Psychometric properties of the Depression Anxiety Stress Scales (DASS) in clinical samples. Behav Res Ther 35: 79–89.
77. McArdle JJ (1988) Dynamic but structural equation modeling of repeated measures data. In Nesselroade JR, Cattel RB, editors. Handbook of multivariate experimental psychology. New York: Plenum Press. pp. 561–614.
78. McArdle JJ (2009) Latent variable modeling of differences and changes with longitudinal data. Annu Rev Psychol 60: 577–605.
79. Christ O, Schmidt P, Schlüter E, Wagner U (2006) Analyse von Prozessen und Veränderungen: Zur Anwendung autoregressiver latenter Wachstumskurvenmodelle [The Analysis of Processes and Changes: Applying Autoregressive Latent Trajectory Models]. Z Sozialpsychol 37: 173–184.

80. Grimm KJ (2007) Multivariate longitudinal methods for studying developmental relationships between depression and academic achievement. Int J Behav Dev 31: 328–339.
81. Ferrer E, McArdle JJ (2003) Alternative structural models for multivariate longitudinal data analysis. Struct Equ Modeling 10: 493–524.
82. McArdle JJ, Hamagami F (2001) Latent difference score structural models for linear dynamic analyses with incomplete longitudinal data. In Collins LM, Sawyer AG, editors. New methods for the analysis of change. Washington, DC: American Psychological Association. pp. 139–175.
83. Berking M, Neacsiu A, Comtois KA, Lineham MM(2009) The impact of experiential avoidance on the reduction of depression in treatment for borderline personality disorder. Behav Res Ther 47: 663–670.
84. Hawley LL, Ho, Zuroff DC, Blatt SJ (2006) The relationship of perfectionism, depression, and therapeutic alliance during treatment for depression: Latent difference score analysis. J Consult Clin 74: 930–942.
85. Jajodia A, Borders A (2011) Memory Predicts Changes in Depressive Symptoms in Older Adults: A Bidirectional Longitudinal Analysis. J Gerontol B Psychol Sci Soc Sci 66: 571–581.
86. Lindwall M, Larsman P, Hagger MS (2011) The reciprocal relationship between physical activity and depression in older European adults: A prospective cross-lagged panel design using SHARE data. Health Psychol 30: 453–462.
87. McArdle JJ, Prindle JJ (2008) A latent change score analysis of a randomized clinical trial in reasoning training. Psychol Aging 23: 702–719.
88. Tasca GA, Lampard AM (2012) Reciprocal influence of alliance to the group and outcome in day treatment for eating disorders. J Couns Psychol 59: 507–517.
89. McArdle JJ, Grimm KJ (2010) Five steps in latent curve and latent change score modeling with longitudinal data. In van Montfort K, Oud JHL, Satorra A, editors. Longitudinal research with latent variables. Heidelberg, Germany: Springer. pp. 245–273.
90. Hu L, Bentler PM (1998) Fit indices in covariance structure modeling: Sensitivity to underparameterized model misspecification. Psychol Methods 3: 424–453.
91. Hu L, Bentler PM (1999) Cutoff criteria for fit indexes in covariance structure analysis: Conventional criteria versus new alternatives. Struct Equ Modeling 6: 1–55.
92. MacCallum RC, Browne MW, Sugawara HM (1996) Power analysis and determination of sample size for covariance structure modeling. Psychol Methods 1: 130–149.
93. Enders CK, Bandalos DL (2001) The relative performance of full information maximum likelihood estimation for missing data in structural equation models. Struct Equ Modeling 8: 430–457.
94. Muthén LK, Muthén BO (2012) MPlus User's Guide. Seventh ed. Los Angeles, CA: Muthén & Muthén.
95. Cohen J (1988) Statistical power analysis for the behavioral sciencies. 2nd ed. Hillsdale, NJ: Erlbaum.
96. Ehring T, Tuschen-Caffier B, Schnülle J, Fischer S, Gross JJ (2010) Emotion regulation and vulnerability to depression: Spontaneous versus instructed use of emotion suppression and reappraisal. Emotion 10: 563–572.
97. Gross JJ, Muñoz RF (1995) Emotion regulation and mental health. Clin Psychol-Sci Pr 2: 151–164.
98. Hollon SD, Muñoz RF, Barlow DH, Beardslee BR, Bell CC, et al. (2002) Psychosocial intervention development for the prevention and treatment of depression: Promoting innovation and increasing access. Biol Psychiat 52: 610–630.
99. Werner K, Gross JJ (2010) Emotion regulation and psychopathology: A conceptual framework. In Kring AM, Sloan DM, editors. Emotion regulation and psychopathology: A transdiagnostic approach to etiology and treatment. New York, NY: Guilford Press. pp. 13–37.
100. Ellard KK, Fairholme CP, Boisseau CL, Farchione TJ, Barlow DH (2010) Unified Protocol for the Transdiagnostic Treatment of Emotional Disorders: Protocol Development and Initial Outcome Data. Cogn Behav Prac 17: 88–101.
101. American Psychiatric Association (2000) Diagnostic and Statistical Manual of Mental disorders: DSM-IV-TR. 4th ed. Washington DC: American Psychiatric Association.
102. Clarke DM, Cook KE, Coleman KJ, Smith GC (2006) A Qualitative Examination of the Experience of 'Depression' in Hospitalized Medically Ill Patients. Psychopathology 39: 303–312.
103. Bar-Haim Y, Lamy D, Pergamin L, Bakermans-Kranenburg MJ, van Ijzendoorn MH (2007) Threat-related attentional bias in anxious and nonanxious individuals: a meta-analytic study. Psychol Bull 133: 1–24.
104. Haug TT, Mykletun A, Dahl AA (2004) The association between anxiety, depression, and somatic symptoms in a large population: The HUNT-II study. Psychosom Med 66: 845–851.
105. Lieb R, Meinlschmidt G, Araya R (2007) Epidemiology of the Association Between Somatoform Disorders and Anxiety and Depressive Disorders: An Update. Psychosom Med 69: 860–863.
106. Lazarus RS (1991) Emotion and Adaptation. New York, NY: Oxford University Press.
107. Grawe K (2004) Psychological therapy. Cambridge, MA: Hogrefe & Huber.
108. Grawe K (2007) Neuropsychotherapy: How the neurosciences inform effective psychotherapy. Counseling and psychotherapy investigating practice from scientific, historical, and cultural perspectives. Mahwah, NJ: Lawrence Erlbaum Associates Publishers.
109. Teasdale JD, Barnard PJ (1993) Affect, cognition, and change: Remodeling depressive thought. Hove, U.K.: Lawrence Erlbaum Associates.
110. Diedrich A, Grant M, Hofmann SG, Hiller W, Berking M (2014) Self-compassion as an emotion regulation strategy in major depressive disorder. Behav Res Ther 58: 43–51.
111. Appelhans BM, Luecken LJ (2006) Heart rate variability as an index of regulated emotional responding. Rev Gen Psychol 10: 229–240.
112. Geiser C, Eid M, Nussbeck FW, Courvoisier DS, Cole DA (2010) Multitrait-multimethod change modelling. AStA Adv Stat Anal 94: 185–201.
113. Ebert DD, Christ O, Berking M (2013) Entwicklung und Validierung eines Fragebogens zur emotionsspezifischen Selbsteinschätzung emotionaler Kompetenzen (SEK-ES). [Development and validation of a self-report instrument for the assessment of emotion-specific regulation skills]. Diagnostica 59: 17–32.

4

Distinct Facial Processing Related Negative Cognitive Bias in First-Episode and Recurrent Major Depression: Evidence from the N170 ERP Component

Jiu Chen[1], Wentao Ma[2], Yan Zhang[2], Xingqu Wu[2], Dunhong Wei[2], Guangxiong Liu[2], Zihe Deng[2], Laiqi Yang[2]*, Zhijun Zhang[1]*

1 Neurologic Department of Affiliated ZhongDa Hospital, Neuropsychiatric Institute and Medical School of Southeast University, Nanjing, Jiangsu Province, China, **2** Center for Mental Disease Control and Prevention, Third Hospital of the People's Liberation Army, Baoji, Shaanxi Province, China

Abstract

Background: States of depression are associated with increased sensitivity to negative events. For this novel study, we have assessed the relationship between the number of depressive episodes and the dysfunctional processing of emotional facial expressions.

Methodology/Principal Findings: We used a visual emotional oddball paradigm to manipulate the processing of emotional information while event-related brain potentials were recorded in 45 patients with first episode major depression (F-MD), 40 patients with recurrent major depression (R-MD), and 46 healthy controls (HC). Compared with the HC group, F-MD patients had lower N170 amplitudes when identifying happy, neutral, and sad faces; R-MD patients had lower N170 amplitudes when identifying happy and neutral faces, but higher N170 amplitudes when identifying sad faces. F-MD patients had longer N170 latencies when identifying happy, neutral, and sad faces relative to the HC group, and R-MD patients had longer N170 latencies when identifying happy and neutral faces, but shorter N170 latencies when identifying sad faces compared with F-MD patients. Interestingly, a negative relationship was observed between N170 amplitude and the depressive severity score for identification of happy faces in R-MD patients while N170 amplitude was positively correlated with the depressive severity score for identification of sad faces in F-MD and R-MD patients. Additionally, the deficits of N170 amplitude for sad faces positively correlated with the number of depressive episodes in R-MD patients.

Conclusion/Significance: These results provide new evidence that having more recurrent depressive episodes and serious depressive states are likely to aggravate the already abnormal processing of emotional facial expressions in patients with depression. Moreover, it further suggests that the impaired processing as indexed by N170 amplitude for positive face identification may be a potentially useful biomarker for predicting propagation of depression while N170 amplitude for negative face identification could be a potential biomarker for depression recurrence.

Editor: Ulrich von Hecker, Cardiff University, United Kingdom

Funding: This study was supported by the Special Research Fund for Traditional Chinese Medicine in Chinese Army (Grant no. 10ZYX108); the Key Program for Clinical Medicine and Science and Technology: Jiangsu Provence Clinical Medical Research Center (Grant no. BL2013025); the National Natural Science Foundation of China (Grant no. 91132000). The funders had no role in study design, data collection and analysis, decision to publish, or preparation of the manuscript.

Competing Interests: The authors have declared that no competing interests exist.

* Email: yanglaiqi6666@163.com (LY); janemengzhang@vip.163.com (ZZ)

Introduction

Depression is a commonly occurring mental disease [1]. The first study of the cognitive theories of depression [2] indicated that cognitive processing can be affected by the unconscious negative or pessimistic schemata activated by stressful events, which include selection, encoding, perception, and interpretation of actual experiences [3,4]. The depressive effect is thought to be due to the negative schemata, which lies dormant until activated by stressful life events [2,4]. However, previous studies have demonstrated that negative cognition comes into being only during depressive episodes [5], and the cognitive processing bias for negative stimuli plays a key role in its onset [6]. Other supporting evidence suggests that depressive states are classically related to increased sensitivity to negative events [7]. This hypersensitivity may be further enhanced with each recurrent depressive episode.

Gotlib and Neubauer have demonstrated that these negative schemata influence information processing by elevating the salience of negative events and by decreasing the salience of positive events [8]. Accordingly, for positive social stimuli, patients with major depression DISORDER (MDD) were less likely to identify mild happy expressions as more intense than neutral and negative expressions, relative to controls [9]. Using emotional stimuli, numerous studies have indicated that patients with MDD have an attentional bias that is specific to sad faces and an impaired inhibition of attending to negative social information [7,10,11]. However, little is known about how effective facial emotional stimuli are during perceptual processing and whether they may lead to a better understanding of mood-related attention bias in depression, particularly in recurrent depression. An in-depth understanding of the specific time course of cognitive processing during the perceptual processes of emotional stimuli can help to describe which specific cognitive processes are influenced by mood-related biases.

Recently, a study from the Canadian National Population Health Survey has reported that the recurrence of major depressive episodes strongly depends on the number of previous episodes [12]. Several pieces of neuroimaging evidence also suggest that the altered striatal connectivity may be affected by the number of depressive episodes, thus contributing to depressive recurrence risk [13]. First episode major depression patients (F-MD) had smaller left hippocampal volumes, left-right asymmetry [14] and larger amygdala volumes [15]. Numerous cross-sectional epidemiological studies have shown that the severity of depression is positively associated with the number of episodes, and that stressful life events during mild and long-term periods may reinforce depressive recurrent risk [16,17]. Previous studies have indicated that recurrent major depression patients (R-MD) have more serious cognitive impairment compared to F-MD patients. Examples of such cognitive impairment are autobiographical memory [18], verbal memory performance [19], executive function [20] and mental representation processing [21]. Also, recurrence chronically modifies access to emotive memories [18]. Moreover, previous studies have demonstrated that R-MD patients have an increased oxidative stress [22] and higher serum neopterin levels [23] compared to F-MD patients. Taken together, the evidence from these studies suggest that R-MD patients present with a more serious impairment compared with F-MD patients, and the recurrence of depressive episodes may reinforce the damage severity. Very little is known, however, about the relationship between the abnormal neural processing of emotional facial expressions and the number of depressive episodes. Furthermore, the differences between cognitive processing biases for negative faces between F-MD and R-MD patients are still poorly understood.

Event-related evoked potential (ERP) measurements, a powerful non-invasive approach that have a time resolution in the millisecond range and allow assessment of cognitive brain function, have been widely used to investigate individuals' information processing of different cognitive schemata [24]. ERP measurements are a type of long-latency evoked potentials extracted from ongoing electrical cerebral background activity by averaging related procedures to reflect human information processing [25]. In accordance with these experimental manipulations, the measurements can then identify and characterize impairments that may exist in pathological states. The amplitude of the electrophysiological response reflects the intensity of the internal information processing, while its latency represents the timing of that process.

Different electrophysiological components are considered to be associated with different cognitive functions. The N170 component, which is a negative-going component and arose from occipito-temporal brain generators, was first reported by Bentin et al. (1996) [26]. Subsequently, numerous ERP studies have demonstrated that the N170 component is sensitive to facial emotional expressions. For example, Batty and Taylor used unfamiliar faces expressing the six basic emotions and neutral faces, and showed that ERP measurements report global effects of emotion from 90 ms, while latency and amplitude differences for emotional expressions are found from 140 ms. This suggests that the N170 component may represent rapid processing of emotional expressions [27]. Using an emotional faces task, Blau et al. and Japee et al. demonstrated that the N170 response shows a strong modulation by emotional facial expression [28,29]. Recently, Wronka and Walentowska used an emotional faces task to discriminate emotional expressions and also demonstrated that N170 amplitude was modulated by facial emotional expressions [30]. Furthermore, in these previous studies, all of the researchers have consistently indicated that if the faces are presented as the attentional focus and the subjects are required to direct their attention to the facial expressions, N170 amplitude is modulated by facial emotional expressions [31–34]. Taken together, the evidence from these studies shows that the N170 amplitude and latency modulation can be used as a neurophysiological indicator of the cognitive processing of emotional faces. Moreover, the onset of the N170 effect can be used as a chronopsychophysiological marker for the onset of the processing of emotional expressions. To sum, the N170 component is an ideal brain marker to assess possible cortical markers of emotional face processing in F-MD and R-MD patients.

The objective of our current study is to compare the neural processing of emotional facial expressions by patients with a first episode and recurrent depression to that of healthy control subjects using the ERP technique. Based on the previous studies, we predict that patients with MDD will present with an impairment of emotion processing. We also predict that there will be a difference between F-MD and R-MD patients. The F-MD group will likely have longer N170 latencies and lower N170 amplitudes to three emotional faces relative to the HC group. The R-MD group will likely have lower N170 amplitudes for happy and neutral faces, but higher N170 amplitudes for sad faces relative to the HC group. Moreover, we further predict that there will be a correlation between the number of depressive episodes and the altered processing of emotional faces. The new information we discover regarding the repeated physiopathologic mechanism for depression will be extremely valuable for clarifying diagnoses, advising disease treatments and planning clinical trials.

Materials and Methods

Ethics statement

All procedures were approved by the Human Participants Ethics Committee of the Baoji Third Hospital of the People's Liberation Army and written informed consent was obtained from all participants prior to entry into the study. Ability to provide informed consent was assessed first by the participant's referring clinician who was not associated with the study and an additional study physician prior to inclusion in the study. None of the participants had significant cognitive impairment which would interfere with their ability to provide informed consent. All potential participants who declined to participate or otherwise did not participate were eligible for treatment and were not disadvantaged in any other way by not participating in the study.

Subjects

From inpatients (all of whom were Chinese Han and right-handed) at Center for Mental disease Control and Prevention of Baoji Third Hospital of the People's Liberation Army in China, we recruited 45 F-MD patients (21 males and 24 females) and 40 R-MD patients (18 males and 22 females); see Table 1 (subjects were aged 18–65 years; mean age: F-MD group: 30.6±11.3 years; R-MD group: 32.8±13.6 years). Psychiatric diagnoses were

Table 1. Demographics and clinical measures of depressed patients and HC subjects.

Items	F-MD (N=45)	R-MD (N=40)	HC (N=46)	F values (χ^2)	p values
Age (years)	30.6(11.3)	32.8(13.6)	31.1(10.8)	0.736	0.830
Gender (males/females)	21/24	18/22	22/24	0.043	0.214
Education (years)	12.6(3.0)	13.1(3.3)	13.8(2.1)	1.003	0.672
$HDRS_{17}$	22.6(7.9)[b]	23.8(8.9)[c]	2.5(1.3)	8.322	0.010*
MMSE scores	25.1(1.3)[a b]	21.5(2.5)[c]	29.0(2.2)	6.242	0.013*
AVLT-DR	3.8(1.2)[a b]	1.9(1.5)[c]	7.8(2.3)	7.660	0.007*
TMT-A (seconds)	78.3(32.6)[a b]	88.6(38.3)[c]	67.4(16.4)	9.603	0.000*
TMT-B (seconds)	212.4(121.4)[a b]	258.6(143.2)[c]	175.3(63.2)	10.312	0.000*
SDMT	34.8(12.3)[a b]	23.9(10.6)[c]	39.6(13.2)	9.328	0.000*
DST	11.3(2.2)[b]	10.0(2.1)[c]	12.5(2.6)	4.463	0.031*
CDT	7.3(1.7)[b]	7.2(1.3)[c]	9.1(1.4)	3.204	0.040*
Number of episode	1.0(0.0)	3.6(2.0)	NA	NA	NA
First	45(100%)	-			
Second	-	16(40.0%)			
Third	-	10(25.0%)			
Fourth	-	8(20.0%)			
Fifth	-	5(12. 5%)			
Sixth	-	1(2.5%)			
Age at onset (years)	28.1(2.1)	28.3(4.6)	NA	NA	NA
Duration of illness (years)	0.6(0.3)[a]	3.5(1.1)	NA	NA	NA
Duration of current episode (weeks)	28.2(6.2)[a]	31.0(8.1)	NA	NA	NA
Antidepressant comedication	38(84.4%)	40(100%)	NA	NA	NA

Notes: Abbreviation: F-MD: first episode of major depression; R-MD: recurrent episodes of major depression; HC: Healthy controls; NA: not applicable; $HDRS_{17}$: 17 items the Chinese Hamilton Depression Rating Scale; MMSE: Mini mental state exam; AVLT-DR: Auditory verbal learning test- delayed recall; TMT-A: Trail making test-A; TMT-B: Trail making test-B; SDMT: Symbol digit modalities test; DST: Digit span test; CDT: Clock drawing test.
*Significant differences were found among first episode depression patients and recurrent depression patients and HC subjects. *P* values were obtained by ANOVA analysis except for gender (chi square test). a–c: post-hoc analysis (LSD test for demographic information and Bonferroni correction for multiple comparison) further revealed the source of ANOVA difference (a: first episode patients vs. recurrent patients; b: first episode patients vs. HC subjects; c: recurrent patients vs. HC subjects).

determined by at least two psychiatrists who agreed on the diagnosis based on the DSM-V criteria [1] for major depression.

Illness durations ranged from 2 months to 30 years (mean illness duration: F-MD group: 0.6±0.3 years; R-MD group: 3.5±1.1 years). Patients' education ranged from 8 years to 22 years (mean years of education: F-MD group: 12.6±3.0 years; R-MD group: 13.1±3.3 years). The severity of depression was evaluated with the 17-item Hamilton Depression Rating Scale (HDRS) [35]. A minimum score of 22.4 was required to participate. All patients received the same antidepressant medication (serotoninergic antidepressive treatment) and the same psychological treatment (psychotherapy interviews and group therapy) [4]. All subjects were clinically stable at the time of testing.

For comparison, 46 healthy control subjects (HC, 22 males and 24 females) without any history of psychiatric illness were matched to the patients in the F-MD and R-MD groups according to age, gender and education (subjects were aged 18–65 years; mean age: 31.1±10.8 years). Exclusion criteria for the patients and the control subjects were a history of substantial head injury, seizures, neurological diseases, dementia, impaired thyroid function, corticoid use or alcohol or substance abuse or dependence. **Table 1** provided group information about age, gender, and education.

Procedures

The experiment was performed with E-Prime 2.0 software (Psychology Software Tools Inc., Pittsburgh, USA). The experimental procedure used an "emotional oddball paradigm" [24,25]. Stimuli consisted of six faces that were selected from a highly standardized set of pictures developed by the Psychology Department of the Chinese Academy of Sciences. The faces had neutral, happy and sad expressions [36]. Standard faces always presented neutral expressions, whereas deviant faces were either the same face displaying an emotion (happy or sad) or a different neutral face (change in identity).

Subjects were confronted with a total of 16 blocks that were defined by 100 stimuli (e.g., 80 frequent stimuli with face A neutral; five deviant face A happy, five deviant face A sad and 10 face B neutral). During the ERP recording, subjects sat on a chair in a quiet, dimly–lit, sound-proof room with their head restrained in a chin rest and placed at 1 m from the 17″ computer screen (refresh rate 75 Hz). Stimuli subtended a visual angle of 3°×4°. Similar to previous reports [37,38], faces were presented for 100 ms in order to assure conscious perception of the faces. A black screen was displayed as an intertribal interval and lasted randomly between 1300 and 1600 ms. The subjects had 1500 ms to answer after the stimulation onset [25]. The participants had to quickly point out the occurrence of a deviant face among the presentation of standard faces by pressing a button with their right index finger. The order of the 16 blocks varied across participants. Reaction time (RT) and accuracy were recorded automatically for each trial.

EEG acquisition and analysis

Electroencephalogram (EEG) data acquisition was carried out continuously throughout the experiment. The EEG data were acquired using a BrainAmp MR portable ERP system (Brain Products GmbH, Munich, Germany) with 32 scalp electrodes. Electrodes were placed according to the extended international 10–20 system [39]. Two ear electrodes served as reference electrodes in off-line analyses, and the AFz electrode was used for grounding. The vertical electro-oculogram (VEOG) and horizontal electro-oculogram (HEOG) were recorded with bipolar channels from sites above the midpoint of the left eye and 10 mm from the right lateral canthus in order to control the interference of eye blinks with the EEG-signal. The EEG was band-pass filtered from 0.1 to 100 Hz, amplified with a gain of 20 and data was stored on a computer disk at the sample rate of 500 Hz. The EEG signal was analyzed using Brain Vision Analyzer software (Brain Products GmbH, Munich, Germany). Offline, the signal was digitally filtered (high pass = 0.1 Hz, low pass = 30 Hz). EEG signals with amplitude larger than ±70 μV were interpreted as artifacts and rejected. To calculate the ERP, epochs of EEG were averaged off–line, and time was locked to stimulus onset from 200 ms pre–stimulus to 800 ms post stimulus relative to a 200 ms pre–stimulus baseline. Only trials leading to correct responses were included. The mean number of epochs included in each ERP average varied between 73.2 and 128.6 for the various types of stimuli used.

Statistical analyses

The statistical analyses were conducted with SPSS 17.0 software (SPSS Inc., Chicago, IL, USA). The analysis of variance (ANOVA) and chi-square test were used to compare the demographic data and neuropsychological test performances between patients and HC subjects. Accuracy and RTs were also analyzed. After rejecting responses with RTs shorter than 200 ms and longer than 1200 ms, a mean RT of correct responses in each stimulus condition was calculated for each subject. The data for accuracy and RTs were analyzed by separate 3×3 ANOVAs with Group (F-MD, R-MD, and HC) as one between-subjects factor, target expression (happy, neutral, and sad) as within-subject factors.

The peak amplitude and peak latency of the N170 response were identified within a time window of 130–210 ms after the onset of the target stimulus [28,40]. The quantification was restricted to the data from the lateral occipital channels P7 and P8. All ERP data were analyzed by a 3×3×2 repeated–measure ANOVA with Group (F-MD, R-MD, and HC) as one between-subjects factor, target expression (happy, neutral, and sad), and electrode location (P7 vs. P8 for N170) as within-subject factors. Post hoc comparisons were analyzed by Bonferroni test.

To investigate the behavioral significance of altered amplitude and latency of event-related N170 potential, the linear regression model with a step-wise analysis was used. This allowed us to examine the relationships between the amplitude and latency of N170, the $HDRS_{17}$ score and behavioral data in each group, and between the amplitude and latency of N170 and the number of episodes in the R-MD group. The statistical significance threshold was set at $P<0.05$.

Results

Demographic and neuropsychological characteristics

Demographic characteristics were shown in **Table 1**. No significant differences in age, gender, and years of education were noted between all groups (all Ps>0.05). Compared with HC subjects, the F-MD and R-MD groups showed the significant declines in muilt-domains of cognitive function, including episodic memory (i.e., AVLT -DR), executive function (i.e., TMT-A and -B), perceptual speed (i.e., SDMT), working memory (i.e., DST) and visuo-spatial cognition (i.e., CDT) (all Ps<0.05). Compared with F-MD patients, R-MD patients showed significantly lower MMSE, AVLT -DR, SDMT, and higher TMT-A and -B scores (all Ps<0.05).

Behavioral results

Reaction times. There was a significant main effect of group in F-MD patients (mean = 1026±312 ms). The F-MD group was slower compared with both the R-MD (mean = 964±362 ms) and HC groups (mean = 842±252 ms) (F (2, 128) = 14.83, $P<0.001$). A significant main effect of target expression was also observed (F (2, 128) = 8.26, $P = 0.030$). The interaction of group×target expression was significant (F (2, 128) = 24.62, $P<0.001$).

Post hoc comparisons showed that F-MD patients had slower RTs for happy, neutral and sad faces relative to HC subjects (t's> 4.03, P's<0.004). R-MD patients had slower RTs for happy and neutral faces, but shorter RTs for sad faces relative to HC subjects (t's>6.23, P's<0.001). R-MD patients also had shorter RTs for sad faces compared with F-MD patients ($t(83) = 2.92$, $P = 0.005$) (Figure 1).

Accuracy. There was a significant group effect on accuracy in R-MD patients (mean = 80.2±10.3%). Accuracy was lower than both the F-MD group (mean = 85.8±10.8%) and the HC group (mean = 92.7±5.2%) (F (2, 128) = 22.06, $P<0.001$). No significant main effect of target expression was found (F (2, 128) = 1.64, $P = 0.063$). The interaction of group×target expression was significant (F (2, 128) = 3.25, $P = 0.024$).

Post hoc comparisons showed that the F-MD and R-MD groups had lower accuracy for happy and neutral faces relative to HC group (t's>3.26, P's<0.008). However, the R-MD group had greater accuracy for sad faces compared with the F-MD and HC groups (t's>2.32, P's<0.016).

Electrophysiological results

N170 amplitude. There was a significant main effect of group on lower amplitudes in the R-MD group (mean = −6.82±2.40 μV). Amplitudes were lower when compared with those of the F-MD (mean = −7.65±3.26 μV) and HC groups (mean = −10.16±2.82 μV) (F (2, 124) = 12.38, $P<0.001$). A significant main effect of target expression was observed (F (2, 124) = 9.63, $P<0.001$). No significant main effect of electrode location was found (F (1, 124) = 1.22, $P = 0.096$). The interaction of group×target expression was highly significant (F (2, 124) = 13.02, $P<0.001$).

Post hoc comparisons showed that the F-MD group had lower amplitudes for happy, neutral and sad faces relative to the HC group (t's>3.26, P's<0.005). The R-MD group had lower amplitudes for happy and neutral, but higher amplitudes for sad faces relative to the HC group (t's>3.08, P's<0.005). Also, the R-MD group had higher amplitudes for sad faces compared to the F-MD group ($t(168) = 3.88$, $P = 0.004$). In the HC subjects, amplitudes for happy faces were significantly higher than those of neutral and sad faces (t's>2.73, P's<0.008), and amplitudes for neutral faces were significantly higher than those for sad faces

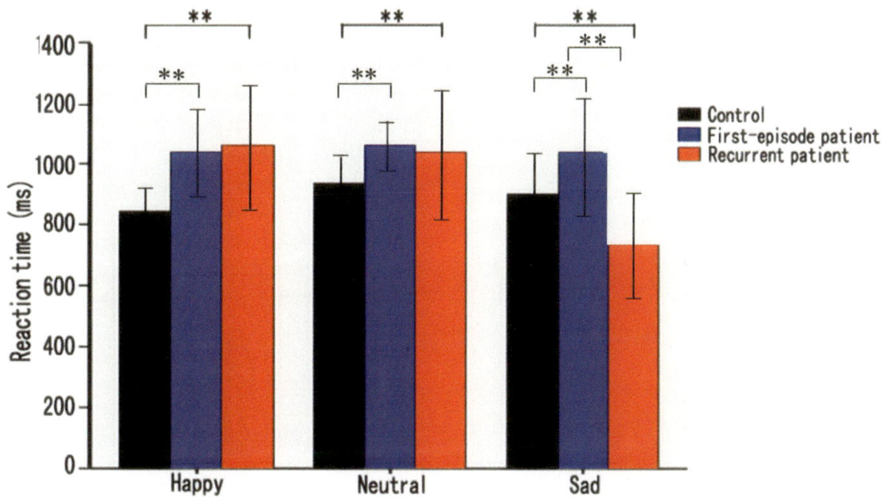

Figure 1. Mean reaction time (ms) for first episode and recurrent depression patients and healthy controls in happy, neutral, and sad face task.

($t(91) = 2.89$, $P = 0.007$). In both F-MD and R-MD groups, amplitudes for sad faces were significantly higher than those of happy and neutral faces (t's>3.65, P's<0.007), but no significant differences in amplitudes were found between happy and neutral faces (P's>0.05) (Figure 2).

N170 latency. There was a significant main effect of group on longer latencies in the R-MD patients (mean = 201.62±28.16 ms). Latencies were longer when compared with those of the F-MD (mean = 192.07±31.42 ms) and the HC groups (mean = 173.85±21.09 ms) (F (2, 124) = 6.92, $P = 0.025$). A significant main effect of target expression was observed (F (2, 124) = 5.38, $p = 0.031$). No significant main effect of electrode location was found (F (1, 124) = 0.78, $P = 0.126$). The interaction of group×target expression was significant (F (2, 124) = 8.85, $P <$ 0.001).

Post hoc comparisons showed that F-MD and R-MD groups had longer latencies for happy, neutral and sad faces relative to the HC group (t's>3.23, P's<0.008), and the R-MD group had longer latencies for happy and neutral faces but shorter for sad faces compared with the F-MD group (t's>3.60, P's<0.006). In HC subjects, latencies for happy faces were significantly shorter than those of neutral and sad faces (t's>3.02, P's<0.010). In F-MD patients, none of the within-group comparisons showed significant differences (P's>0.05). In R-MD patients, latencies for sad faces were significantly shorter than those of happy and neutral faces (t's>4.23, P's<0.004), but no significant differences in latencies were found between happy and neutral faces (P's>0.05) (Figure 2).

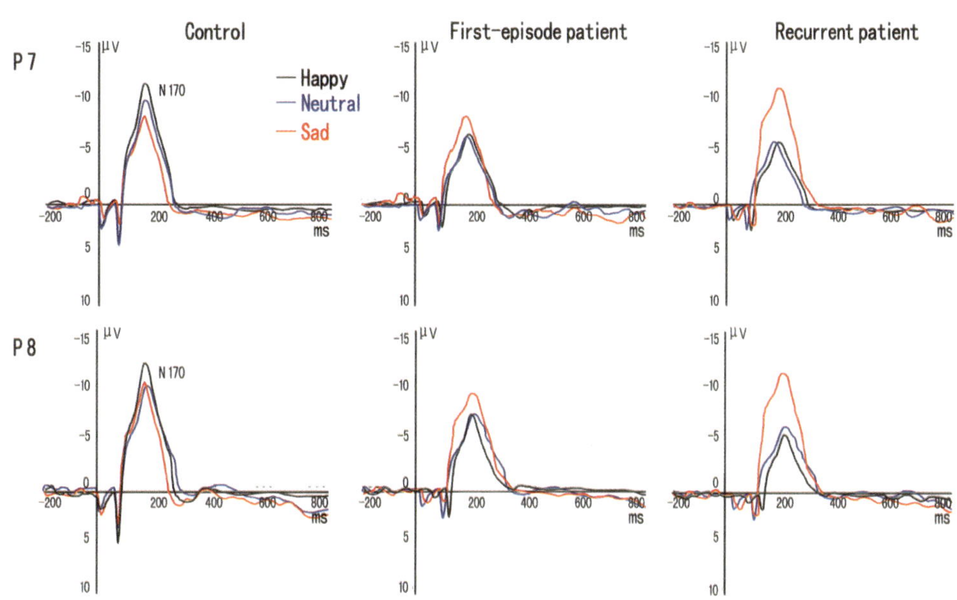

Figure 2. Grand-averaged event-related potential (ERP) waveforms of the N170 components elicited by happy (black line), neutral (blue line), and sad (red line) face pictures at P7 and P8 electrodes in first episode and recurrent depression patients and controls.

The relationship between $HDRS_{17}$, behavioral performance, number of episodes and ERP data

The multivariate regression analysis demonstrated that the deficits of N170 amplitude for happy and sad faces closely correlated with $HDRS_{17}$ scores in R-MD patients (F (1, 39) = 12.02, $P<0.001$, negative relationship for happy faces; F (1, 39) = 16.92, $P<0.001$, positive relationship for sad faces) (Figure 3). The correlation between N170 amplitude for sad faces and $HDRS_{17}$ score confirmed a markedly negative relationship in F-MD patients (F (1, 44) = 7.68, $P<0.001$) (Figure 3). However, no correlations were evident with respect to behavioral performance in the F-MD and R-MD groups (P's>0.05). Interestingly, the multivariate regression analysis demonstrated that the deficits of N170 amplitude for only sad faces positively correlated with the number of episodes in R-MD patients (F (1, 39) = 14.36, $P<0.001$) (Figure 3). Additionally, no correlations were found between $HDRS_{17}$ scores, behavioral performance, number of episodes or the deficits of N170 latency in the F-MD and R-MD groups (P's> 0.05). Furthermore, control subjects had no correlations between N170 index, behavioral performance or cognitive scores (all P's> 0.05).

Discussion

To our knowledge, our study is the first to investigate the relationship between the abnormal neural processing of emotional facial expressions and the number of depressive episodes in patients. Our study further confirms that the electrophysiological processing of emotional facial expressions is altered in patients with depressive disorders. Our new data also provides new insights into understanding the unconscious negative cognitive bias, which may be an important biomarker for depression recurrence.

Our study reports that F-MD and R-MD patients had slower RTs and lower accuracies for identifying happy and neutral faces relative to HC subjects. This data suggests that their processing for happy and neutral faces is impaired. These results corroborated and expanded the previously described emotional processing deficits in clinical depression [41–43]. A noticeable exception was that R-MD patients had shorter RTs and higher accuracies for sad faces compared with the F-MD and HC groups. These results suggest that R-MD patients employ specific processing schemata for negative faces and rely on different processing mechanisms for the happy and neutral faces. In fact, R-MD patients are more excited for sad faces and may exaggerate the negative emotion [9,44]. Taken together, the specific cognitive bias for sad faces by R-MD patients may be a consequence of focus on their inner world (negative emotion) [33], which may be strongly associated with interpersonal dysfunction in their clinical manifestation.

Our study also showed that F-MD and R-MD patients had reduced N170 amplitudes and longer N170 latencies for identification of happy and neutral faces. These data suggest dysfunctional emotional processing that includes the speed and strength of processing. These findings were also consistent with previous depression studies that showed impaired facial processing [4,7,45,46]. Depressed patients have impaired performance with only positive stimuli [18]. Furthermore, patients with depressive disorders show reduced intensity and frequency of facial expressions with positive hedonic stimuli or specific physiological reactivity [47]. Several neuroimaging studies have also indicated that reduced amygdala activation in response to positive stimuli in depression may be linked to anhedonic symptoms caused by inappropriate salience attribution to positive information [48,49]. Taken together, the evidence suggests that N170 impairment during facial processing may underlie one of the hallmark features of depression - anhedonic symptoms. It may also lead to a better understanding of interpersonal difficulties that are related to depression [42,50], since patients utilize facial expressions as important indicators to manage their own behavior and to evaluate the attitudes of others.

Interestingly, our study indicated that R-MD patients had higher N170 amplitudes for sad faces compared to the F-MD and HC groups and shorter N170 latencies for sad faces compared with the F-MD group. This positive ERP in the R-MD group seems directly related to negative items and can be correlated with the bias for negative information [51,52]. These findings were similar to previous depression reports that suggest faces expressing more sadness tend to be chosen as displaying greater intensity than happy and neutral faces. This may be due to the fact that sad faces are more arousing to R-MD patients than faces expressing other emotions when compared with the two other groups [52]. However, the negative cognitive bias was not found in F-MD patients, opposite of the R-MD patients who processed different emotional faces with a remarkably unconscious cognitive bias. This result suggests that R-MD patients have a specific emotional processing mechanism for negative faces, distinguishing them from F-MD patients. It further suggests that the unconscious negative cognitive bias may predict a sequential progression in F-MD patients, which could be strongly associated with the neuropathologic spread of depression. However, additional longitudinal studies will be needed to determine whether the unconscious negative cognitive bias in F-MD patients is specifically associated with the disease's progression.

Our current study also investigated the relationship between $HDRS_{17}$ score, behavioral data and ERP indexes. The data revealed a negative relationship between N170 amplitude and severity of depression for happy face recognition, while N170 amplitude was positively correlated with severity of depression for sad face recognition in R-MD patients. Collectively, these findings suggest that propagation of depression may intensify reductions in happy emotions while reinforcing negative emotions in R-MD patients. It is possible that the heightened perception of negative events may lead depressed individuals to feel worse or worthless about themselves and the whole outer world. Simultaneously, their lower mood can hinder their perception of happy events. Thus, they focus more on their inner world, which may be strongly associated with interpersonal dysfunction in their clinical manifestation [53]. However, only a negative relationship for sad face recognition was found in F-MD patients, suggesting that repeated episodes of depression may aggravate the deficits in emotional processing for happy faces and eventually lead to a lower mood [43]. Impaired positive emotional processing as indexed by N170 amplitude may be a useful and important biomarker of potential progression of depression [54].

In this study, the relationship between the amplitude and latency of N170 and the number of depressive episodes was also examined to confirm whether the unconscious negative bias in depression is a marker for stable cognitive vulnerability and possibly related to the recurrence of depression. Our results indicated that the N170 amplitudes for sad face recognition were significantly positively correlated with the number of depressive episodes, indicating that the emotional processing of sad faces differs with episode occurrence [4,12]. As a result, it should be suggested that the hypersensitive perception of negative social stimuli is a stable cognitive vulnerability predictor associated with depression recurrence [7]. With episode repetition, patients generate specifically related mechanisms that result in negative bias reinforcement. The mechanisms can propagate depression through decreases in social reinforcement and social support that

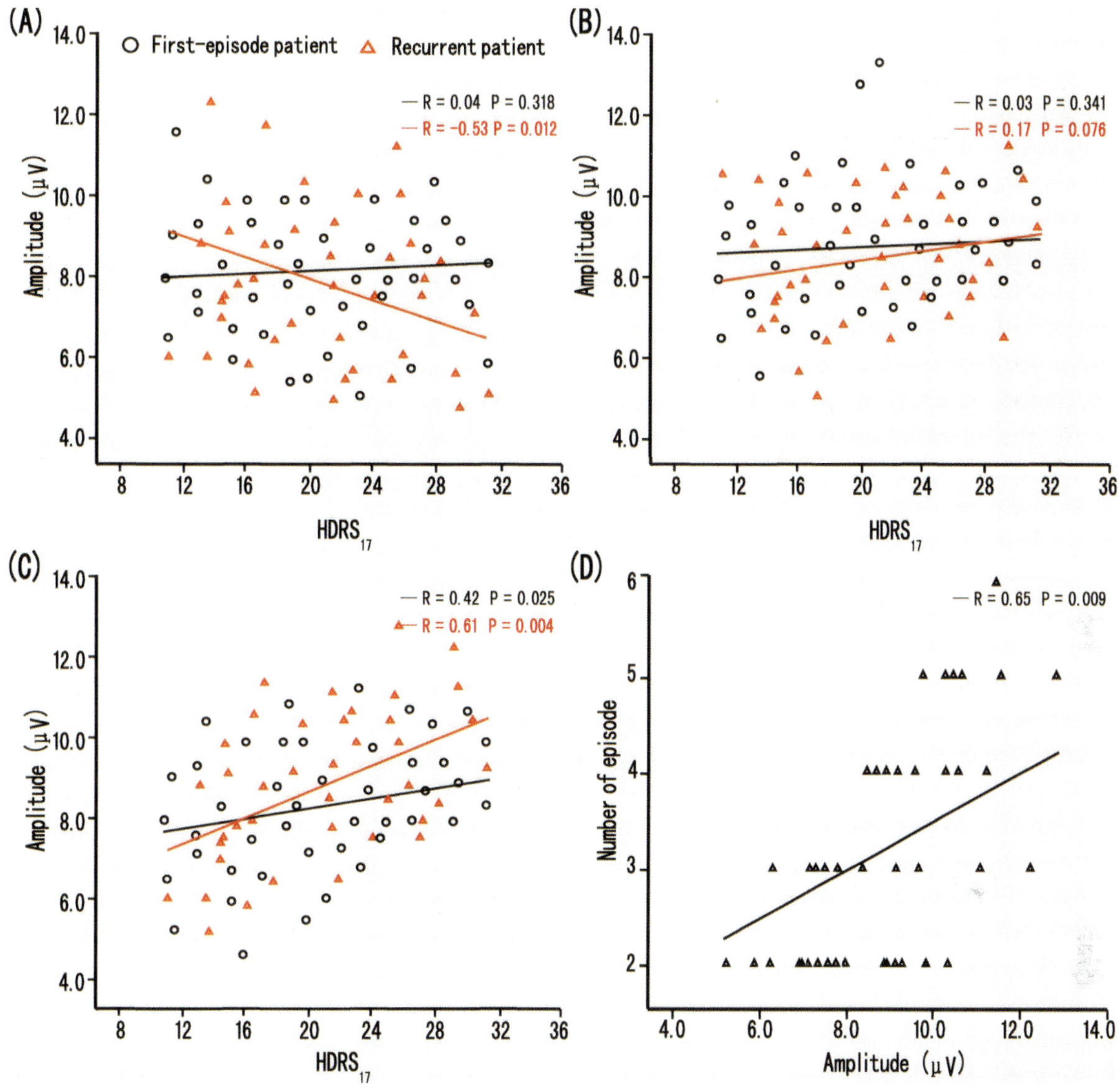

Figure 3. Correlation of clinical variables and the amplitude of event-related N170 potential in F-MD and R-MD patients. (A, B, C) Scattergrams representing the correlations between the groups and the N170 amplitude elicited by happy (A), neutral (B) and sad (C) facial pictures in F-MD (black line) and R-MD (red line) patients. (D) Scattergrams representing the correlations between the number of patient episodes and the N170 amplitude elicited by sad facial pictures in R-MD patients. Amplitude data are merged from P7 and P8 electrodes.

include negative feedback seeking, excessive reassurance seeking and interpersonal avoidance [4,50]. Taken together, the evidence suggests that the unconscious negative cognitive bias may predict the recurrence of depression, and that the impaired negative emotional processing indexed by N170 amplitude may be a useful and important biomarker of potential depression recurrence.

There are, of course, limitations to this study. First, the sample size is relatively small in this study, which could affect the explanation of our results. Second, some of the depressed patients had mild anxiety symptoms, which could have influenced the results. Additionally, all patients were receiving antidepressant medication during the task. This could have influenced the behavioral or ERP performances of the patient groups. Finally, there are limitations imposed by the cross-sectional design of this study. Prospective longitudinal studies that assess changes in these complex relationships over time are needed. These future studies will help determine whether or not the changes in these parameters can be used as potential biomarkers for identifying individuals at high risk of recurrence and may clarify the diagnosis, or predict outcome in future studies.

Conclusion

The current study provides novel insight into the relationship between the abnormal neural processing of emotional facial expressions and the number of patients' depressive episodes. Our findings have important clinical implications for a more principled understanding of repeated physiopathological mechanisms of depression. Moreover, they further suggest that impaired emotional processing as indexed by N170 amplitude of positive and negative faces may be a useful biomarker for predicting the propagation and recurrence of depression. It will be a more significant and interesting contribution if future studies examine the relationship between the number of previous depressive episodes and the impaired emotional processing from the abnormal brain structure by functional magnetic resonance imaging technique.

Acknowledgments

We thank all psychiatric nurses and doctors for their help in this study.

Author Contributions

Conceived and designed the experiments: JC LY ZZ. Performed the experiments: ZD YZ. Analyzed the data: JC WM DW. Contributed reagents/materials/analysis tools: XW GL. Contributed to the writing of the manuscript: JC.

References

1. American Psychiatric Association (APA) (2013) Diagnostic and Statistical Manual of Mental Disorders, 5th Edition, DSM-V. APA, Arlington, VA.
2. Beck A, Rush A, Shaw B, Emery G (1979) Cognitive therapy of depression. New York: Guilford Press.
3. Just N, Abramson L, Alloy L (2001) Remitted depression studies as tests of the cognitive vulnerability hypotheses of depression onset: a critique and conceptual analysis. Clin Psychol Rev 1: 63–83.
4. Nandrino JL, Dodin V, Martin P, Henniaux M (2004) Emotional information processing in first and recurrent major depressive episodes. J Psychiatr Res 5: 475–484.
5. Blackburn I, Roxborough H, Muir W, Glabus M, Blackwood D (1990) Perceptual and physiological dysfunction in depression. Psychol Med 1: 95–103.
6. Mathews A, MacLeod C (2005) Cognitive vulnerability to emotional disorders. Annu Rev Clin Psychol 1: 167–195.
7. Dai Q, Feng Z (2012) More excited for negative facial expressions in depression: evidence from an event-related potential study. Clin Neurophysiol 11: 2172–2179.
8. Gotlib IH, Neubauer DL (2000) Information processing approaches to the study of cognitive biases in depression. In: Johnson, S.L., Hayes, A.M. (Eds.), Stress, Coping and Depression. Erlbaum, Mahwah, pp. 117–143.
9. Yoon KL, Joormann J, Gotlib IH (2009) Judging the intensity of facial expressions of emotion, depression-related biases in the processing of positive affect. J Abnorm Psychol 181: 223–228.
10. Hankin BL, Gibb BE, Abela JRZ, Flory K (2010) Selective attention to affective stimuli and clinical depression among youths: role of anxiety and specificity of emotion. J Abnorm Psychol 119: 491–501.
11. Zhong MT, Zhu XZ, Yi JY, Yao SQ, Atchley AA (2011) Do the early attentional components of ERPs reflect attentional bias in depression? It depends on the stimulus presentation time. Clin Neurophysiol 122: 1371–1381.
12. Bulloch A, Williams J, Lavorato D, Patten S (2014) Recurrence of major depressive episodes is strongly dependent on the number of previous episodes. Depress Anxiety 1: 72–76.
13. Meng C, Brandl F, Tahmasian M, Shao J, Manoliu A, et al. (2014) Aberrant topology of striatum's connectivity is associated with the number of episodes in depression. BrainPt 2: 598–609.
14. Kronmüller KT, Schröder J, Köhler S, Götz B, Victor D, et al. (2009) Hippocampal volume in first episode and recurrent depression. Psychiatry Res 1: 62–66.
15. Frodl T, Meisenzahl EM, Zetzsche T, Born C, Jäger M, et al. (2003) Larger amygdala volumes in first depressive episode as compared to recurrent major depression and healthy control subjects. Biol Psychiatry 4: 338–344.
16. Roca M, Armengol S, García-García M, Rodriguez-Bayón A, Ballesta I, et al. (2011) Clinical differences between first and recurrent episodes in depressive patients. Compr Psychiatry 1: 26–32.
17. Mitchell PB, Parker GB, Gladstone GL, Wilhelm K, Austin MP (2003) Severity of stressful life events in first and subsequent episodes of depression: the relevance of depressive subtype. J Affect Disord 3: 245–252.
18. Nandrino JL, Pezard L, Posté A, Réveillère C, Beaune D (2002) Autobiographical Memory in Major Depression A Comparison between First-Episode and Recurrent Patients. Psychopathology 6: 335–340.
19. Fossati P, Harvey PO, Le Bastard G, Ergis AM, Jouvent R, et al. (2004) Verbal memory performance of patients with a first depressive episode and patients with unipolar and bipolar recurrent depression. J Psychiatr Res 2: 137–144.
20. Karabekiroğlu A, Topçuoğlu V, Gimzal Gönentür A, Karabekiroğlu K (2010) Executive function differences between first episode and recurrent major depression patients. Turk Psikiyatri Derg 4: 280–288.
21. Chen J, Yang LQ, Zhang ZJ, Ma WT, Wu XQ, et al. (2013) The association between the disruption of motor imagery and the number of depressive episodes of major depression. J Affect Disord 2: 337–343.
22. Stefanescu C, Ciobica A (2012) The relevance of oxidative stress status in first episode and recurrent depression. J Affect Disord 1–3: 34–38.
23. Celik C, Erdem M, Cayci T, Ozdemir B, Ozgur Akgul E, et al. (2010) The association between serum levels of neopterin and number of depressive episodes of major depression. Prog Neuropsychopharmacol Biol Psychiatry 2: 372–375.
24. Kim EY, Lee SH, Park G, Kim S, Kim I, et al. (2013) Gender Difference in Event Related Potentials to Masked Emotional Stimuli in the Oddball Task. Psychiatry Investig 2: 164–172.
25. Campanella S, Rossignol M, Mejias S, Joassin F, Maurage P, et al. (2004) Human gender differences in an emotional visual oddball task: an event-related potentials study. Neurosci Lett 1: 14–18.
26. Bentin S, Allison T, Puce A, Perez E, McCarthy G (1996) Electrophysiological Studies of Face Perception in Humans. J Cogn Neurosci 6: 551–565.
27. Batty M, Taylor MJ (2003) Early processing of the six basic facial emotional expressions. Cogn Brain Res 3: 613–20.
28. Blau VC, Maurer U, Tottenham N, McCandliss BD (2007) The face-specific N170 component is modulated by emotional facial expression. Behav Brain Funct 3: 7.
29. Japee S, Crocker L, Carver F, Pessoa L, Ungerleider LG (2009) Individual differences in valence modulation of face-selective M170 response. Emotion 9: 59–69.
30. Wronka R, Walentowska W (2011) Attention modulates emotional expression processing. Psychophysiology 48: 1047–1056.
31. Caharel S, Courtay N, Bernard C, Lalonde R, Rebai M (2005) Familiarity and emotional expression influence an early stage of face processing: an electrophysiological study. Brain Cogn 59: 96–100.
32. Ibáñez A, Gleichgerrcht E, Hurtado E, González R, Haye A, et al. (2010) Early neural markers of implicit attitudes: N170 modulated by intergroup and evaluative contexts in IAT. Front Hum Neurosci 4: 188.
33. Dai Q, Feng ZZ (2011) Deficient distracter inhibition and enhanced facilitation for emotional stimuli in depression: an ERP study. Int J Psychophysiol 79: 249–258.
34. Calvo MG, Beltrán D (2014) Brain lateralization of holistic versus analytic processing of emotional facial expressions. Neuroimage 92C: 237–247.
35. Zheng YP, Zhao JP, Phillips M, Liu JB, Cai MF, et al. (1988) Validity and reliability of the Chinese Hamilton Depression Rating Scale. Br J Psychiatry 152: 660–664.
36. Wang Y, Luo YJ (2005) Standardized and assessment of face expression of undergraduate students. Chin J Clin Psychol (in Chinese) 13: 396–398.
37. Hurtado E, Haye A, González R, Manes F, Ibáñez A (2009) Contextual blending of ingroup/outgroup face stimuli and word valence: LPP modulation and convergence of measures. BMC Neurosci 10: 69.
38. Ibáñez A, Hurtado E, Riveros R, Urquina H, Cardona JF, et al. (2011) Facial and semantic emotional interference: behavioral and cortical responses to the dual valence association task. Behav Brain Funct 7: 8.
39. Jasper HH (1958) The ten-twenty electrode system of the International Federation. Electroencephalogr Clin Neurophysiol 10: 371–375.
40. Hietanen JK, Astikainen P (2013) N170 response to facial expressions is modulated by the affective congruency between the emotional expression and preceding affective picture. Biol Psychol 2: 114–124.
41. Joormann J, Gotlib IH (2006) Is this happiness I see? Biases in the identification of emotional facial expressions in depression and social phobia. J Abnorm Psychol 115: 705–714.
42. Joormann J, Gotlib IH (2007) Selective attention to emotional faces following recovery from depression. J Abnorm Psychol 116: 80–85.
43. Demenescu LR, Kortekaas R, den Boer JA, Aleman A (2010) Impaired attribution of emotion to facial expressions in anxiety and major depression. PLoS ONE 12: e15058.
44. Leppanen JM (2006) Emotional information processing in mood disorders: a review of behavioral and neuroimaging findings. Curr Opin Psychiatry 19: 34–39.
45. Campanella S, Falbo L, Rossignol M, Grynberg D, Balconi M, et al. (2012) Sex differences on emotional processing are modulated by subclinical levels of alexithymia and depression: a preliminary assessment using event-related potentials. Psychiatry Res 1–2: 145–153.
46. Rossignol M, Philippot P, Crommelinck M, Campanella S (2008) Visual processing of emotional expressions in mixed anxious-depressed subclinical state: an event-related potential study on a female sample. Neurophysiol Clin 5: 267–275.
47. Sloan DM, Strauss ME, Wisner KL (2001) Diminished response to pleasant stimuli by depressed women. J Abnorm Psychol 3: 488–493.
48. Arnone D, McKie S, Elliott R, Thomas EJ, Downey D, et al. (2012) Increased amygdala responses to sad but not fearful faces in major depression: relation to mood state and pharmacological treatment. Am J Psychiatry 8: 841–850.
49. Stuhrmann A, Dohm K, Kugel H, Zwanzger P, Redlich R, et al. (2013) Mood-congruent amygdala responses to subliminally presented facial expressions in major depression: associations with anhedonia. J Psychiatry Neurosci 4: 249–258.
50. Joiner T (2000) Depression's vicious scree: self-propagatory and erosive factors in depression chronicity. Clin Psychol Sci Pract 7: 203–218.
51. Dietrich D, Emrich H, Waller C, Wieringa B, Johannes S, et al. (2000) Emotion/cognition-coupling in word recognition memory of depressive patients: an event-related potential study. Psychiatry Res 96: 15–29.
52. Vanderhasselt MA, De Raedt R, Dillon DG, Dutra SJ, Brooks N, et al. (2012) Decreased cognitive control in response to negative information in patients with

remitted depression: an event-related potential study. J Psychiatry Neurosci 4: 250–258.
53. Gotlib IH, Krasnoperova E, Yue DN, Joormann J (2004) Attentional biases for negative interpersonal stimuli in clinical depression. J Abnorm Psychol 1131: 127–135.
54. Kujawa A, Hajcak G, Torpey D, Kim J, Klein DN (2012) Electrocortical reactivity to emotional faces in young children and associations with maternal and paternal depression. J Child Psychol Psychiatry 2: 207–215.

5

Relationship between Coping with Interpersonal Stressors and Depressive Symptoms in the United States, Australia, and China: A Focus on Reassessing Coping

Tsukasa Kato*

Toyo University, Department of Social Psychology, Bunkyo-ku, Tokyo, Japan

Abstract

Objective: Reassessing coping involves efforts to wait patiently for an appropriate opportunity to act or for a change or improvement in the situation, and can be observed in individuals encountering a stressful relationship event. It was hypothesized that reassessing coping would be negatively associated with depressive symptoms.

Methods: A cross-sectional Web-based survey was conducted in order to test this hypothesis by examining relationships between coping strategies including reassessing coping, distancing coping and constructive coping for stressful relationship events and depressive symptoms. Participants were 1,500 individuals recruited from the general populations of the United States, Australia, and China.

Results: Structural equation modeling analysis revealed that scores on coping strategies predicted depressive symptom scores in the samples from all three countries with medium or large effect sizes. Further, the beta values for reassessing coping scores were negative and significant in all samples, indicating that the hypothesis was supported for each of the population samples surveyed. In addition, distancing coping, which reflects strategies that attempt to actively damage, disrupt, and dissolve a stressful relationship, was associated with high levels of depressive symptoms.

Conclusions: Reassessing coping for interpersonal stressors was be negatively associated with depressive symptoms in sample from general populations of the United States, Australia, and China.

Editor: Judith Homberg, Radboud University, Netherlands

Funding: This research was supported by the Japan Society for the Promotion of Science (Grant-in-Aid for Scientific Research C-25380948) and the founding of support is external to the authors' organization (http://www.jsps.go.jp/). The funders had no role in study design, data collection and analysis, decision to publish, or preparation of the manuscript.

Competing Interests: The author has declared that no competing interests exist.

* Email: mtsukasa@hotmail.com

Introduction

Several researchers [1–4] have proposed mechanisms by which interpersonal stressors increase the risk of depression and provided evidence for their relationships. The World Health Organization [5] states that certain mental and behavioral disorders, such as depression and anxiety, can result from failing to cope adaptively with a stressor. According to the transactional theory proposed by Lazarus et al. [6,7], coping is defined as "constantly changing cognitive and behavioral efforts to manage specific external and/or internal demands that are appraised as taxing or exceeding the resources of the person" (p. 141). This theory hypothesizes that coping behavior affects psychological functioning, including depressive symptoms, and has been supported by numerous studies [6].

Kato [8] defined interpersonal stressors as "stressful episodes between two or more people that involve quarrels, arguments, negative attitudes or behavior, an uncomfortable atmosphere during a conversation or activity, and concern about hurting others' feelings" (p. 100); he proposed three types of coping strategies, based on the transactional theory, for dealing with interpersonal stressors. According to research on how college students and workers deal with interpersonal stressors, the following coping strategies were identified: reassessing coping, distancing coping, and constructive coping. Although coping strategies individuals employ and the effects on psychological distress are dependent on the nature of the stressors [6,7], conventional research has measured and categorized coping strategies for interpersonal stressors using a broadly applicable coping scale [8], such as the Ways of Coping Questionnaire (WCQ) [9]. Therefore, Kato's approach [8] presented unique coping strategies for interpersonal stressors. Thus, focusing on these three coping strategies proposed by Kato [8], in particular the strategy of reassessing coping, we examined the relationships between coping strategies for interpersonal stressors and depressive symptoms in general populations of the United States, Australia, and China.

Reassessing coping

Reassessing coping refers to efforts to wait patiently for an appropriate opportunity to act or for a change or improvement in the situation [8]. This type of coping is an active strategy that involves exercising self-control, avoiding premature action, and waiting until an appropriate opportunity arises. Therefore, reassessing coping is distinct from avoidant coping, which involves avoiding stressful problems or situations. Previous studies have found a non-significant negative correlation between reassessing coping and avoidant coping [8]. Kato [10] stated that reassessing coping enables people to take time to deal with stressful relationships, attain a better grasp of the situation, control their emotions, and consider appropriate countermeasures. Additionally, reassessing coping can influence other individuals or parties involved within the stressful relationship, helping to change their mental state, and thus permitting them to adopt a calmer, more accepting attitude toward the stressful relationship as well. In short, reassessing coping increases the likelihood that the situation will improve.

Thus, some studies have suggested that reassessing coping attenuates psychological distress in response to stressful relationships. For example, in a sample of college students, reassessing coping was negatively associated with depressive symptoms, anxiety, and general distress [8]. Correlations between reassessing coping and good psychological functioning, including experiencing fewer depressive symptoms, have been reported by other studies conducted among full-time workers in dealing with workplace interpersonal stress [10] and among hospital nursing staff in relationships with patients as stressors [11]. Moreover, a previous study [8] showed that reassessing coping incrementally predicted depressive symptoms beyond the effects of other popular coping strategies (i.e., 8 strategies of the WCQ) and conflict management styles (i.e., 5 styles categorized by the dual-concern model [12,13]) on depressive symptoms.

Although the aforementioned findings on the effects of reassessing coping on depressive symptoms were obtained through research performed specifically in Japan, several studies suggest that these findings may be supported for Western and other populations. For example, clinical interventions based on mindfulness [14–16], detached mindfulness [17], or meta-cognitive awareness [18], propose these strategies as primary skill that individuals should develop. These skills, which allow distancing oneself from negative emotions when they are evoked [16], have been shown to reduce psychological distress and promote well-being [for reviews, 17,19]. Thus, it is likely that distancing oneself from stressful situations represents a coping strategy that could reduce depressive symptoms. Therefore, we hypothesized that reassessing coping would be associated with a lower level of depressive symptoms in populations of other countries as well.

In the current study, we focused on reassessing coping among three coping strategies proposed by Kato [8], because no other coping style has proven to be effective in reducing psychological dysfunction including depressive symptoms in interpersonal stress. For example, Penley et al.'s [20] meta-analytic review of 11 coping types found that all coping styles were either negatively or non-significantly related to physical or psychological health outcomes with respect to interpersonal relationships as stressors.

Distancing coping

Distancing coping reflects strategies that attempt to actively damage, disrupt, and dissolve a stressful relationship (e.g. avoiding contact with the person and ignoring the person); that is, distancing in this coping style means intentionally breaking off relations with another individual involved within the stressful relationship. Therefore, this coping strategies differs from the concept of distancing used in mindfulness-based clinical interventions.

Distancing coping may lead to poor interpersonal relationships [8], and the deterioration of these relationships can produce psychological and physiological dysfunctions [for a review, 21]. Distancing coping was indeed found to be positively correlated with depressive symptoms, anxiety, burnout, insomnia, and general psychological distress in a study involving Japanese students [8], workers [10,11], and hospital nursing staffs [11]. Therefore, we hypothesized that distancing coping would be associated with a higher level of depressive symptoms in populations of other countries as well.

Constructive coping

Another strategy, constructive coping, involves efforts that actively seek to improve, maintain or sustain a relationship without aggravating others (e.g. reflecting on one's own conduct and trying to understand the other person's feelings) and emphasizes respecting and living in harmony with others. Previous studies in Japanese samples have found positive but no-significant correlations between constructive coping and depressive symptoms [8,10]. Likewise, some studies [22,23] have indicated no significant correlation between coping strategies similar to constructive coping and depressive symptoms but positive. Other studies on coping strategies similar to constructive coping [24] have found that such coping is significantly associated with increased psychological distress. Therefore, we hypothesized that there would be positive or no-significant correlation between constructive and depressive symptoms.

Cross-cultural differences in coping strategies

In the present study, we also examined cross-cultural differences in the frequency with which reassessing coping is used, as individuals from different cultures are known to adopt different coping strategies [for a review, 25]. For instance, Triandis [26] suggested that the following characteristics are distinctive of collectivistic cultures: over cautiousness, hypervigilance, avoidance of decisions and interpersonal conflicts, and increased likelihood of using silence, ambiguity, and indirect messages during communication_ all of which, according to Kato [8], are included in reassessing coping. Constructive coping may also include characteristics of collectivistic cultures as they emphasize respecting and living in harmony with others, and how one behaves is often based on what one perceives to be the thoughts, feelings, and actions of others [26]. Oyserman et al.'s meta-analysis [27] in various societies revealed that collectivism was lower in Australia, but higher in China, as compared to the United States. Therefore, we hypothesized that reassessing coping and constructive coping would be most frequently used in China, followed by the United States, and Australia.

We selected the United States and Australian samples as representing from individualistic cultures and the Chinese sample as a collectivistic cultures for a Web-based survey. The United States and China are the most highly populated countries among individualistic and collectivistic cultures, respectively. Australia has been dominated by immigration that reflects a multicultural mix representing the globe, and more than a quarter of the Australian population was born in other countries.

Gender differences in coping strategies

Gender differences in coping have not yet been established conclusively; however, women use more coping strategies in general than men [for a review, 28]. Women also encounter higher levels of stressful events related to interpersonal relationships [for reviews, 29,30] and are more likely to respond more sensitively [for a review, 4,30]. Therefore, women may attempt to use more coping strategies in general also for interpersonal stressors than men. As a result, we hypothesized that women would employ distracting coping and constructive coping more frequency than men. As reassessing coping is a waiting strategy without approach to another individual involved within the stressful relationships, we hypothesized that gender differences in this particular form of coping would be absent in the current study. In fact, no significant gender difference in reassessing coping was found in Japanese samples [8].

Methods

Participants

United States sample. This sample comprised 246 men and 254 women aged 18 to 79 years (mean age 45.4, $SD = 15.3$). Approximately 78.6% were Caucasian, 7.2% were African American, 5.6% were Asian American, 4.8% were Hispanic, and 3.6% were of other ethnicities; one person preferred not to say. Further, about 51.4% of the participants were married, 31.2% had never been married, and 17.4% were divorced, separated, or widowed.

Australian sample. The Australian sample included 239 men and 261 women aged 18 to 79 years (mean age 45.4, $SD = 14.8$). Approximately 55.8% were Caucasian, 29.2% were European Australian, 7.8% were Asian Australian, and 6.6% were of other ethnicities; six persons preferred not to say. In addition, approximately 54.2% were married and 32.2% had never been married, while 13.6% were divorced, separated, or widowed.

Chinese sample. Individuals in this sample included 263 men and 237 women aged 19 to 76 years (mean age 40.1, $SD = 11.9$). Approximately 98.0% were Chinese, and 2% were of other ethnicities. In terms of marital status, 87.0% were married, 11.6% had never been married, and 1.4% were divorced, separated, or widowed.

Procedure

All participants were recruited through a Web-based survey. Data were collected by the polling organization Rakuten Research (Tokyo, Japan), through their Web panel (see http://research.rakuten.co.jp/en/) of over 4.01, 0.83, and 1.43 million members in the United States, Australia, and China, respectively, who had registered and received one ID per person.

The details of the survey were sent to potential participants, who ranged in age from 18 to 79 years, through an e-mail in early December 2013. If potential participants agreed to participate in this survey, they clicked on another link to view the survey, which began once they entered their ID. Participants could not skip any questionnaire items. The data were collected so that a sample was almost evenly divided by gender and age in each country. A chi-square test showed that no significant differences in gender between the three samples were found at $p < .05$. A Kruskal-Wallis rank analysis revealed that the median age in the Chinese sample was significantly lower than in the United States and Australian samples, but no significant difference between was United States and Australian was found at $p < .05$. The project, including the Web-based survey, was approved by the Institutional Ethics Committee of the Department of Social Psychology at Toyo University in Japan.

Measures

Coping with interpersonal stressors. The Interpersonal Stress Coping Scale (ISCS) [8], which was designed to measure coping strategies for interpersonal stressors, was used. The ISCS consists of three 5-item subscales evaluating reassessing coping (e.g., taking a pragmatic view of the matter, deciding not to take the matter too seriously), distancing coping (e.g., avoiding contact with the person, ignoring the person), and constructive coping (e.g., reflecting on one's own conduct, trying to understand the other person's feelings). A previous study [8] reported that confirmatory factor analyses (CFAs) showed good fit to the three-factor model for the ISCS, but poor fit to other models (e.g., one-factor model and some two factor models). The score of each of the three strategies is associated with the theoretically related constructs [8]. The validity for the ISCS score was previously established only in Japanese samples. Cronbach's alphas for scores on reassessing, distancing, and constructive coping were.805 (95% CI [.780,.828]),.839 (95% CI [.823,.854]), and.733 (95% CI [.699,.762]), respectively [8]; the number of independent alphas was eight ($N = 3{,}686$).

The instructions were as follows: "Please recall the specifics of your own experiences of stress due to interpersonal relationships. These may include quarreling with others, being talked about behind your back, feeling awkward while speaking, and worrying if you have hurt someone's feelings. Please read each item and indicate to what extent you used that strategy in the situations you encountered." Participants rated the extent to which they used each item on a 4-point Likert scale ranging from 0 (*did not use*) to 3 (*used a great deal*). In the present study, trait coping strategies were measured.

Depressive symptoms. The Center for Epidemiologic Studies' Depression Scale (CES-D) [31], a 20-item self-report scale, was used to measure depressive symptoms in this study. Development of the CES-D was originally based on the American population [31]; however, the validity and reliability of CES-D scores have also been established in a number of other populations, including those of Australia [32] and China [33]. Participants rated each item according to their experiences within the past week on a 4-point Likert scale ranging from 1 (*rarely or none of the time*) to 4 (*most or all of the time*).

Data analysis

First, three measurement invariances of the ISCS (3 factors, 5 items per factor) across the three samples were tested using a mean and covariance structure (MACS) analysis, based on CFA models, in order to compare mean ISCS subscale scores: configural invariance (equivalence of factor structure across groups), metric invariance (equivalence of factor loadings across groups), and invariance in uniqueness (equivalence of error variances across groups). Configural invariance served as a baseline model. Scalar invariance (equivalence of intercepts across groups) was not tested because it was unclear as to whether observed mean differences reflected lack of measurement invariance or simple actual differences [34].

Based on guidelines proposed by Hu and Bentler [35], root-mean-square error of approximation (RMSEA) values of.06 or lower, standardized root-mean-square residual (SRMR) values of.08 or lower, and comparative fit index (CFI) values of.95 or greater were considered good fits; CFI values greater than.90 were deemed acceptable [35]. A change in CFI (ΔCFI) value equal to or less than.01 served as a practical indicator of substantial improvement in fit [36]. Although chi-square statistics (i.e., χ^2 and $\Delta\chi^2$) are known to be sensitive to sample size, we provided these statistics as they have traditionally been used as indicators of goodness-of-fit for CFA.

Second, our hypothesis on the relationship between three coping strategies and depressive symptoms was tested using a multiple group analysis, which enabled cross-cultural and gender comparisons of the relationship. Structural equation modeling (SEM) was conducted using the Amos 22 software [37].

Results

Measurement invariances of the ISCS

The MACS was conducted to test the measurement invariances of the ISCS. Goodness-of-fit statistics pertaining to the three models are shown in Table 1. The RMSEA and SRMR values for the three models were less than the cutoff criteria of.06 and.08, respectively; the CFI values were greater than the cutoff criterion of.90, which indicated acceptable fit. ΔCFI values of −.004 and −.004 were both less than the cutoff criterion of.01 [36]. These results suggested that the three-factor model for the ISCS had the same factor structure, with similar factor loadings and error variances across all three samples.

Cross-cultural differences in coping with interpersonal stress

Means, standard deviations, and alpha coefficients for all variables are shown in Table 2. To test cross-cultural differences with regard to each coping strategy, 2 (gender) × 3 (countries) analyses of variance (ANOVAs) were conducted, with the ISCS scores for each coping strategy as the dependent variable. The ANOVA on reassessing coping revealed that only the main effect of country was significant ($F(2, 1494) = 48.35$, $p < .001$, $\eta_p^2 = .061$); however, the interaction between gender and country ($F(2, 1494) = 2.92$, $p = .054$, $\eta_p^2 = .004$) as well as the main effect of gender ($F(1, 1494) = 0.06$, $p = .81$, $\eta_p^2 = .001$) were not significant at $p < .05$. Furthermore, Bonferroni post-hoc tests showed that reassessing coping scores were significantly higher in China ($M = 8.66$, $SD = 2.65$) than in the United States ($M = 7.57$, $SD = 3.21$) and Australia ($M = 6.81$, $SD = 3.16$), in that order.

In the ANOVA on distancing coping, significant main effects of gender ($F(1, 1494) = 4.12$, $p < .05$, $\eta_p^2 = .003$) and country ($F(2, 1494) = 3.06$, $p < .05$, $\eta_p^2 = .004$), but no significant interaction ($F(2, 1494) = 0.04$, $p = .096$, $\eta_p^2 = .001$) were observed. Bonferroni post-hoc tests revealed that distancing coping scores for women ($M = 5.78$, $SD = 3.68$) were significantly higher than those for men ($M = 5.40$, $SD = 3.43$), whereas differences between the three countries were not significant.

The ANOVA on constructive coping also revealed significant main effects of gender ($F(1, 1494) = 14.70$, $p < .001$, $\eta_p^2 = .010$) and country ($F(2, 1494) = 39.82$, $p < .001$, $\eta_p^2 = .051$) but no significant interaction ($F(2, 1494) = 0.52$, $p = .595$, $\eta_p^2 = .001$). Through Bonferroni post-hoc tests, constructive coping scores were found to be significantly higher in China ($M = 8.05$, $SD = 2.95$) than in the United States ($M = 7.23$, $SD = 3.55$) and Australia ($M = 6.26$, $SD = 3.22$), in that order. Additionally, women ($M = 7.47$, $SD = 3.40$) scored significantly higher than men ($M = 6.89$, $SD = 3.23$) on this type of coping.

Coping strategies and depressive symptoms

To test our hypothesis on the relationship between reassessing coping and depressive symptoms, a multiple group analysis, which enabled cross-cultural comparisons of the relationship, was conducted using maximum likelihood estimation (see Figure 1). For all samples, the R^2 values were significant at the $p < .001$ level

Table 1. Goodness-of-fit Indexes for the three-factor model for the ISCS.

Model	χ^2	df		CFI	RMSEA	SRMR	$\Delta\chi^2$	Δdf	ΔCFI
Configural invariance	849.36	261	***	.915	.039	.052			
Metric invariance	905.74	285	***	.911	.038	.053	56.38	24	.004
Invariance in uniqueness	1154.62	327	***	.911	.041	.059	305.26	66	.004

*** $p < .001$.

Table 2. Means, standard deviations, and alphas for scores of each coping strategy and depressive symptoms.

Variable		United States				Australia				China			
		n	Mean	SD	α	n	Mean	SD	α	n	Mean	SD	α
Reassessing coping	Men	246	7.86	3.03	.66	239	6.64	3.32	.75	263	8.60	2.56	.65
	Women	254	7.30	3.35	.73	261	6.96	3.00	.70	237	8.73	2.75	.70
Distancing coping	Men	246	5.70	3.71	.83	239	5.22	3.74	.85	263	5.30	2.81	.75
	Women	254	6.11	4.19	.88	261	5.52	3.89	.86	237	5.70	2.70	.71
Constructive coping	Men	246	6.93	3.35	.79	239	5.80	3.19	.78	263	7.83	2.83	.76
	Women	254	7.51	3.71	.83	261	6.67	3.19	.77	237	8.30	3.07	.79
Depressive symptoms	Men	246	36.22	11.16	.91	239	34.65	11.21	.92	263	35.32	9.26	.88
	Women	254	38.72	13.51	.93	261	36.70	11.98	.93	237	35.85	9.81	.90

(United States: R^2 =.19, F (3,496) = 39.50, Cohen's f^2 =.24; Australia: R^2 =.18, F (3,496) = 35.41, Cohen's f^2 =.21; China: R^2 =.26, F (3,496) = 58.80, Cohen's f^2 =.36), indicating that significant proportions of the variance in depressive symptom scores were accounted for by scores of each coping strategy (see Table 3). The beta weights for reassessing coping scores in all samples were significant and negative in the SEM analysis with depressive symptom scores (United States: $\beta = -.28$, $p<.001$; Australia: $\beta = -.28$, $p<.001$; China: $\beta = -.28$, $p<.001$). There were no significant differences in coping scores between all samples at the $p<.05$ level (z = 0.32, 0.43, and 0.11; p = .37,.33, and.46; United States vs. Australia, United States vs. China, and Australia vs. China).

Again, a multiple group analysis was conducted to examine gender differences in the relationship between reassessing coping and depressive symptoms (see Table 3). For genders, the R^2 values were significant at the $p<.001$ level (women: R^2 =.17, F (3,748) = 51.52, Cohen's f^2 =.21; men: R^2 =.24, F (3,744) = 77.13, Cohen's f^2 =.31). The beta weights for reassessing coping scores in genders were significant and negative (women: $\beta = -.23$, $p<.001$; men: $\beta = -.35$, $p<.001$). There were no significant gender differences in the beta-weight at the $p<.05$ level (z = 1.61, p =.054).

Meanwhile, the beta weights for distancing coping scores in all country samples were significant and positive (the United States: β =.41, $p<.001$; Australia: β =.39, $p<.001$; China: β =.46, $p<.001$). The beta-weight difference in distancing coping between the Australian and Chinese samples was significant (z = 2.05, $p<.05$), but the differences between the United States and Australian (z = 0.55, p =.29) and the United States and Chinese (z = 1.49, p =.068) samples were not. Moreover, the beta weights for distancing coping scores in both women and men were significant and positive (women: β =.39, $p<.001$; men: β =.45, $p<.001$). No significant gender difference in the beta-weight was found (z = 0.84, p =.20).

The beta weights for constructive coping scores in both the United States and Australian samples were significant and positive (United States: β =.13, $p<.01$; Australia: β =.15, $p<.001$; China: β =.04, p =.43); however, these beta values were small. The beta-weight difference in constructive coping between the Australian and Chinese samples was significant (z = 1.91, $p<.05$), but the differences between the United States and Australian (z = 0.44, p =.33) and the United States and Chinese (z = 1.48, p =.07) samples were not. In addition, the beta weight for constructive coping scores was significant and positive in men (β =.17, $p<.001$), but not in women (β =.07, p =.08). No significant gender difference in the beta-weight was shown (z = 1.62, p =.053).

Discussion

The hypothesis that reassessing coping with interpersonal stressors is associated with lower levels of depressive symptoms was tested for each sample in the United States, Australia, and China via a cross-sectional Web-based survey. The SEM analysis revealed that significant proportions of the variance in depressive symptom scores were accounted for by participants' scores on all three coping strategies for interpersonal stress in every sample. The effect sizes were medium or large; according to Cohen [38], small, medium, and large effect sizes correspond to f^2 values of.02,.15, and.35, respectively. In all samples, the beta values for reassessing coping were significant and negative, indicating that our hypothesis was supported. Until now, the effects of reassessing coping on psychological distress have been demonstrated only with specific samples in Japan [8,10,11]. However, our result showed

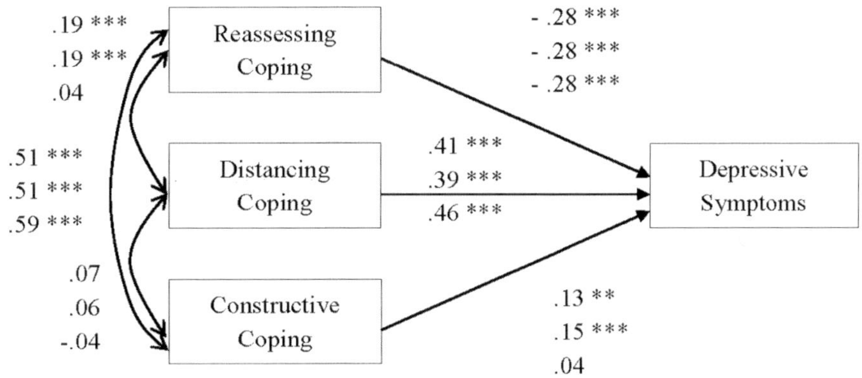

Figure 1. Path coefficients (β: Standardized partial regression coefficients) in structural equation modeling. The upper, center, and lower values are the beta weights in the United States, Australian, and Chinese samples, respectively. Three asterisks (***) and two asterisks (**) are $p<.001$ and $p<.01$, respectively.

that reassessing coping is associated with reduced depressive symptoms also in three populations with different sociocultural values (e.g., collectivistic vs. individualistic). These findings have potential implications for many individuals dealing with interpersonal stressors_the most frequently encountered stressors in daily life that strongly influence levels of depressive symptoms [39]. Consequently, when learning how to cope with interpersonal stressors, reassessing coping may be crucial to reduce their negative effects on depressive symptoms.

On the other hand, distancing coping was significantly associated with a higher level of depressive symptoms in each country. This result was consistent with previous studies in Japanese samples [8,10,11] and our hypothesis. In addition, the beta values for this strategy were relatively high (β =.41,.39, and.46) in all of the countries we surveyed. Distancing coping may be a maladaptive strategy in a number of countries. If so, stress management that reduces the use of distancing coping may help in attenuating psychological distress, including depressive symptoms.

Constructive coping was significantly associated with a higher level of depressive symptoms in the United States and Australian samples, but no significant association was found in the Chinese sample. Although our beta values in the United States and Australian samples were small, our findings in these samples were consisted with previous studies in Western cultures [24] that examined relationships between coping strategies similar to constructive coping and psychological distress. The result in the Chinese sample was consistent with those in Japanese samples [8,10,11], in which positive but non –significant correlations between constructive coping and depressive symptoms. The effects of constructive coping on depressive symptoms as well as the frequency of use may differ between cultures. However, previous research as well as the current study have not presented the rationale and its evidence for the effects of constructive coping on depressive symptoms or psychological distress; future research should uncover the mechanisms for the effects of constructive coping before any cultural and gender differences are discussed.

Our findings on cross-cultural differences in reassessing and constructive coping indicated that individuals in China scored highest on this approach toward coping with interpersonal stressors, followed by those in the United States and in Australia. These results were consistent with our hypothesis. Therefore, reassessing and constructive coping may be associated with characteristics of collectivistic cultures. These cross-cultural differences in coping strategies for interpersonal stress may be elaborated through further research on understanding cultural differences and counseling research on interpersonal relationships.

Our hypothesis on gender difference in constructive and distancing coping, that women would employ constructive coping more frequently than men, was supported. Others [4,30] have interpreted gender differences in depression and depressive symptoms by differences in how women and men those in respond to interpersonal stressors. Our findings and future research may contribute to advance research on gender differences in depression.

Several limitations to the present study need to be mentioned. Our findings, obtained through a cross-sectional Web-based survey, need to be interpreted with some caution because this method may produce issues associated with Web-administered surveys as well as limitations with regard to conclusions. Several researchers have asserted a number of methodological issues related to Internet studies [for a review, 40]. However, Gosling et al. [40] suggested that many of these were preconceptions, after comparing a large Internet sample ($N = 361{,}703$) with a set of 510 published, traditional samples. For example, Internet samples were more diverse than traditional samples with respect to socioeconomic status and geographic location. Furthermore, there was little support for the belief that Internet users were unusually maladjusted; instead, there was evidence that Internet-based findings were not adversely affected by non-serious respondents and were consistent with those drawn from traditional methods of research. Therefore, our data collected through a Web-based survey were useful in understanding reassessing coping with interpersonal stress, although some caution may need to be exercised in the interpretation of the present findings.

Next, our data were gathered through self-reported measures via a cross-sectional design, although a previous study on reassessing coping by Kato [8] employed a longitudinal approach. Causality between coping strategies and depressive symptoms cannot be established from our findings on their associations. According to the transactional theory proposed by Lazarus and colleagues [6,7], coping behavior affects psychological functioning, including depressive symptoms. This theory's validity and utility have been supported by numerous studies [6]. Therefore, in the current study, coping strategies might be causal factors, and depressive symptoms, their probable outcomes. Nevertheless, attention should be directed toward interpretations of a causal relationship between coping behavior and depressive symptoms, even with longitudinal data obtained through further research on the topic.

Table 3. Structural equation modeling analyses predicting depressive symptoms scores from scores of each coping strategy.

Predictor							95% CL	
	R^2	B	SE B	β	t		LL	UL
United States	.19	***	$N = 500$					
Reassessing coping		− 1.10	0.18	−.28	−5.94	***	−1.46	−0.73
Distancing coping		1.29	0.13	.41	10.05	***	1.04	1.55
Constructive coping		0.46	0.16	.13	2.77	**	0.13	0.78
Australia	.18	***	$N = 500$					
Reassessing coping		−1.01	0.18	−.28	−5.73	***	−1.36	−0.67
Distancing coping		1.19	0.13	.39	9.46	***	0.95	1.44
Constructive coping		0.56	0.17	.15	3.28	***	0.22	0.90
China	.26	***	$N = 500$					
Reassessing coping		−0.99	0.17	−.28	−5.74	***	−1.33	−0.65
Distancing coping		1.57	0.13	.46	11.84	***	1.31	1.83
Constructive coping		0.12	0.15	.04	0.78		−0.18	0.43
Women	.17	***	$N = 752$					
Reassessing coping		−0.87	0.16	−.23	−5.57	***	−1.17	−0.56
Distancing coping		1.26	0.11	.39	11.62	***	1.05	1.48
Constructive coping		0.25	0.14	.07	1.77		−0.03	0.53
Men	.24	***	$N = 748$					
Reassessing coping		−1.20	0.13	−.35	−8.98	***	−1.46	−0.93
Distancing coping		1.39	0.10	.45	13.83	***	1.19	1.58
Constructive coping		0.56	0.13	.17	4.49	***	0.31	0.81

The all samples composed
*** $p < .001$, ** $p < .01$.

In the current study, we did not define or measure the type of interpersonal relationship (e.g., significant other, acquaintance, and professional relationship) where participants encountered interpersonal stressors. The effects of reassessing coping on depressive symptoms may depend on the degree of closeness between people in a relationship. These issues should be taken into consideration when interpreting our findings.

Despite these limitations, our hypothesis that reassessing coping is negatively associated with depressive symptoms was supported by a Web-based survey of representative in the United States, Australia, and China. We also observed that distancing coping was associated with a high level of depressive symptoms in all countries. In addition to these findings, our data indicated the existence of cross-cultural differences in coping strategies for interpersonal stress. The findings of our study may enable individuals to better deal with distressing interpersonal relationships that they may be experiencing in their daily lives.

Author Contributions

Conceived and designed the experiments: TK. Performed the experiments: TK. Analyzed the data: TK. Contributed reagents/materials/analysis tools: TK. Wrote the paper: TK.

References

1. Hames JL, Hagan CR, Joiner TE (2013) Interpersonal processes in depression. Annu Rev Clin Psychol 9: 355−377.
2. Hammen C (2009) Adolescent depression: stressful interpersonal contexts and risk for recurrence. Curr Dir Psychol Sci 18: 200−204.
3. Joiner TE, Coyne JC, editors (1999) The interactional nature of depression: advances in interpersonal approaches. Washington, DC: American Psychological Association.
4. Rudolph KD (2009) The interpersonal context of adolescent depression. In: Nolen-Hoeksema S, Hilt L, editors. Handbook of depression in adolescence. NY: Routledge. pp. 377−418.
5. World Health Organization (2001) The World health report 2001: mental health: new understanding, new hope. Switzerland: World Health Organization.
6. Lazarus RS (1999) Stress and emotion: A new synthesis. New York: Springer.
7. Lazarus RS, Folkman S (1984) Stress, appraisal, and coping. New York: Springer.
8. Kato T (2013) Assessing coping with interpersonal stress: development and validation of the Interpersonal Stress Coping Scale in Japan. Int Perspect Psychol 2: 100−115.
9. Folkman S, Lazarus RS (1988) Manual for the ways of coping questionnaire. Palo Alto, CA: Consulting Psychologists Press.
10. Kato T (2014) Coping with workplace interpersonal stress among Japanese employees. Stress Health, first published online, March 18. doi: 10.1002/smi.2566
11. Kato T (2014) Coping with interpersonal stress and psychological distress at work: comparison of hospital nursing staff and salespeople. Psychol Res Behav Manage 7: 31−36.
12. Thomas KW (1976) Conflict and conflict management. In: Dunnette MD, editor. Handbook of industrial and organizational psychology. Chicago, IL: Rand McNally College Publishing Company. pp. 889−938. London: Psychological Press.
13. van de Vliert E (1997) Complex interpersonal conflict behaviour: theoretical frontiers.
14. Linehan M (1993) Skills training manual for treating borderline personality disorder. New York: Guilford.
15. Kabat-Zinn J (1990) Full catastrophe living: using the wisdom of your body and mind to face stress, pain and illness. New York: Delacorte.
16. Segal ZV, Williams JM, Teasdale JD (2002) Mindfulness-based cognitive therapy for depression: a new approach to preventing relapse. New York: Guilford.
17. Wells A (2005) Detached mindfulness in cognitive therapy: a metacognitive analysis and ten techniques. J Ration-Emot Cognit-Behav Ther 23: 337−355.
18. Teasdale JD, Moore RG, Hayhurst H, Pope M, Williams S et al (2002) Metacognitive awareness and prevention of relapse in depression: empirical evidence. J Consult Clin Psychol 70: 275−287.
19. Keng S, Smoski MJ, Robins CJ (2011) Effects of mindfulness on psychological health: a review of empirical studies. Clin Psychol Rev 31: 1041−1056.
20. Penley JA, Tomaka J, Wiebe JS (2002) The association of coping to physical and psychological health outcomes: a meta-analytic review. J Behav Med 25: 551−603.
21. Viswesvaran C, Sanchez JI, Fisher J (1999) The role of social support in the process of work stress: a metaanalysis. J Vocat Behav 54: 314−334.
22. Kramer BJ (1993) Expanding the conceptualization of caregiver coping: the importance of relationship focused coping strategies. Fam Relat 42: 383−391.
23. Kayser K, Sormanti M, Strainchamps E (1999) Women coping with cancer: the influence of relationship factors on psychological adjustment. Psychol Women Q 23: 725−739.
24. Seiffge-Krenke I (2006) Coping with relationship stressors: the impact of different working models of attachment and links to adaptation. J Youth Adolesc 35: 25−39.
25. Wong PTP, Wong LCJ, editors (2006) Handbook of multicultural perspectives on stress and coping. New York: Springer.
26. Triandis HC (1995) Individualism and collectivism. Boulder, CO: Westview Press.
27. Oyserman D, Coon HM, Kemmelmeier M (2002) Rethinking individualism and collectivism: evaluation of theoretical assumptions and meta-analyses. Psychol Bull 128: 3−72.
28. Tamres LK, Janicki D, Helgeson VS (2002) Sex differences in coping behavior: a meta-analytic review and an examination of relative coping. Pers Soc Psychol Rev 6: 2−30.
29. Shih JH, Eberhart NK (2010) Gender differences in the associations between interpersonal behaviors and stress generation. J Soc Clin Psychol 29: 243−255.
30. Rudolph KD (2002) Gender differences in emotional responses to interpersonal stress during adolescence. J Adolesc Health 30: 3−13.
31. Radloff LS (1977) The CES-D Scale: a self-report depression scale for research in the general population. Appl Psychol Meas 1: 385−401.
32. McCallum J, Mackinnon A, Simons L, Simons J (1995) Measurement properties of the Center for Epidemiological Studies Depression Scale: an Australian community study of aged persons. J Gerontol: Soc Sci 50B: S182−S189.
33. Zhang B, Fokkema M, Cuijpers P, Juan L, Smits N et al (2011) Measurement invariance of the Center for Epidemiological Studies Depression scale (CES-D) among Chinese and Dutch elderly. BMC Med Res Meth 11: 74−83.
34. Raju NS, Laffitte LJ, Byrne BM (2002) Measurement equivalence: a comparison of methods based on confirmatory factor analysis and item response theory. J Appl Psychol 87: 517−529.
35. Hu L, Bentler PM (1999) Cutoff criteria for fit indexes in covariance structure analysis: conventional criteria versus new alternatives. Struct Equ Modeling 6: 1−55.
36. Cheung GW, Rensvold RB (2002) Evaluating goodness-of-fit indexes for testing measurement invariance. Struct Equ Modeling 9: 233−255.
37. Arbuckle JL (2013) Amos 16.0 [Computer software]. Spring House, PA: Amos Development Corporation.
38. Cohen J (1988) Statistical power analysis for the behavioral sciences (2nd ed.). Hillsdale, NJ: Erlbaum.
39. Maybery DJ, Graham D (2001) Hassles and uplifts: including interpersonal events. Stress Health 17: 91−104.
40. Gosling SD, Vazire S, Srivastava S, John OP (2004) Should we trust Web-based studies? a comparative analysis of six preconceptions about Internet questionnaires. Am Psychol 59: 93−104.

6

Estimating the Inbreeding Depression on Cognitive Behavior: A Population Based Study of Child Cohort

Mohd Fareed*, Mohammad Afzal*

Human Genetics and Toxicology Laboratory, Section of Genetics, Department of Zoology, Faculty of Life Sciences, Aligarh Muslim University, Aligarh, Uttar Pradesh, India

Abstract

Background: Cognitive ability tests are widely assumed to measure maximal intellectual performance and predictive associations between intelligence quotient (IQ) scores and later mental health problems. Very few epidemiologic studies have been done to demonstrate the relationship between familial inbreeding and modest cognitive impairments in children.

Objective: We aimed to estimate the effect of inbreeding on children's cognitive behavior in comparison with non-inbred children.

Methodology: A cohort of 408 children (6 to 15 years of age) was selected from inbred and non-inbred families of five Muslim populations of Jammu region. The Wechsler Intelligence Scales for Children (WISC) was used to measure the verbal IQ (VIQ), performance IQ (PIQ) and full scale IQ (FSIQ). Family pedigrees were drawn to access the family history and children's inbred status in terms of coefficient of inbreeding (F).

Results: We found significant decline in child cognitive abilities due to inbreeding and high frequency of mental retardation among offspring from inbred families. The mean differences (95% C.I.) were reported for the VIQ, being −22.00 (−24.82, −19.17), PIQ −26.92 (−29.96, −23.87) and FSIQ −24.47 (−27.35, −21.59) for inbred as compared to non-inbred children ($p>0.001$). The higher risk of being mentally retarded was found to be more obvious among inbred categories corresponding to the degree of inbreeding and the same accounts least for non-inbred children ($p<0.0001$). We observed an increase in the difference in mean values for VIQ, PIQ and FSIQ with the increase of inbreeding coefficient and these were found to be statistically significant ($p<0.05$). The regression analysis showed a fitness decline (depression) for VIQ ($R^2=0.436$), PIQ ($R^2=0.468$) and FSIQ ($R^2=0.464$) with increasing inbreeding coefficients ($p<0.01$).

Conclusions: Our comprehensive assessment provides the evidence for inbreeding depression on cognitive abilities among children.

Editor: Hemachandra Reddy, Oregon Health & Science University, United States of America

Funding: The authors have no support or funding to report.

Competing Interests: The authors have declared that no competing interests exist.

* Email: mohdfareedk@gmail.com (MF); afzal1235@rediffmail.com (MA)

Introduction

The evolution of human brain and cognitive function is driven by different networking or feedback processes underlying genetic and environmental system. Cognitive behavior being an important part of neuroscience that has emerged from quantitative genetic research with intriguing findings and immense implications. Several genetic and epidemiological studies worldwide have documented the risk factors associated with child's mental health. Cognitive impairments among children, being very much common in developing countries, pose a great challenge in context of medical and public health. Early-onset of cognitive impairment, also known as intellectual disability (ID), commonly referred to as mental retardation (with an IQ below 70), is characterized by significant limitations both in intellectual functioning and the adaptive behavior of the child, which originates before the age of 18 years [1].

A recent study has documented nation-wide cognitive abilities being significantly and substantially correlated with a wide range of phenomena such as educational, economic, political, demographic, sociological, epidemiological, geographic and climatic variables [2]. Although gender based differences in cognitive abilities have been frequently reported and correlated with many factors, there is substantial social and cultural variability in gender equality which is known to be one of the strongest predictor of sex-typed cognitive abilities [3]. Several studies have reported the socio-demographic characteristics such as socioeconomic status (SES), literacy and educational attainment associated with cognitive abilities [4–7]. Moreover, quantitative genetic research has revealed surprising findings as most of the environmental measures in social and behavioral sciences show significant and substantial genetic influence [8–11].

Quantitative genetic research consistently shows substantial genetic influence on individual cognitive differences in spatial, memory and verbal abilities [12,13]. The variation in normal human cognition is related to many factors and the sum total of all genetic effects is not likely to be greater than 50% for many types of cognition [14]. Moreover, genes and gene-environment interactions provide substantial pathways for parsing cognitive processes. The two key genetic conceptsS pleiotropy (in which one gene affects many traits) and polygenicity (in which many genes affect a trait) suggest that there is genetic input into the brain structure and function which is general, not modular [15]. With the sequencing of the human genome, it has become possible to identify widespread sequence variations with subsequent heritable risks for common diseases or traits [16]. Approximately, more than 20,000 genes can be considered to play a role in the nurture, plasticity and maintenance of the central nervous system (CNS), although many of these will also play roles in other organ systems as well [17]. The expedition for gene defects underlying cognitive impairment or ID has been much focused on the X-chromosome since the late 19th century, which has ended with molecular elucidation of the fragile X syndrome, the most common form of X-linked ID [18]. Recently, the X-linked recessive gene defects have been revealed to account for about 10 to 12% of the ID seen among the males [19], probably lesser than the erstwhile conjecture [20]. This leaves substantial room for autosomal impact over cognitive impairment, arising either from recessive or dominant gene defects. Still, compared with X-linked ID (XLID), the molecular elucidation of the autosomal recessive ID (ARID) has lagged far behind, which provide ample scope for rather different homozygosity studies.

Inbreeding (consanguineous marriages among humans) produces homozygous offspring, since the mating of pairs occurs between genetically closely related individuals. The phenomenon of inbreeding or endogamy, increases the level of homozygotes for autosomal recessive genetic disorders and generally leads to decreased fitness of a population known as inbreeding depression which provides a major focus in clinical studies [21]. The inbreeding depression that results from such consanguineous mating is mostly a consequence of additive effect of recessive alleles in the homozygous condition [22]. Parental consanguinity has been associated with increased risk of adverse prenatal outcomes including stillbirths, low birth weight, preterm delivery, abortion, infant and child mortality, congenital birth defects, cognitive impairments, malformations and many other complex disorders [12–32]. A study has revealed that the overall incidence of congenital malformations was 2.5 times higher amongst the children of inbred families when compared to that of non-inbred families [33]. Consanguinity has been associated with significant decline in mean values for height, weight and body mass index (BMI) and the subsequent depression on children growth, much influenced in proportion to their inbreeding coefficients with least variation for non-genetic factors [21]. Inbreeding is also thought to predispose offspring to neuropsychological disorders such as hereditary Parkinsonism [34]. Several studies have identified parental consanguinity as an important risk factor for mental retardation or ID [26,27,35], and it has been shown that inbreeding is correlated with reduced cognitive performance [36].

The determination of major medical conditions in early childhood due to consanguinity is an important component of clinical genetic studies. The populations of India and other South Asian countries, which have many Muslim communities, offer great opportunities for studying the influence of socio-cultural and genetic variability on consanguinity and child health. North Indian populations and those from Jammu and Kashmir (J&K) have historical, linguistic, cultural, and socio-religious significance for the Indian subcontinent [37]. The incidence of consanguineous marriages ranges from 35% to 50% among the populations under study. One of our recent studies taken among the same populations showed higher frequency of homozygosity for Rhesus protein genes than that found elsewhere in the Indian subcontinent [38]. The present study, done for the first time in Jammu region, can amount to making a preliminary effort toward realization of genetic hazards due to inbreeding. Such a study is of great help for genetic counseling and the basics of genetic epidemiology in the region. The aim of the present study was to explore the effect of inbreeding among children from northernmost part of Indian subcontinent for cognitive abilities (IQ) in comparison with non-genetic factors. Analysis of pedigree was done to estimate the coefficient of inbreeding (F), followed by the observation of cognitive impairment trends among children from Muslim populations of inbred and non-inbred families.

Methods

Ethics Statement

The study was approved by the Institutional Ethics Committee of Jawaharlal Nehru Medical College (JNMC), Aligarh Muslim University, India. We obtained informed written consent from the parents, caretakers, or guardians on behalf of minors/children participants involved in our study.

Population and Study design

The Muslim populations were selected in our survey from Rajouri and Poonch Districts of J&K for two reasons: firstly, consanguineous marriages are favored among Muslim families, while the Hindu and Sikh religions avoid marriages among close relatives; secondly nearly 70% of the total population is Muslim in the region surveyed. In order to select the subjects for their IQ studies, preliminary visits to the areas were made and it was found that more than 75% (approx.) population lives in villages, which is mainly due to topographical feature of the area (hilly region), which thus makes it less urbanized. We also observed the culture and beliefs related with marriages among different populations. The castes and tribes were very rigid, favoring marriages among close relatives or those within the caste, which in turn also increases the rate of inbreeding.

The study was conducted during April 2013 through July 2013 and a total of 408 children (6 to 15 years of age) were selected randomly on *a priori* basis from five Muslim populations viz., Gujjar and Bakarwal (n = 97), Mughal (n = 72), Malik (n = 86), Syed (n = 65) and Khan (n = 88). The age group of the children selected was 6 to 15 years. Children from non-consanguineous marriages (either belonging to the same family or from other families of the same population) served as control. Only the first two parity-order children were taken. Those having prolonged illness or suffering from congenital defects were excluded. Children with no schooling were also excluded. Figure 1 depicts the steps involved in the recruitment process. The details of sample size and variables under study are presented in Table 1.

Parental background

The parental background characteristics were assessed in two dimensions: the residence (rural or urban) and the socioeconomic status (SES; low, medium and high). The indigenous adapted Kuppuswamy's socioeconomic status scale [39] was used in this study (Table 2). The parental SES was based on three domains: education, occupation and household income. SES was assessed for both the parents (i.e., mother and father) and mean scores on

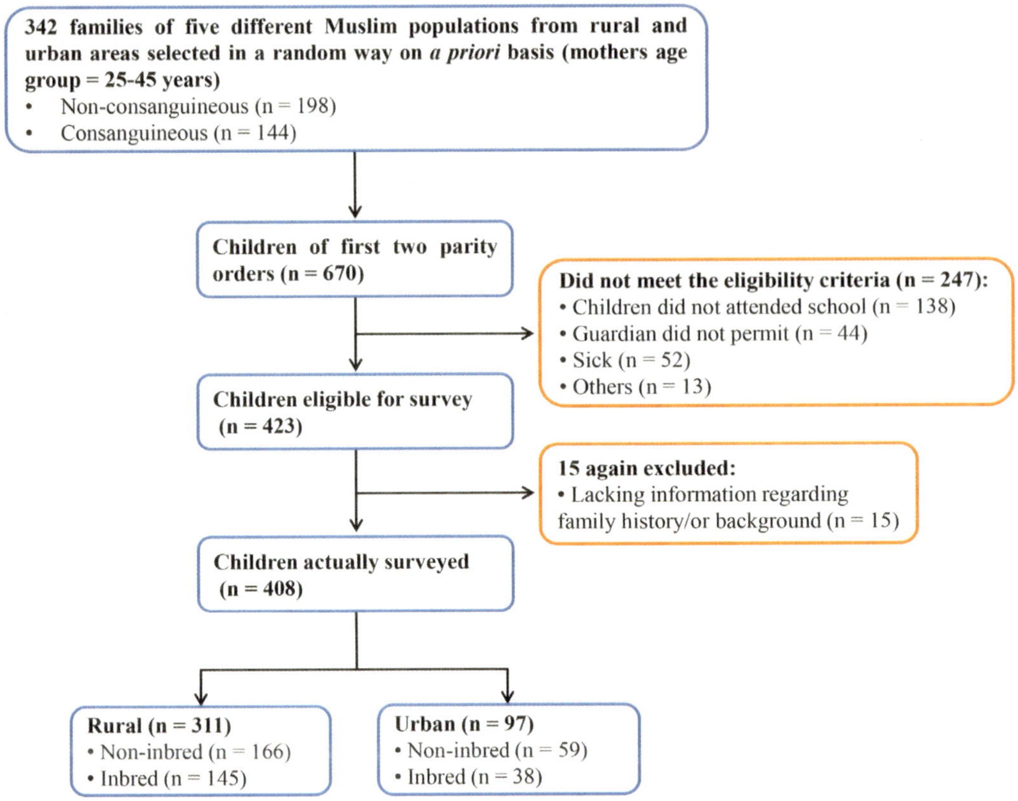

Figure 1. Study design. Flowchart depicting the steps involved in the recruitment process.

the whole were taken for complete parental SES. On the basis of scores, we categorised SES into three classes: 26–29 as high, 11–25 as medium and <10 as low. All the information was recorded in a standardised questionnaire.

Pedigree analysis

Genealogical information (family pedigrees) up to five generations back (volunteered by the parents) helped in ascertaining the consanguinity persuasion of their marriage and thus, child's inbreeding status was determined. The information provided by the parents was cross checked by seeking help from the elder members of the family. In case of ambiguity such data were omitted.

Wright's path relationship method for calculating the coefficient of inbreeding (F) was used for all mating types following the order: double first cousin ($F = 0.125$) > first cousin ($F = 0.0625$) > first cousin once removed ($F = 0.03125$) > second cousin ($F = 0.0156$). In non-consanguineous families or for the distant marriages, the coefficient of inbreeding was effectively zero ($F = 0.000$) [21].

Measures

The Wechsler's Intelligence Scales exists in two forms, Wechsler's Adult Intelligence Scale (WAIS) and Wechsler's Intelligence Scales for Children (WISC). For determining the IQ of children below 16 years, the WISC test system is used. We used Indian adapted WISC-III (3rd edition), which is made up of a battery of ten subtests consisting of five verbal and five performance tests as follows:

Verbal IQ tests

(a) *Information:* General knowledge based questions.

(b) *Comprehension:* Questions based on social situations or common concepts.

(c) *Arithmetic:* Orally administered arithmetic questions.

(d) *Vocabulary:* Examinee was asked to define a provided word.

(e) *Digit span:* Children were orally given sequences of numbers and asked to repeat them, either as heard or in reverse order.

Performance IQ tests

(a) *Picture completion:* Children were shown artwork of common objects with a missing part, and asked to identify the missing part by pointing and/or naming.

(b) *Block design:* Children have to put together red and white blocks in a pattern according to the model displayed. This was timed, and some of the more difficult puzzles result into the award of bonus scores for speed.

(c) *Object assembly:* Children were provided with pieces of four different objects such as man, horse, auto and human face. For perfect performance, full scores as well as bonus is given. Imperfect performance like inverting or omitting pieces leads to negative marking.

(d) *Mazes:* Children were shown the samples and with the help of pencil a demonstration was given. The test was discontinued if two consecutive failures were found.

(e) *Coding:* Children under 8 years of age could mark rows of shapes with different lines according to a code, whereas children over eight transcribe a digit-symbol code. The task was time-limited, again with a bonus for speed.

Table 1. Details of sample size and selection of categories in the study.

Factors	Categories	Non-inbred	Inbred	Total (n)
Residence	Rural	166 (53.38%)	145 (46.62%)	311
	Urban	59 (60.82%)	38 (39.18%)	97
SES	High	52 (61.90%)	32 (38.10%)	84
	Medium	111 (54.15%)	94 (45.85%)	205
	Low	62 (52.11%)	57 (47.89%)	119
Population	Gujjar and Bakarwal	55 (56.70%)	42 (43.30%)	97
	Mughal	41 (56.94%)	31 (43.06%)	72
	Malik	47 (54.65%)	39 (45.35%)	86
	Syed	35 (53.85%)	30 (46.15%)	65
	Khan	47 (53.41%)	41 (46.59%)	88
Age (in years)	6	27 (56.25%)	21 (43.75%)	48
	7	21 (55.26%)	17 (44.74%)	38
	8	35 (57.38%)	26 (42.62%)	61
	9	10 (55.56%)	08 (44.44%)	18
	10	35 (58.33%)	25 (41.67%)	60
	11	14 (56.00%)	11 (44.00%)	25
	12	24 (46.15%)	28 (53.85%)	52
	13	11 (50.00%)	11 (50.00%)	22
	14	22 (68.75%)	10 (31.25%)	32
	15	26 (50.00%)	26 (50.00%)	52
Gender	Male	105 (55.85%)	83 (44.15%)	188
	Female	120 (54.55%)	100 (45.45%)	220
	Combined	225 (55.15%)	183 (44.85%)	408

Values presented as number and percentage (in parentheses) against different categories.
Total sample size 408, n = number of subjects.

Each of the above subtests consists of many items, each item carries a quantum of raw score (1, 2, 3, and so on) upon completion within a given fraction of time (in seconds). The sum total of these scores gives a raw subset score, which was then converted into IQ score by using WISC manual. The means of the subsets of the two categories (verbal and performance), gives VIQ and PIQ and the overall mean (of VIQ and PIQ) gives FSIQ. Table 3 presents the classification of the subjects on the basis of their FSIQs on WISC-III manual. The medium of the test was English as no Urdu or Hindi versions were available. So the verbal tests were translated into Urdu by the author, with slight alterations in their cultural reference wherever necessary. Such alterations were kept to a minimum (two occasions), one each in information and comprehension. Alterations in the performance subsets were not needed.

Procedure

The subjects were approached through their parents and their name, age, sex, class and school attended with parental consanguinity were entered in the record form. The children were asked questions from the questionnaire as per instructions given in the manual and their answers were then recorded on the schedule. Each child performed the test individually in a quiet room at their home, which lasted for about one hour depending

Table 2. Characteristics of socioeconomic status (SES) scale used in the study.

Education	Score	Occupation	Score	Income	Score
Profession or honours	07	Profession	10	≥30375	12
Graduate or post graduate	06	Semi-profession	06	15188–30374	10
Intermediate or post high school	05	Clerical, shop-owner, farmer	05	11362–15187	06
High school certificate	04	Skilled worker	04	7594–11361	04
Middle school certificate	03	Semi-skilled worker	03	4556–7593	03
Primary school certificate	02	Unskilled worker	02	1521–4555	02
Illiterate	01	Unemployed	01	≤1520	01

Table 3. Classification of intelligence based on WISC-III scores.

IQ score	Classification
130 and above	Very Superior
120–129	Superior
110–119	High Average
90–109	Average
80–89	Low Average
70–79	Borderline
55–69	Mild Mental Retardation
40–54	Moderate Mental Retardation

upon the intelligence and/or cooperation from the candidate. The VIQ and PIQ subtests were performed in a sequence as per guidelines. Timing was noted with a stop-watch. While giving the tests, full rapport was established with the child and every effort was made to engage his attention. Unnecessary interference by parents or by brothers/sisters and others in the household was avoided. Some encouraging words were also used and appreciating gestures were made to keep the enthusiasm of the child. Those who ran away after sitting for a while were approached later, while those who began to cry or kept mum were omitted. The scoring was done immediately after the test. The raw scores thus collected, were later converted into scaled scores with the help of the WISC-III manual.

Statistical analysis

Statistical analysis was conducted using SPSS software 17.0 version (SPSS, Chicago, IL, USA) and GraphPad InStat 3.0 (USA). Data are presented as mean±SD and mean±SE for comparing the results using different variables (residence, SES, age, gender and inbreeding). For FSIQ categories (scores range: ≥ 130 to 40–54), chi-square (χ^2) test was used to determine the significant differences. The differences in mean values among inbred categories from the non-inbred (as controlled) children for VIQ, PIQ and FSIQ (95% Confidence Interval) were analyzed using post-hoc tests (Bonferroni and Tukey HSD) and p-value $<$ 0.05 was considered for the level of significance. ANOVA-test for four factor analysis on VIQ, PIQ and FSIQ was used and p-values were compared for significant results. Regression analysis was done to estimate inbreeding depression on VIQ, PIQ and FSIQ and 'R^2' values were observed at $p<0.01$. The inbreeding depression on cognitive abilities (VIQ, PIQ and FSIQ) was calculated using average coefficient of inbreeding (α) and percentage of depression in trait for 'α' [21,27,40] as follows:

$$\text{Average coefficient of inbreeding } (\alpha) = \frac{n\times 0.125 + n\times 0.0625 + n\times 0.03125 + n\times 0.0156 + \ldots(n\times 0.000)}{N}\times 100 \quad (1)$$

$$\%\text{ Mean depression in trait for } '\alpha' = \frac{\overline{X}(\text{Non-inbred}) - \overline{X}(\text{Inbred})}{\overline{X}(\text{Non-inbred})}\times 100 \quad (2)$$

$$\%\text{ Depression in trait due to 1\% increase of } '\alpha' = \frac{\%\text{ Mean depression in trait for } '\alpha'}{\text{Average coefficient of inbreeding } (\alpha)}\times 1 \quad (3)$$

In the first equation, 'n' indicates number of individuals multiplied with inbreeding coefficients (F) for each of the inbreeding category. The F-value = 0.000 indicates simply non-inbred individuals while N is sum total of the individuals. The $\overline{X}$ in the second indicates the mean value of the trait.

Results

Descriptive characteristics of cognitive abilities with inbreeding

Figure 2 presents an overview of the normal distribution for cognitive abilities (VIQ, PIQ and FSIQ) among inbred and non-inbred children. The frequency polygon for inbred children showed a shift toward low cognitive abilities as compared to non-inbred group (i.e., increased frequency of mental illness among inbred as compared to non-inbred children). We found a significant difference for VIQ, PIQ and FSIQ between inbred and non-inbred children (at $p<0.0001$, using ANOVA). The mean difference (95% CI) in terms of VIQ −22.00 (−24.82, −19.17), PIQ −26.92 (−29.96, −23.87) and FSIQ −24.47 (−27.35, −21.59) for inbred children compared with non-inbred children were found to be statistically significant ($p<0.001$, using Tukey-Kramer Comparisons Test).

Figure 3 shows the range and distribution of IQ, assessing the cognitive ability differences among inbred and non-inbred children for different factors. The inbred subjects lie largely toward average to borderline IQ scores, not passing the ambit of superior IQs in case of all factors. The overall picture showed inbred subjects exhibit a cognitive shift toward low IQ, while non-inbred group presented the balanced distribution with a turn toward high cognitive abilities.

Cognitive differences among inbred and non-inbred children

Figure 4 presents the differences in cognitive abilities among inbred and non-inbred children across different factors. The inbred children showed significant decline in mean values as compared to non-inbred group for all the factors ($p<0.001$). Despite the fact, non-inbred subjects showed slight differences in their intelligence for residence (urban > rural) and SES (high > medium > low), yet their effect remained non-significant among inbred subjects, which indicate the cognitive ability being strongly suppressed as a result of inbreeding. Factors other than inbreeding, like population, age and sex showed inconsequential differences. This provides the indication of inbreeding depression (a genetic component) having much influence over cognitive parameters than other factors.

Factor analysis for cognitive abilities

Table 4 presents summary statistics based on ANOVA test for factor analysis. To investigate the strong cognitive predictor, we hypothesized two models (Model I and Model II). In both the models, age and inbreeding were taken as common and constitute a total of four factors, to predict the level of significance for each factor. In model I, inbreeding was found significant whereas population, sex and age presented non-significant association with VIQ, PIQ and FSIQ. In model II, again only inbreeding was

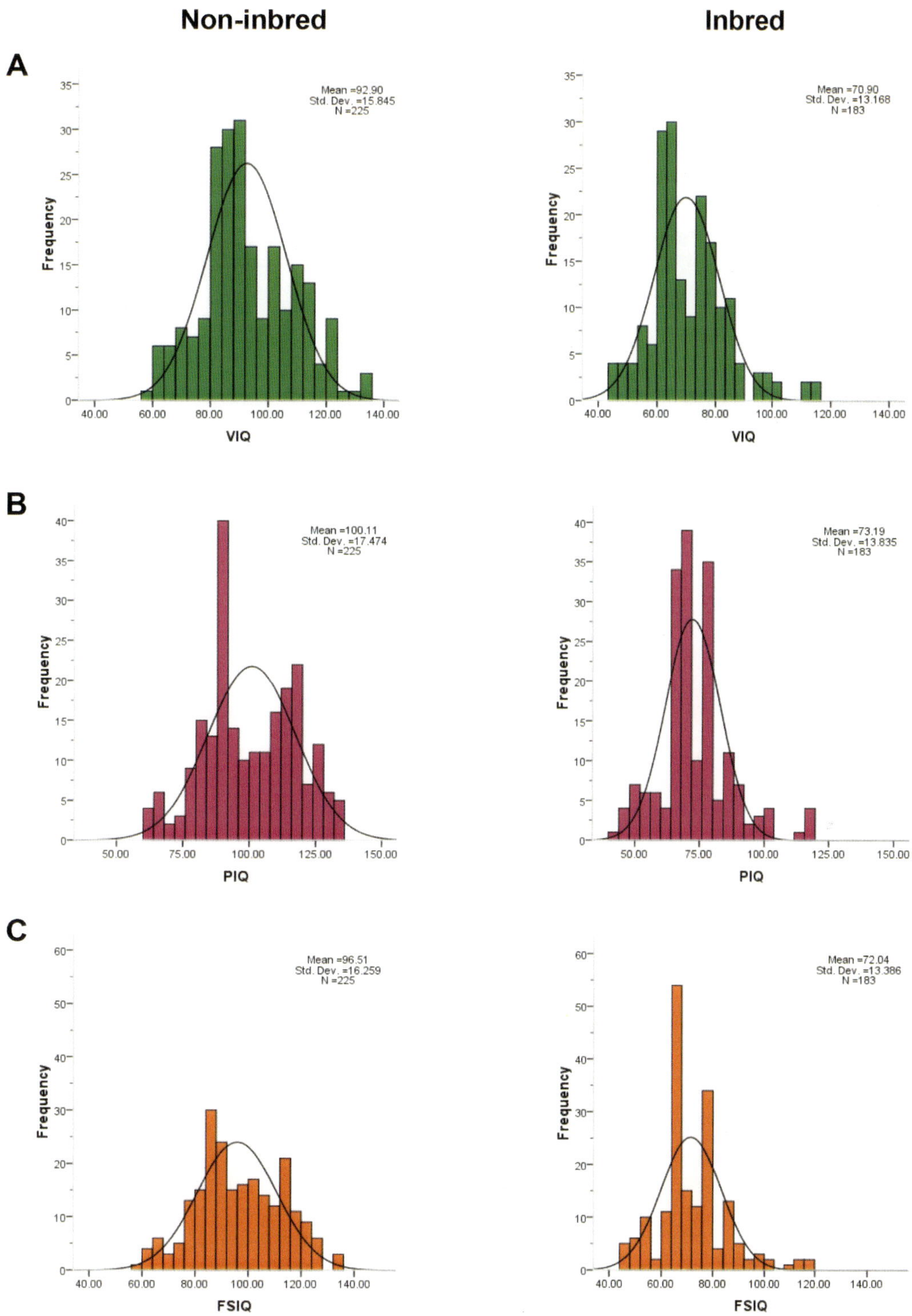

Figure 2. Normal distribution of cognitive abilities among inbred in comparison with non-inbred children. Differences in normal distributions of inbred in comparison with non-inbred children for VIQ, PIQ and FSIQ show highly significant results (at $p<0.0001$, using One-way Analysis of Variance). The mean difference (95% CI) for VIQ −22.00 (−24.82, −19.17), PIQ −26.92 (−29.96, −23.87) and FSIQ −24.47 (−27.35, −21.59) among inbred groups in comparison with non-inbred found to be statistically significant (at $p<0.001$, using Tukey-Kramer Comparisons Test). The non-inbred shows a regular pattern, whereas frequency distributions among inbred children represent a shift toward lower values and sparsity toward the high average or superior IQs.

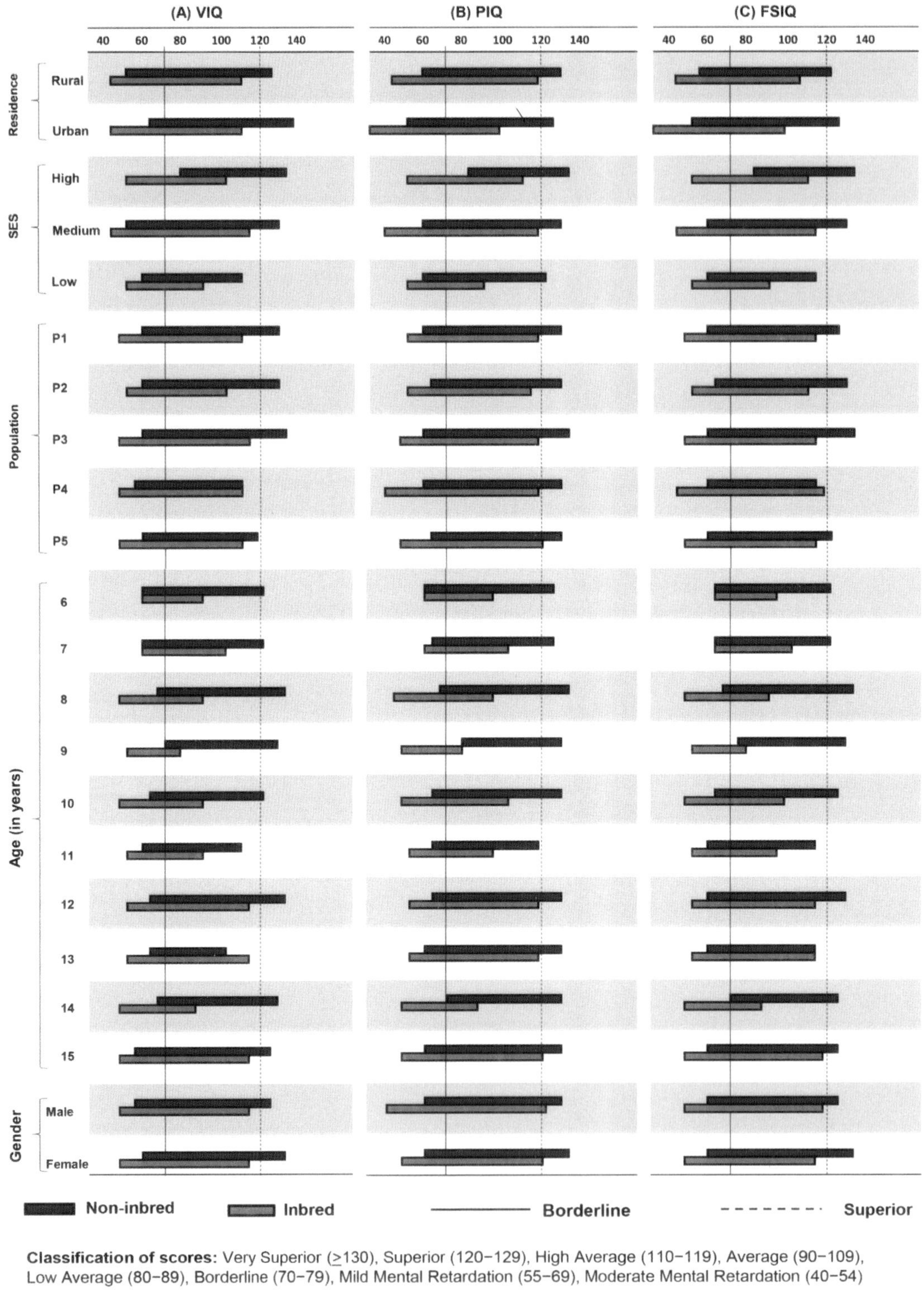

Figure 3. Range distribution of cognitive abilities for different factors. The IQ range has been established with minimum and maximum values observed for each category. Among all factors, inbred subjects exhibit a range shift toward low IQ, not crossing the superior IQ which is the indication of inbreeding load on the child's cognitive abilities to have elevated levels of mental illness. Factors, like residence, SES and population (except age and sex) show significant differences though overall effect yet remained incompetent in comparison with inbreeding. The populations presented as, P1 = Gujjar and Bakarwal, P2 = Mughal, P3 = Malik, P4 = Syed, P5 = Khan.

found as a prominent factor significantly associated with all cognitive tests whereas residence, SES and age were remained insignificant. These two models strongly support the cogent impact of inbreeding on cognitive abilities of children.

Inbreeding coefficient step-up and cognitive abilities

Table 5 presents the mean difference in cognitive abilities among inbred children as compared to control group (i.e., non-inbred children). With the increase of inbreeding coefficient (i.e.,

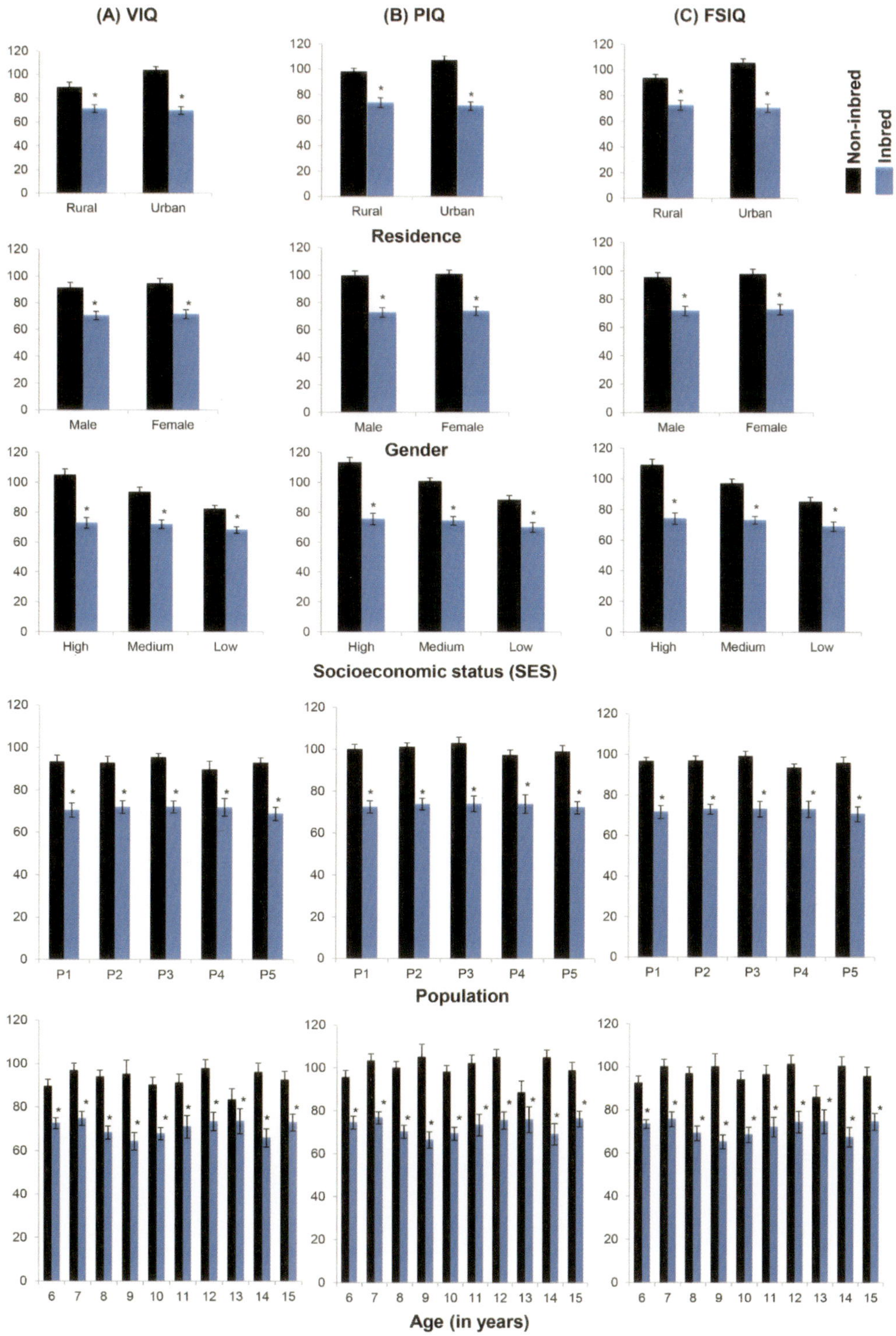

Figure 4. Cognitive abilities among inbred and non-inbred children. The results presented as mean±SEM. The significant decline in mean values observed for VIQ, PIQ and FSIQ among inbred children in comparison with non-inbred group. *The difference in mean values of inbred from non-inbred children for each factor is found to be statistically significant ($p<0.05$, using student's t-test). Populations presented as, P1 = Gujjar and Bakarwal, P2 = Mughal, P3 = Malik, P4 = Syed, P5 = Khan.

the inbred categories; $F=0.0156$ to 0.125), there was found a persuasive decline in mean values for cognitive parameters in comparison with non-inbred group ($F=0.00$). The mean difference in VIQ, PIQ and FSIQ showed a significant inflation with the increase of the degree of inbreeding ($p<0.05$, using post-hoc tests) and followed the order: double first cousin > first cousin > first cousin once removed > second cousin > non-inbred. This indicates the risk for cognitive impairments or ID was more common among the subjects having greater value of inbreeding coefficients.

Table 4. ANOVA results of four factor analysis based on mean values of verbal, performance and full scale IQ.

	Model I						Model II					
	Source	**df**	**ss**	**ms**	**F-value**	**p-value**	**Source**	**df**	**ss**	**ms**	**F-value**	**p-value**
VIQ												
	Population	04	546.08	136.52	0.0645	0.9917	Residence	01	1084.5	1084.5	0.9987	0.3316
	Gender	01	4.43	4.43	0.0021	0.7017	SES	02	3268.973	1634.4865	1.5052	0.2501
	Age	09	13325.65	1480.62	0.6998	0.9639	Age	09	8002.68	889.18	0.8188	0.6072
	Inbreeding	01	27954.30	27954.30	13.2126	0.0018***	Inbreeding	01	14721.29	14721.29	13.5575	0.0018***
	Within Groups	19	40198.71	2115.72			Within Groups	17	18459.34	1085.84		
PIQ												
	Population	04	350.81	87.70	0.02926	0.9982	Residence	01	191.9005	191.9005	0.1264	0.7266
	Gender	01	6.11	6.11	0.00203	0.8428	SES	02	4424.3895	2212.1947	1.4573	0.2605
	Age	09	14002.61	1555.84	0.51911	0.9645	Age	09	8671.4005	963.4889	0.6347	0.753
	Inbreeding	01	39858.22	39858.22	13.2988	0.0017***	Inbreeding	01	21173.8995	21173.8995	13.9491	0.0016***
	Within Groups	19	56945.08	2997.11			Within Groups	17	25804.901	1517.9353		
FSIQ												
	Population	04	464.86	116.21	0.04619	0.9956	Residence	01	546.69	546.69	0.42709	0.5222
	Gender	01	1.59	1.59	0.00063	0.8167	SES	02	3828.1561	1914.07805	1.4953	0.2522
	Age	09	12555.44	1395.05	0.5545	0.9802	Age	09	8091.6296	899.0699	0.70239	0.6991
	Inbreeding	01	33628.87	33628.87	13.3668	0.0017***	Inbreeding	01	17808.3793	17808.3793	13.9127	0.0017***
	Within Groups	19	47801.26	2515.85			Within Groups	17	21760.1104	1280.0065		

Model I = Population × Gender × Age × Inbreeding, Model II = Residence × SES × Age × Inbreeding.
df = degrees of freedom; ss = sum of squares; ms = means square; SES = socioeconomic status.
In Model I, the population, gender, and age based differences are found to be non-significant for all cognitive tests.
In Model II, the residence, SES and age are found to be insignificant.
Inbreeding is found to be significant for all cognitive parameters in both the models.
***Statistically significant at $p<0.001$.

The frequency distribution (in percentage) of children based on FSIQ scores for each category was examined (Figure 5). The line graph presents the significant difference ($p<0.0001$) in frequency distribution of FSIQs among inbred categories correlated with non-inbred group. For mental retardation (FSIQ = 55–69 or 40–54), the lowest frequency was observed in case of non-inbred children, whereas inbred children with higher inbreeding coefficients presented higher frequency of mental retardation. The line graph for inbred subjects gets flattened toward high FSIQ scores (i.e., high average, superior, and very superior), whereas it showed the high frequency peaks toward lower FSIQ scores (i.e., borderline and mental retardation).

Inbreeding depression on cognitive behavior

Besides the differences in percentage and mean values for VIQ, PIQ and FSIQ for different factors, we found relatively similar trend in regression model with increasing inbreeding coefficients (Figure 6). The regression slope shows a fitness decline with the increase of inbreeding coefficient. The observed linear decline in fitness for VIQ ($R^2 = 0.436$), PIQ ($R^2 = 0.468$) and FSIQ ($R^2 = 0.464$) were found to be statistically significant ($p<0.01$). Moreover, regression analysis showed Pearson correlation 'r' for VIQ, PIQ and FSIQ as −0.660, −0.684 and −0.681, respectively, all of which were statistically significant at $p<0.01$. The negative sign for r-value indicates the depression in cognitive tests with the increasing levels of inbreeding. The regression analysis strongly supports the evidence of inbreeding depression on child's verbal, performance and full intellectual skills.

Table 6 presents the summary statistics for average coefficient of inbreeding and percentage of inbreeding depression on cognitive parameters. The average coefficient of inbreeding was almost the same for all of the factors except SES. The average coefficient of inbreeding among the subjects followed the order: low > medium > high SES families. This suggests that children from higher SES tend to have low inbreeding ($\alpha = 1.93$), which is due to parental education and awareness for marriage choice, being not much confined to social norms, whereas lower SES depicts the children from higher inbreeding level ($\alpha = 3.06$), suggesting a lower awareness or lack of education as well as adherence to social beliefs among parents for marrying within families/castes. The percentage depression for all IQ values among children in case of high inbreeding coefficients provide greater risk of being mentally retarded (or ID).

Discussion

Parental consanguinity leads to inbreeding which often result into genetic drift, and hence may swiftly give rise to evolutionary consequence to pose the most immediate risk [41]. Inbreeding exposes the action of deleterious recessive alleles and reduces fitness in terms of loss of heterozygosity [22]. The increased homozygosity (due to inbreeding) implies lower genetic variation that may lead to the expression of recessive alleles, or loss of hybrid vigor, of essential genes for the traits and thus may lead to the cause of depression (fitness decline) among inbred populations [21]. The harmful effects of inbreeding were first documented and quantified in detail by Charles Darwin, who carried out experiments on 57 plant species that involved self-fertilization (inbreeding) and outcrossing between unrelated groups. Darwin's experiments supported his hypothesis that self-fertilization must be strongly disadvantageous for the progeny produced– it lowered vigor and fertility in most of his species studied [42]. Further, inbreeding experiments carried out in maize plant has exposed the cause of depression in growth and vigor among selfed generations [43]. Increased frequency of polydactyly has also been reported among inbred strains of guinea pigs [44]. The majority of studies done on human beings support the relationship between inbreeding and the increased risk for recessive and many other

Table 5. Mean differences in cognitive abilities among inbred categories in comparison with non-inbred.

Dependent Variable	F	Mean±SD	Mean Difference±SE (95% CI)
VIQ	0.00	92.89±15.84	
	0.0156	86.77±13.92	−6.12±2.58 (−0.97, 13.21)
	0.03125	78.87±6.20	−14.02±3.08* (5.56, 22.46)
	0.0625	67.66±7.57	−25.23±1.59* (20.85, 29.61)
	0.125	58.62±13.90	−34.27±2.79* (26.60, 41.94)
PIQ	0.00	100.11±17.47	
	0.0156	90.38±14.18	−9.72±2.82* (1.99, 17.46)
	0.03125	80.53±7.16	−19.57±3.36* (10.36, 28.78)
	0.0625	69.79±7.18	−30.31±1.74* (25.53, 35.08)
	0.125	60.43±16.34	−39.67±3.05* (31.31, 48.04)
FSIQ	0.00	96.51±16.25	
	0.0156	88.57±13.99	−7.93±2.64* (0.68, 15.18)
	0.03125	79.70±6.51	−16.80±3.15* (8.16, 25.44)
	0.0625	68.72±7.15	−27.78±1.63* (23.31, 32.25)
	0.125	59.52±14.99	−36.98±2.86* (29.14, 44.82)

Results for mean differences in verbal, performance and full scale IQ of inbred groups (F = 0.0156 to 0.125) from non-inbred (F = 0.000) obtained by using post-hoc tests (Bonferroni and Tukey HSD).
The values for mean difference show significant increase (indicating inbreeding depression) with the increase of the coefficient of inbreeding (F).
Negative sign represents the decrease in mean difference from control one (i.e., non-inbred).
F = Coefficient of inbreeding, CI = Confidence Interval (Lower bound, Upper bound), SE = standard error.
*Significantly different from control (i.e., non-inbred) at $p<0.05$.

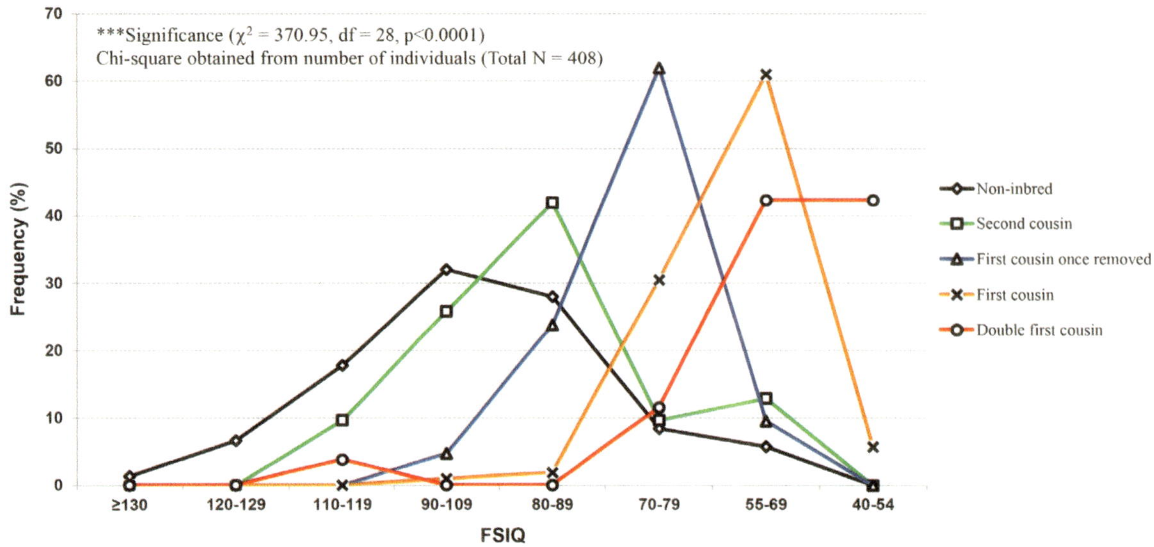

Figure 5. FSIQ comparisons in respect to the degree of inbreeding. The results depict the percentage frequency distribution of FSIQ in relation to coefficient of inbreeding. The non-inbred children display high frequency peaks on left side (presenting high FSIQ values) and downturn toward low FSIQ scores. On the other hand, elevated peaks are observed for low FSIQ scores (on right side) with the increase of inbreeding coefficient (F = 0.0156 to 0.125) and flattened toward high FSIQ scores, providing the evidence for inbreeding depression on children FSIQ.

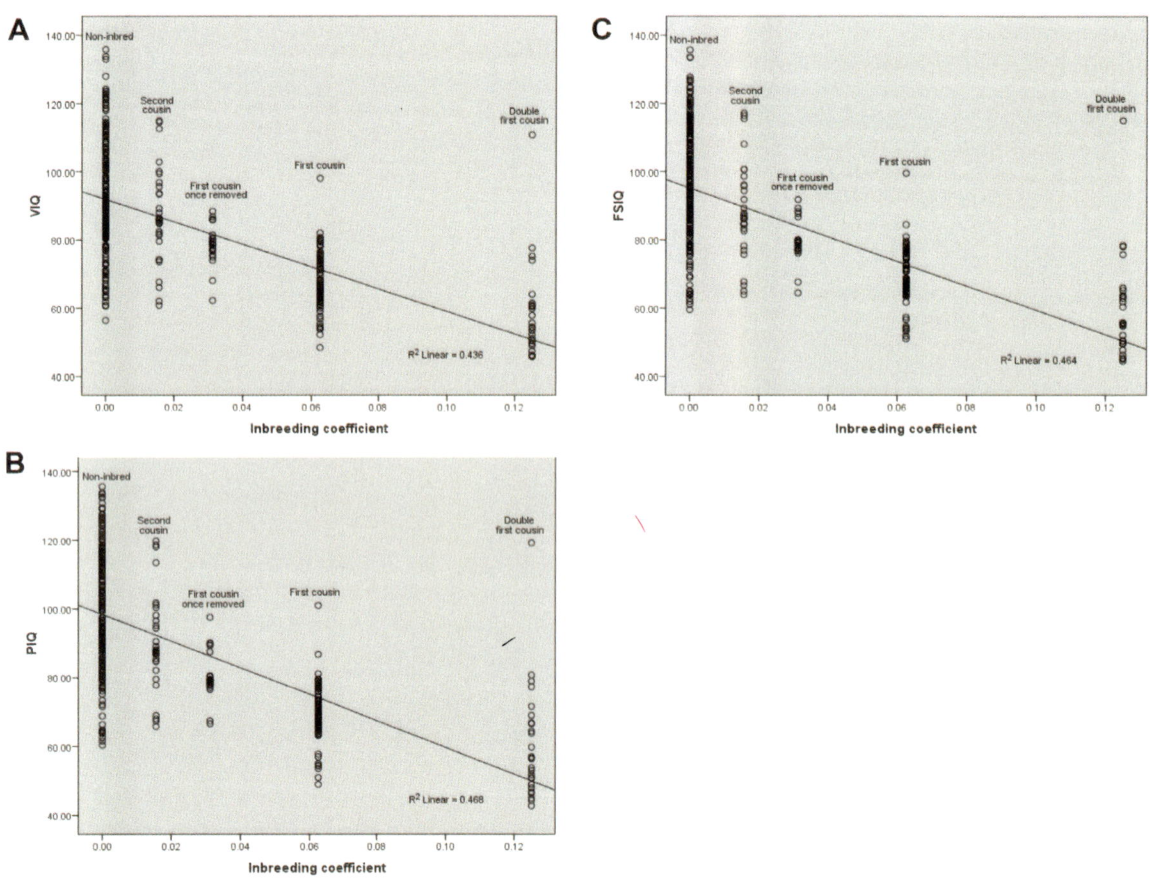

Figure 6. Inbreeding depression on cognitive abilities. The regression analysis presents almost similar trend for VIQ, PIQ and FSIQ. The slope depicts fitness decline (regression slope) with increase of inbreeding coefficient (F). The observed linear decline in fitness for cognitive parameters; (A) VIQ (R^2 = 0.436), (B) PIQ (R^2 = 0.468) and (C) FSIQ (R^2 = 0.464) are found to be significant. Pearson correlation 'r' for VIQ, PIQ and FSIQ are −0.660, −0.684 and −0.681 respectively, and found to be statistically significant ($p<0.01$). The negative values indicate the decreasing trend for cognitive abilities due to inbreeding.

Table 6. Average coefficient of inbreeding and percentage inbreeding depression on cognitive abilities.

Factors	Categories	Average coefficient of inbreeding (α)	% Depression in VIQ for α	% Depression in VIQ due to 1% increase of inbreeding coefficient	% Depression in PIQ for α	% Depression in PIQ due to 1% increase of inbreeding coefficient	% Depression in FSIQ for α	% Depression in FSIQ due to 1% increase of inbreeding coefficient
Residence	Rural	2.78	20.12	7.23	24.56	8.83	22.45	8.07
	Urban	2.17	32.63	15.03	33.37	15.37	33.01	15.21
SES	High	1.93	30.41	15.75	33.23	17.21	31.86	16.51
	Medium	2.69	22.96	8.53	26.14	9.71	24.62	9.15
	Low	3.06	17.11	5.59	20.67	6.75	18.94	6.19
Population	Gujjar and Bakarwal	2.53	24.34	9.62	27.52	10.87	24.56	9.71
	Mughal	2.32	22.41	9.65	26.99	11.63	24.79	10.68
	Malik	2.61	24.43	9.36	28.04	10.76	26.34	10.09
	Syed	2.71	19.78	7.29	24.02	8.86	21.99	8.11
	Khan	3.01	25.86	8.59	26.94	8.95	26.42	8.77
Age (in years)	Combined (6–15)	2.64	23.67	8.96	26.89	10.18	25.35	9.61
Sex	Male	2.71	22.81	8.41	27.01	9.96	25.01	9.22
	Female	2.57	24.42	9.51	26.81	10.43	25.68	9.99

Almost all the factors shows the same trend of inbreeding depression viz. PIQ > FSIQ > VIQ, though there is a significant difference among the categories of each factor.

complex traits. The pioneers of human inbreeding, Schull and Neel [45,46] while studying children of atomic bomb survivors in Japan after the World War II, found higher mortality, increased rate of genetic disorders, and many other health related hazards, more often among inbred children in comparison with the non-inbred group. The relative abundance of recessive disorders among inbred communities of many Arab countries has been associated clearly with the practice of consanguinity [23,47].

In the present study, coefficient of inbreeding (a measure of homozygosity) has been calculated through standard pedigree method. Higher value of inbreeding coefficients presents more homozygosity and respective cognitive behaviors have been studied. Based on the same hypothesis, a number of recommendations (such as large population size, different degrees of inbreeding against control groups and well-developed statistical methodology) have been suggested for the optimal design of experiments to study genetic drift and inbreeding as well as correction of data for general environmental effects [48]. A recent study has provided an evidence of inbreeding depression on growth parameters of children with higher frequencies of underweight (BMI <18.5 kg/m^2) cases with increasing inbreeding coefficients [21]. The regression based fitness-related model has been used to quantify the inbreeding depression on cognitive behavior. Similarly, inbreeding load with increased inbreeding coefficients has also been made clear in earlier studies [21,22,49,50].

This study is one of the first attempts with details of inbreeding coefficients and elaborate statistics to examine the effects of inbreeding on the cognitive abilities of children among the indigenous Muslim populations of Jammu region (Northern India). Our results showed a significant decline in cognitive abilities of children due to inbreeding and higher frequency of mental retardation observed among offspring of inbred families, whereas children from non-consanguineous families display higher values of VIQ, PIQ and FSIQ scores and consequently low frequency of mental retardation or ID. Various studies on consanguineous marriages and other forms of inbreeding have cited a discernible reduction in cognitive abilities, with increased mental illness in the offspring of such unions [26,51–53]. A familial study has reported the incidence of mental retardation among the children of first-cousins being four times greater than that in the control group [54]. The study of Morton [51] has revealed that the offspring of first-cousins had over five time's higher risk of mental retardation when compared to that of the control. The study concluded that decline in IQ or increase in the frequency of mental retardation were consistent with rare recessive alleles associated with around 325 loci, whose likelihood of being transmitted to offspring increases with the relatedness of the parents. The present study differs in several aspects from a previous study conducted among the Ansari Muslims of Bhagalpur [26], as it overcomes the limitations with inclusion of details of inbreeding categories, SES, also five Muslim populations and elaborate statistical models.

Our confirmatory factor analysis, based on ANOVA for the three cognitive domains: VIQ, PIQ and FSIQ, showed significant result in context of inbreeding. Other factors like SES, residence, population, age and gender were found insignificant. Nevertheless, SES and residence have shown significant differences in the mean values of cognitive abilities (Figure 4), though the effects were not sufficient to observe significant effect of inbreeding. This explains the heritability of cognitive abilities was much more influenced by genetic factors (i.e., inbreeding) with least environmental effects. A Dutch twin study has also addressed the changing genetic contribution with age, which displayed the shared environment estimates (c^2) contributed toward continuity while change in cognition, and the unique environment contributed to change in development [55]. Parental SES and chaos in the home accounted for about 10% or even less of the total variance in the test scores, indicating that they mediate some of the c^2 effect, but most of that variance still remained unexplained [56]. One of the most recent study has showed a lesser variability in body mass parameters for demographic factors, which may be due to different populations confined to same geographical and environmental conditions explaining the greater extent of their genetic differences [21]. The heritability of intelligence might not be the same for every level of social backgrounds and may be modified by SES [57]. A recent study has revealed that the variation in the intelligence levels among children may be attributed to a greater extent, to individual genetic differences, with almost diminished environmental differences [58].

Figure 7 presents an overview depicting the pathways specifying the factors involved in cognitive impairment with special emphasis on inbreeding. Our simpler model presents the major sources of variance underlying the complex cognitive behavior. It is noteworthy that we have assumed inbreeding, as well as the environmental and social factors for the same cohort to make them rather fit to predict the intelligence more effectively. The phenomenon of inbreeding, undoubtly, is one of the most potent factors to contribute to cognitive behaviors, and also the underlying genetic mechanism. Though heritability of cognitive differences is becoming increasingly clear, the exact nature of the genetic polymorphisms implied by this heritability is still unclear [59]. A recent study based on single nucleotide polymorphism (SNP) predicted that elimination of minor allele leads to no deleterious effect on cognitive ability for a few generations of inbreeding [60].

The recent most techniques provide comprehensive tool to explore the nature and genetics of recessive cognitive disorders [61]. The first homozygosity mapping among Iranian consanguineous families with identification of 8 novel gene loci has revealed heterogeneity of non-syndromic autosomal recessive ID (NS-ARID) [62]. To identify the causative mutation, hundreds of genes were required to be screened among these families, and the gap of knowledge has recently been filled with systematic Sanger sequencing method that led to identification of numerous novel genes for NS-ARID [63]. The next generation sequencing (NGS) has revolutionized the genetic dissection of ID with the identification of gene defects related to ARID and other cognitive disorders. The use of whole-exome enrichment sequencing (WES), a high-throughput NGS technique, has been able to identify for the first time a homozygous variant of *TECR* gene on chromosome 19p13 in a large consanguineous family with NS-ID [64]. In populations where parental consanguinity is common, not all the recessive conditions persist due to autozygous changes, there might be other defects like compound heterozygosity or mutations in intronic, promoter, or other non-coding sequences that could not be detected by WES approach. To unravel the molecular basis of cognitive disorders, candidate gene hunting approach provides substantial novel genes to identify their mechanistic processes. The recently attempted deep sequencing methods reported quite novel candidate genes which are therefore, known to be very attractive candidates for study of synapse- or brain-specific functions, while others involve the basic cellular processes which have been well studied in ID analysis such as DNA transcription and translation, protein degradation, mRNA splicing, energy metabolism and fatty-acid synthesis or turnover [65].

Our study reveals that the extent to which consanguinity affects IQ is proportional to the degree of inbreeding. On the basis of the

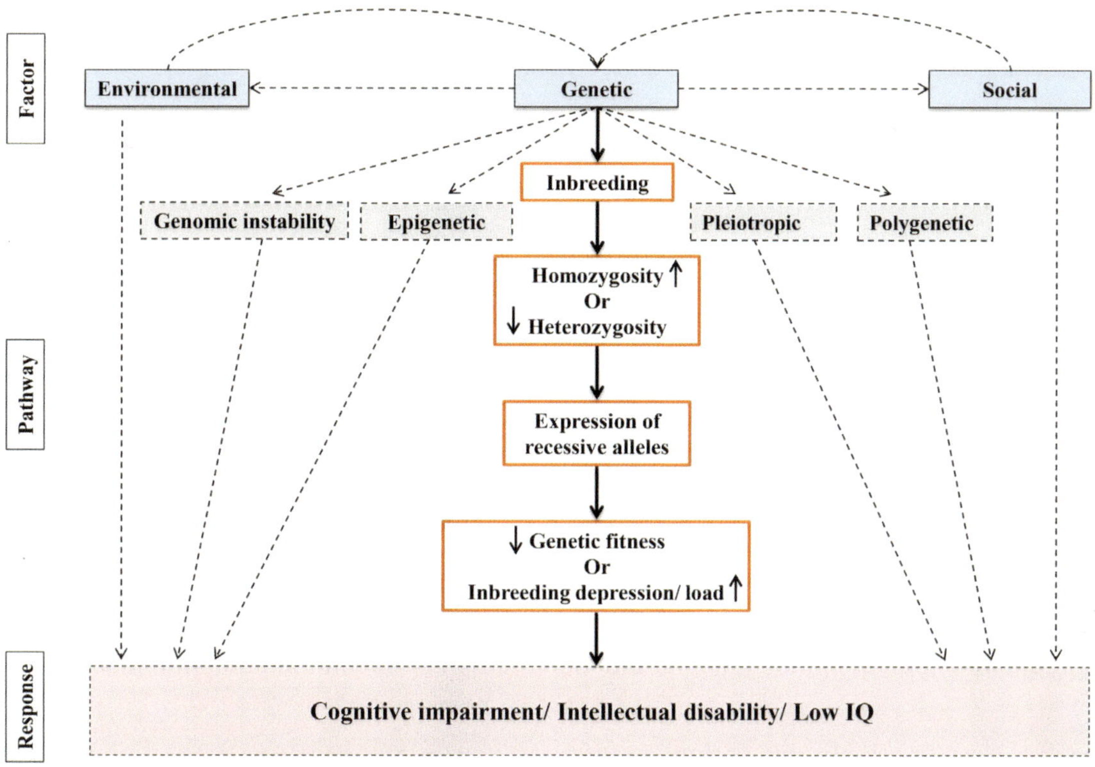

Figure 7. Pathways specifying factors involved in cognitive impairment. The flowchart briefly explains the factors (i.e., environmental, social and genetic) causing cognitive impairment. These factors are inter-related directly or through indirect mechanisms. There are many sub-pathways of each factor, not mentioned here. Inbreeding (due to consanguineous marriages) is also overwhelmed by geography, environment and social norms. Inbreeding increases the homozygosity which in turn results into the expression of autosomal recessive genes that may be one of the causes for abnormal brain development and function.

cognitive study (VIQ, PIQ and FSIQ) outcomes, the offspring of double first-cousins exhibited, on an average, significantly higher inbreeding load (on test scores) than those of first-cousins, which in turn, keep on decreasing with the lowering of inbreeding coefficients and the least of depression being observed among offspring of non-consanguineous parents. Such increasing depression with respect to inbreeding were also reported in previous studies [36,51,55,66–68].

Strengths and Limitations

Our study has immense strengths, though with a few limitations. Firstly, our cohort presents less variation in cognitive abilities for demographic factors, depicting different populations confined to the same environmental conditions. This leaves substantial room for larger study covering different national or geographical regions. A recent study based on national IQs has presented potential significance for demographic, epidemiological and climatic factors [2].

Secondly, the selection of subjects, methodology and statistical analysis can be attempted in a proper way to find out the significant results. ANOVA based factor assessment followed by post-hoc tests provides enough information and the regression analysis provides best measure of cognitive depression in proportion to the degree of inbreeding. However, other statistical tools like oblique rotation method and goodness of fit models can be used as cognitive predictors [69].

Thirdly, standard pedigree information has been used to determine the inbreeding coefficient (F), the extent of inbreeding is related to the amount of ancestry that is shared by the parents of an inbred individual. The pedigree analysis approach adds strength to this study with several advantages: (a) provides natural mating patterns, (b) give accurate estimates of individual inbreeding and its effects and (c) having easy comparisons among studies [41]. However, considerations of more serious methods to study the genetic nature of the recessive cognitive defects such as NGS, WES and candidate gene approaches could provide rather more detailed conclusive proof [61].

Conclusions

In summary, our comprehensive assessment revealed that parental consanguinity and degree of inbreeding was significantly associated with depression in intellectual behaviors among children. Factors other than inbreeding showed little influence, suggesting that genetic component (i.e., inbreeding) was more influential over these parameters under study. Moreover, the depression in cognitive abilities seems to be more prominent due to increase in the degree of inbreeding (F). This study provides new leads for health care providers and health policy makers to train and make people familiar with the assessment of harmful effects of inbreeding on mental health and cognitive efficiency.

Further studies in context of inbreeding, however, need to be investigated to establish a possible causal relationship between cognitive behavior and so-called generalist genes.

Acknowledgments

We thank the Council of Scientific and Industrial Research (CSIR), New Delhi, India, for the award of Senior Research Fellowship (to MF). We are thankful to the Chairman, Department of Zoology, AMU, Aligarh for providing necessary laboratory facilities for this work. We are also thankful to Dr. Mir Kaisar Ahmad, Senior Resident, Department of Clinical Biochemistry, Sher-I-Kashmir Institute of Medical Sciences, Srinagar for his help and suggestions during this study. Thanks are due to the parents of the children without whose cooperation this work could not have been completed.

Author Contributions

Conceived and designed the experiments: MA MF. Performed the experiments: MF. Analyzed the data: MF MA. Contributed reagents/materials/analysis tools: MF MA. Contributed to the writing of the manuscript: MF MA.

References

1. American Psychiatric Association (2013) The diagnostic and statistical manual of mental disorders DSM 5. Bookpoint US.
2. Lynn R, Vanhanen T (2012) National IQs: A review of their educational, cognitive, economic, political, demographic, sociological, epidemiological, geographic and climatic correlates. Intelligence 40: 226–234.
3. Reilly D (2012) Gender, culture, and sex-typed cognitive abilities. PLoS ONE 7: e39904.
4. Hanscombe KB, Trzaskowski M, Haworth CMA, Davis OSP, Dale PS, et al. (2012) Socioeconomic status (SES) and children's intelligence (IQ): in a UK-representative sample SES moderates the environmental, not genetic, effect on IQ. PLoS ONE 7: e30320.
5. Maika A, Mittinty MN, Brinkman S, Harper S, Satriawan E, et al. (2013) Changes in socioeconomic inequality in Indonesian children's cognitive function from 2000 to 2007: a decomposition analysis. PLoS ONE 8: e78809.
6. Brucki SMD, Mansur LL, Carthery-Goulart MT, Nitrini R (2011) Formal education, health literacy and mini-mental state examination. Dement Neuropsychol 5: 26–30.
7. Apolinario D, Brucki SMD, Ferretti REdL, Farfel JM, Magaldi RM, et al. (2013) Estimating premorbid cognitive abilities in low-educated populations. PLoS ONE 8: e60084.
8. Kendler KS, Baker JH (2007) Genetic influences on measures of the environment: a systematic review. Psychol Med 37: 615–626.
9. Plomin R, Bergeman CS (1991) Nature of nurture. Behav Brain Sci 14: 414–427.
10. van der Sluis S, Willemsen G, de Geus EJC, Boomsma DI, Posthuma D (2008) Gene-environment interaction in adults' IQ scores: measures of past and present environment. Behav Genet 38: 348–360.
11. Vinkhuyzen AAE, van der Sluis S, de Geus EJC, Boomsma DI, Posthuma D (2010) Genetic influences on 'environmental' factors. Genes Brain Behav 9: 276–287.
12. Plomin R, DeFries JC (1998) The genetics of cognitive abilities and disabilities. Sci Am 278: 62–69.
13. Butcher LM, Kennedy JKJ, Plomin R (2006) Generalist genes and cognitive neuroscience. Curr Opin Neurobiol 16: 145–151.
14. Bouchard TJ Jr, McGue M (2003) Genetic and environmental influences on human psychological differences. J Neurobiol 54: 4–45.
15. Kovas Y, Plomin R (2006) Generalist genes: implications for the cognitive sciences. Trends Cogn Sci 10: 198–203.
16. Fareed M, Afzal M (2013) Single nucleotide polymorphism in genome-wide association of human population: A tool for broad spectrum service. Egypt J Med Hum Genet 14: 123–134.
17. Goldberg TE, Weinberger DR (2004) Genes and the parsing of cognitive processes. Trends Cogn Sci 8: 325–335.
18. Verkerk AJ, Pieretti M, Sutcliffe JS, Fu YH, Kuhl DP, et al. (1991) Identification of a gene (FMR-1) containing a CGG repeat coincident with a breakpoint cluster region exhibiting length variation in fragile X syndrome. Cell 65: 905–14.
19. Ropers HH, Hamel BC (2005) X-linked mental retardation. Nat Rev Genet 6: 46–57.
20. Herbst DS, Miller JR (1980) Nonspecific X-linked mental retardation II: the frequency in British Columbia. Am J Med Genet 7: 461–469.
21. Fareed M, Afzal M (2014) Evidence of inbreeding depression on height, weight, and body mass index: A population-based child cohort study. Am J Hum Biol doi:10.1002/ajhb.22599.
22. Charlesworth D, Willis JH (2009) The genetics of inbreeding depression. Nat Rev Genet 10: 783–796.
23. Tadmouri GO, Nair P, Obeid T, Al Ali MT, Al Khaja N, et al. (2009) Consanguinity and reproductive health among Arabs. Reprod Health 6: 17.
24. Bener A, Saleh NM, Salameh KMK, Basha B, Joseph S, et al. (2013) Socio-demographic and consanguinity risk factors associated with low birthweight. J Pak Med Assoc 63: 598–603.
25. Stoltenberg C, Magnus P, Skrondal A, Lie RT (1999) Consanguinity and recurrence risk of stillbirth and infant death. Am J Public Health 89: 517–523.
26. Afzal M (1988) Consequences of consanguinity on cognitive behaviour. Behav Genet 18: 583–594.
27. Badaruddoza, Afzal M (1993) Inbreeding depression and intelligence quotient among north Indian children. Behav Genet 23: 343–347.
28. Badaruddoza, Afzal M, Akhtaruzzaman (1994) Inbreeding and congenital heart diseases in a north Indian population. Clin Genet 45: 288–291.
29. Badaruddoza, Afzal M, Ali M (1998) Inbreeding effects on the incidence of congenital disorders and fetal growth and development at birth in north India. Indian Pediatr 35: 1110–1113.
30. Bittles AH (2001) Consanguinity and its relevance to clinical genetics. Clin Genet 60: 89–98.
31. Shieh JTC, Bittles AH, Hudgins L (2012) Consanguinity and the risk of congenital heart disease. Am J Med Genet Part A 158A: 1236–1241.
32. Bittles AH, Black ML (2010) Consanguinity, human evolution and complex diseases. Proc Natl Acad Sci USA 107: 1779–1786.
33. Jaber L, Halpern GJ, Shohat M (1998) The impact of consanguinity worldwide. Community Genet 1: 12–17.
34. Mitsui T, Kawai H, Sakoda S, Miyata M, Saitio S (1994) Hereditary parkinsonism with multiple system degeneration: beneficial effect of anticholinergics, but not of levodopa. J Neurol Sci 125: 153–157.
35. Gustavson KH (2005) Prevalence and etiology of congenital birth defects, infant mortality and mental retardation in Lahore, Pakistan: a prospective cohort study. Acta Paediatr 94: 769–774.
36. Bashi J (1977) Effects of inbreeding on cognitive performance. Nature 266: 440–442.
37. Fareed M, Shah A, Hussain R, Afzal M (2012) Genetic study of phenylthiocarbamide (PTC) taste perception among six human populations of Jammu and Kashmir (India). Egypt J Med Hum Genet 13: 161–166.
38. Fareed M, Hussain R, Shah A, Afzal M (2014) A_1A_2BO and Rh gene frequencies among six populations of Jammu and Kashmir, India. Transfus Apher Sci 50: 247–252.
39. Kumar N, Gupta N, Kishore J (2012) Kuppuswamy's socioeconomic scale: updating income ranges for the year 2012. Indian J Pub Health 56: 103–104.
40. Vandenberg SG (1972) Assortative mating, or who marries whom? Behav genet 2: 127–157.
41. Keller LF, Waller DM (2002) Inbreeding effects in wild populations. Trends Ecol Evol 17: 230–241.
42. Darwin CR (1876) The effects of cross and self-fertilization in the vegetable kingdom. London: John Murray.
43. Jones DF (1924) The attainment of homozygosity in inbred strains of maize. Genetics 9: 405–418.
44. Wright S (1934) An analysis of variability in number of digits in an inbred strain of guinea pigs. Genetics 19: 506–536.
45. Schull WJ, Neel JV (1965) The effects of inbreeding on Japanese children. New York: Harper and Row.
46. Schull WJ, Neel JV (1972) The effects of parental consanguinity and inbreeding in Hirado, Japan. V. Summary and interpretation. Am J Hum Genet 24: 425–453.
47. Saad HA, Elbedou S, Hallaq E, Merrick J, Tenenbaum A (2014) Consanguineous marriage and intellectual and developmental disabilities among Arab Bedouins children of the Negev region in southern Israel: a pilot study. Front Public Health 2: 3.
48. Lynch M (1988) Design and analysis of experiments on random drift and inbreeding depression. Genetics 120: 791–807.
49. Lynch M (1991) The genetic interpretation of inbreeding depression and outbreeding depression. Evolution 45: 622–629.
50. Richards C (2000) Inbreeding depression and genetic rescue in a plant metapopulation. Am Nat 155: 383–394.
51. Morton NE (1978) Effect of inbreeding on IQ and mental retardation. Proc Natl Acad Sci USA 75: 3906–3908.
52. Woodley MA (2009) Inbreeding depression and IQ in a study of 72 countries. Intelligence 37: 268–276.
53. Jensen AR (1983) Effects of inbreeding on mental-ability factors. Pers Individ Dif 4: 71–87.
54. Reed WE, Reed SC (1965) Mental retardation: A family study. Philadelphia: Saunders.
55. Bartels M, Rietveld MJH, Van Baal GCM, Boomsma DI (2002) Genetic and environmental influences on the development of intelligence. Behav Genet 32: 237–249.
56. Petrill SA, Pike A, Price T, Plomin R (2004) Chaos in the home and socioeconomic status are associated with cognitive development in early childhood: environmental mediators identified in a genetic design. Intelligence 32: 445–460.
57. Turkheimer E, Haley A, Waldron M, D'Onofrio B, Gottesman II (2003) Socioeconomic status modifies heritability of IQ in young children. Psychol Sci 14: 623–628.
58. Trzaskowski M, Harlaar N, Arden R, Krapohl E, Rimfeld K, et al. (2014) Genetic influence on family socioeconomic status and children's intelligence. Intelligence 42: 83–88.
59. Deary IJ, Spinath FM, Bates TC (2006) Genetics of intelligence. Eur J Hum Genet 14: 690–700.

60. Power RA, Nagoshi C, Defries JC, Donnelly P, Barroso I, et al. (2014) Genome-wide estimates of inbreeding in unrelated individuals and their association with cognitive ability. Eur J Hum Genet 22: 386–390.
61. Musante L, Ropers HH (2014) Genetics of recessive cognitive disorders. Trends Genet 30: 32–39.
62. Najmabadi H, Motazacker MM, Garshasbi M, Kahrizi K, Tzschach A, et al. (2007) Homozygosity mapping in consanguineous families reveals extreme heterogeneity of non-syndromic autosomal recessive mental retardation and identifies 8 novel gene loci. Hum Genet 121: 43–48.
63. Ropers HH (2010) Genetics of early onset cognitive impairment. Annu Rev Genomics Hum Genet 11: 161–187.
64. Caliskan M, Chong JX, Uricchio L, Anderson R, Chen P, et al. (2011) Exome sequencing reveals a novel mutation for autosomal recessive non-syndromic mental retardation in the TECR gene on chromosome 19p13. Hum Mol Genet 20: 1285–1289.
65. Najmabadi H, Hu H, Garshasbi M, Zemojtel T, Abedini SS, et al. (2011) Deep sequencing reveals 50 novel genes for recessive cognitive disorders. Nature 478: 57–63.
66. Badaruddoza (2004) Effect of inbreeding on Wechsler intelligence test scores among north Indian children. Asia Pac J Public Health 16: 99–103.
67. Agrawal N, Sinha SN, Jensen AR (1984) Effects of inbreeding on Raven matrices. Behav Genet 14: 579–585.
68. Verweij KJH, Abdellaoui A, Veijola J, Sebert S, Koiranen M, et al. (2014) The association of genotype-based inbreeding coefficient with a range of physical and psychological human traits. PLoS ONE 9: e103102.
69. Blankevoort CG, Scherder EJA, Wieling MB, Hortobágyi T, Brouwer WH, et al. (2013) Physical predictors of cognitive performance in healthy older adults: a cross-sectional analysis. PLoS ONE 8: e70799.

Prevalence and Psychosocial Correlates of Depressive Symptoms in Urban Chinese Women during Midlife

Carmen K. M. Wong[1], Jun Liang[2], Man L. Chan[2], Yin H. Chan[2], Laam Chan[2], Kwong Y. Wan[2], Ming S. Ng[2], Dicken C. C. Chan[1], Samuel Y. S. Wong[1], Martin C. S. Wong[1]*

1 Division of Family Medicine and Primary Health Care, JC School of Public Health and Primary Care, The Chinese University of Hong Kong, 4/F, School of Public Health building, Prince of Wales Hospital, Shatin, New Territories, Hong Kong SAR, **2** The Hong Kong Primary Care Research Network, F2029A, Special Block, Tuen Mun Hospital, New Territories, Hong Kong SAR

Abstract

Objective: Depression is common in women with much research focusing on hormonal changes and menopausal symptoms but with little exploration of psychosocial problems in midlife. This study investigates the prevalence of clinically relevant depressive symptoms in midlife Chinese women and its association with psychosocial factors.

Methods: A cross-sectional, community-based household survey of women aged 45 to 64 years of age was conducted in Hong Kong from September 2010 to March 2011. The structured questionnaire included demographic data, educational status, marital status and household income, as well as perceived current stressful events and significant life events in the past 12 months. Information on clinically relevant depressive symptoms was measured by the validated chinese Patient Health Questionnaire (PHQ-9).

Results: A total of 402 participants were recruited in the study period. Of the 393 women who completed the questionnaire, the prevalence of clinically relevant depressive symptoms (PHQ-9 score $\geq$10) was 11.0%. In multiple regression analysis, being single/divorced/separated/widowed, having an educational level of primary school level or below, having multiple chronic diseases, loss of hobby or loss of close social support in the past 12 months in midlife were associated with clinically relevant depressive symptoms.

Conclusions: Correlates of clinically relevant depressive symptoms in midlife Chinese women can be used to identify those at increased risk and potentiate further studies to explore early psychosocial and community interventions.

Editor: Robert Stewart, Institute of Psychiatry, United Kingdom

Funding: The authors have no support or funding to report.

Competing Interests: The authors have declared that no competing interests exist.

* Email: wong_martin@cuhk.edu.hk

Introduction

Women and depression

According to the World Health Organization [1], by the year 2020 depression will be the second most significant condition globally in terms of disability-adjusted life years lost. The lifetime prevalence of major depression ranges from 6–17% [2] and studies have consistently shown dysthymia, minor depression, brief recurrent depression and major depression to be more common in women compared to men. The prevalence of these conditions in women can range from 1.5 to 3 times to that of men [3,4] and such differences may be consistent across life stages as women show higher rates of depression from the age range 11–15 to midlife [5]. Given that there are no gender differences in the course of depression e.g. illness duration, recovery time and recurrence risk [5,6], social environmental factors are likely to have contributed to the early onset and increase in prevalence of depression in women.

Midlife women

The risk of developing depression during the menopausal transition is high and associated with the presence of vasomotor symptoms, greater hormonal variability and changes in health and lifestyle behaviours [7–9]. A large, epidemiologically based study conducted in the US noted differences in psychological and vasomotor symptoms between caucasian and chinese midlife women. Symptoms of muscle and joint pain, and psychological symptoms such as lack of concentration, irritability, insomnia were more prevalent than vasomotor symptoms in Chinese women [9]. These findings were consistent with local and regional studies [10–12]. Although social and cultural factors are likely to play an important role in differences seen in psychological and depressive symptoms in midlife women, there has been little exploration of psychosocial correlates of depressive symptoms in women during their midlife years. In this study, a stratified household interview approach was selected to investigate the prevalence and psychosocial correlates of clinically relevant depressive symptoms in midlife women living within urban communities of Hong Kong.

Material and Methods

Study population and sampling frame

This study was a cross- sectional, population-based household survey of middle aged Chinese women (45 to 64 years old) in Hong Kong. Midlife women of age 45–65 constitute 30% of women in Hong Kong and 16% of the total Hong Kong Chinese population of over 7 million people [13]. Household surveys by cluster sampling has been the most frequently used sampling method as private and public housing blocks make up 99% of the residences of the population [14].

Geographically, Hong Kong is made up of Hong Kong Island, Kowloon and New Territories district, in which 18.0%, 29.8% and 52.2% of the population reside respectively. In this study, the community sample was drawn from the New Territories West district which comprises 1.88 million of the population and comparable to the Hong Kong population in terms of proportion of population of Chinese ethnicity (95.1% vs. 93.6%), post secondary educational attainment (23.9% vs. 25.9%), labour force participation (60.7% vs. 59.7%), median age (40.4 vs. 41.7), proportion never married (31.8% vs. 31.6%), average domestic household (3.0 vs. 2.9), median monthly household income ($20,040 vs. $20,500) and owner occupancy of residence (53.6% vs. 52.1%) [13].

A list of housing blocks in the Kwai Tsing, Tseun Wan, Tuen Mun and Yuen Long district which comprises the New Territories West district was drawn and stratified into private and public housing to avoid over sampling of public housing blocks. A total of three public housing estates and two private housing estates were included. Trained interviewers visited all households identified by computer generated random numbers in the cluster sample. Informed consent was obtained from eligible subjects (women aged 45–64) who agreed to participate in the study. Only one woman from each household was selected using the nearest date of birthday to interview date method. Eligible subjects who were unavailable for the study were visited on two further occasions. Interviews were conducted from the study period September 2010 to March 2011. The overall response rate was 60.0% and 402 participants were successfully interviewed.

Ethics approval

Ethical approval was obtained from the Joint NTWC Clinical Research Ethical Committee (Ref. no.: NTWC/CREC/883/10) before the start of the trial. Written formal consent was obtained and participants were able to withdraw from the survey at any time.

Questionnaire

A structured questionnaire was administered face-to-face by trained interviewers to each participant. The questionnaire included information on socio-demographic data such as age, gender, marital status, educational attainment, employment status, median monthly household income as well as lifestyle history (smoking, alcohol) and medical history (general health, chronic disease and significant life events). The Patient Health Questionnaire (PHQ-9) survey was used to assess clinically relevant depressive symptoms. The PHQ-9 is a nine item depression scale of the PHQ. A score of 5 and above indicate depressive symptoms which are mild and warrant watchful waiting, a score of 10 to 14 indicates clinically relevant moderate depression, which warrant initiation of counselling and/or medication and a score of 15 and above indicates moderately severe symptoms requiring medication. The PHQ-9 has widespread clinical use in primary care clinics in the screening and monitoring of depression and it has been validated in Chinese [15]. The cutoff score of 10 and above has a sensitivity of 88% and a specificity of 88% for major depression [16].

In addition, the survey encompass the 8-question modified Life Event scale to capture important life events that occurred in the previous 12 months [17]. These events included: serious illness or accidents in spouse, death of a close relative or friend, separation from a child, close friend or relative to whom the subject depend on for help, loss of a pet, giving up of an important hobby, experience of serious financial difficulties, move of residence and any other significant events, either good or bad.

Statistical Methods and Analysis

Sample size calculation was based on the assumption of achieving a 5% precision level and a conservative assumption of depression prevalence of 50% to yield the greatest number of subjects. Using $4\times p(1-p)/(\text{precision})^2$ where p = estimated proportion of participants having depressive symptoms, the minimal sample needed was 383 participants.

All data were entered and analyzed in PASW Statistics version 18.0. The primary outcome was the prevalence of depressive symptoms defined as PHQ-9 score ≥ 10. Each of the socio-demographic, lifestyle and clinical variables listed above was consecutively tested against the outcome variable by bivariate analysis. All p-values ≤ 0.05 were regarded as statistically significant in the comparative analysis.

Results

A total of 402 participants were recruited in the study period, of which 393 women completed the questionnaire. Table 1 illustrates the demographic and lifestyle characteristics of the study population.

The mean age of the participating women was 52.5 years (s.d. 5.3) and had been resident in Hong Kong for 29.0 years. Of the 402 women, the majority (81%) were married or in cohabiting relationships, and lived with family members (96%). Educational levels at secondary school level or above was obtained in over half of the women (56%). Approximately half of those interviewed (49%) were housewives without salaried jobs. Overall, women had on average 2 children (mean 2.3, s.d. 1.1). Up to 56% had median household income lower than HK$10,000. The majority of women were non smokers (95%) and non alcohol drinkers (94%). Over half of women rated their general health as fair or poor (52% and 9% respectively) whilst the rest rated their health from good to excellent. Over 60% of women were free from chronic illnesses, whilst 22% suffered from one chronic condition and 17% suffered from two or more conditions. Only 6.0% (n = 24) had a self reported diagnosis of depression or anxiety.

Prevalence of clinically significant depressive symptoms and psychosocial and lifestyle correlates

Using PHQ-9 as the measuring instrument with a cut-off level of 10 points and above, 11.0% of participants (n = 43) suffered from clinically relevant depressive symptoms indicative of major depression. Of those, 18 participants scored 15 points and above indicating severe depressive symptoms.

For socioeconomic factors, being single/divorced/separated/widowed, having an educational level of primary school level or below, having poorer reported general health and having multiple chronic diseases were significantly associated with clinically relevant depressive symptoms. There were no significant associations of depressive symptoms with early to late midlife age groups, living alone, number of children, employment status, monthly

Table 1. Socio-demographic Characteristics.

	N = 402 (%)
Age groups	
45–50 years	164 (40.8%)
51–54 years	96 (23.9%)
55–60 years	104 (25.9%)
61–64 years	38 (9.5%)
Mean age in years (sd)	52.5 (5.3)
Mean duration of residence in Hong Kong (sd)	29.0 (19.2)
Residence	
Living alone	15 (3.9%)
Living with spouse/ parents/ children/ siblings	368 (96.1%)
Marital Status	
Single/Divorced/Separate/Widowed	72 (18.9%)
Married/cohabit	308 (81.1%)
Mean number of children (sd)	2.3 (1.1)
Educational level	
Primary school and below	170 (44.5%)
Secondary school and above	212 (55.5%)
Job	
Full time	53 (23.5%)
Part time	62 (27.4%)
Housewife	111 (49.1%)
Monthly Household income (HK$)	
<10,000	173 (56.2%)
10,000–19,999	32 (10.4%)
≥ 20,000	9 (2.9%)
Not known/ refused to respond	94 (30.5%)
Menopausal Status	
Pre/ Perimenopausal	236 (58.7%)
Postmenopausal	166 (41.3%)
Number of chronic diseases	
0	213 (60.9%)
1	79 (22.6%)
2+	58 (16.6%)
Medical History	
Cardiovascular disease (MI/Stroke)	11 (2.7%)
Hypertension	53 (13.2%)
Diabetes	28 (7.0%)
Depression/Anxiety	24 (6.0%)
General health status	
Excellent	4 (1.0%)
Very good	57 (14.4%)
Good	93 (23.5%)
Fair	207 (52.4%)
Poor	34 (8.6%)
Patient Health Questionnaire (PHQ-9)	
0–4 points	255(64.9%)
5–9 points	95 (24.2%)
10–14 points	25 (6.4%)
15+ points	18 (4.6%)

Table 2. Bivariate associations of those with clinically depressive symptoms (PHQ 10+) and those without (PHQ <10) on socio-demographic characteristics and stressful life events.

	n	Prevalence of depression (n, %)	P- value
Age group			
45–54 years	252	29 (11.5%)	0.631 ($\chi^2=0.231$, df = 1)
55–64 years	141	14 (9.9%)	
Marital Status			
Single/Divorced/Separate/Widowed	72	16 (22.2%)	<0.001 ($\chi^2=12.653$, df = 1)
Married/cohabit	305	24 (7.9%)	
Residence			
Living alone	15	3 (20.0%)	0.223[a]
Living with spouse/parents/children/siblings	365	39 (10.7%)	
Number of children			
None	12	1 (8.3%)	0.594 ($\chi^2=1.041$, df = 2)
1	62	9 (14.5%)	
2+	302	31 (10.3%)	
Educational level			
Primary school and below	170	25 (14.7%)	0.043 ($\chi^2=4.109$, df = 1)
Secondary school and above	209	17 (8.1%)	
Job			
Full time	53	8 (15.1%)	0.323 ($\chi^2=2.262$, df = 2)
Part time	61	4 (6.6%)	
Housewife	111	14 (12.6%)	
Monthly Household income (HK$)			
<10,000	173	24 (13.9%)	0.256 ($\chi^2=1.292$, df = 1)
10,000 +	41	3 (7.3%)	
Smoking status			
Non-smoker	349	36 (10.3%)	0.759 ($\chi^2=0.094$, df = 1)
Current smoker/Past smoker	13	1 (7.7%)	
Drinking status			
Non-drinker	332	33 (9.9%)	0.897 ($\chi^2=0.017$, df = 1)
Current drinker	22	2 (9.1%)	
General health status			
Excellent/Very good/Good	152	4 (2.6%)	<0.001 ($\chi^2=17.164$, df = 1)
Fair/Poor	238	38 (16.0%)	
Menopausal Status			
Pre/Perimenopausal	228	23 (10.1%)	0.524 ($\chi^2=0.406$, df = 1)
Postmenopausal	165	20 (12.1%)	
Number of chronic diseases			
0	210	11 (5.2%)	<0.001 ($\chi^2=36.483$, df = 2)
1	79	7 (8.9%)	
2+	58	19 (32.8%)	
Number of stressful life events			
0–1	272	21 (7.7%)	0.001 ($\chi^2=10.220$, df = 1)
2 or above	117	22 (18.8%)	
Stressful life event			
Serious illness or accident of spouse or partner	31	9 (29.0%)	0.004[a]
Death of close relative or friend	92	15 (16.3%)	0.075 ($\chi^2=3.173$, df = 1)
Separated from close friend or relative whom depend on for help	31	9 (29.0%)	0.003[a]
Loss of pet	20	1 (5.0%)	0.710[a]
Loss of a hobby	70	17 (24.3%)	<0.001 ($\chi^2=14.837$, df = 1)
Serious financial trouble	65	13 (20.0%)	0.010 ($\chi^2=6.650$, df = 1)

Table 2. Cont.

	n	Prevalence of depression (n, %)	P- value
Moving home	13	2 (15.4%)	0.645[a]
Experience in either good or bad important events	103	18 (17.5%)	0.012 ($\chi^2=6.363$, df = 1)
Most concerned issues			
Marriage	8	1 (12.5%)	0.887 ($\chi^2=0.020$, df = 1)
Children	151	15 (9.9%)	0.613 ($\chi^2=0.256$, df = 1)
Finance	82	13 (15.9%)	0.109 ($\chi^2=2.566$, df = 1)
Job	30	6 (20.0%)	0.121[a]
Health	176	20 (11.4%)	0.809 ($\chi^2=0.058$, df = 1)
Others	27	0 (0%)	-

Chi-squared test was applied unless indicated otherwise.
Note: [a] Fisher's exact test.

household incomes, menopausal status, smoking or drinking. Psychosocial correlates of depressive symptoms included having experienced two or more stressful life events in the past 12 months, of which "serious illness or accident of spouse or partner", "separation from close friend or relative", "loss of a hobby", "serious financial trouble" and "experience in either a good or bad important event" was significant. Current worries regarding marriage, children, finance, job or health had no correlation with depressive symptoms (see table 2).

Multivariate model

All variables found to be significantly associated with clinically relevant depressive symptoms were entered into the multivariate logistic regression model. Factors such as not being in a married or cohabiting relationship, having primary school education of lower, having multiple co-morbidity and life events such as "loss of hobby" or "separated from close friend or relative whom depend on for help", was independently associated with having clinically relevant depressive symptoms (see table 3).

Discussion

This was the first household survey conducted in midlife Chinese women to investigate the prevalence and correlates of depressive symptoms with psychosocial factors using a validated screening tool for depressive symptoms.

The prevalence of clinically relevant depressive symptoms in Chinese midlife women was 11.0%. Studies have suggested ethnic differences, in which Chinese midlife women had lower odds than white women to have significant depressive symptoms [18],

Table 3. Multivariate regression model prevalence odds ratio for those with clinically depressive symptoms (PHQ 10+) versus those without (PHQ <10).

Variable	Odds ratio (95% CI)
Marital Status	
Married/Cohabit	1
Single/Divorced/Separate/Widowed	**2.45 (1.04–5.80)[a]**
Educational level	
Secondary school and above	1
Primary school and below	**2.39 (1.07–5.34)[a]**
Number of chronic medical conditions	
0	1
1	1.59 (0.56–4.53)
2 or above	**7.66 (3.04–19.31)[a]**
Stressful life event	
Serious illness or accident of spouse or partner	1.06 (0.33–3.48)
Death of close relative or friend	1.29 (0.53–3.10)
Separated from close friend or relative whom depend on for help	**3.69 (1.11–12.23)[a]**
Loss of a hobby	**2.58 (1.06–6.25)[a]**
Serious financial trouble	1.50 (0.56–3.98)
Experience in either good or bad important events	0.81 (0.33–1.99)

Note: [a] p-value <0.05.

although our study results showed higher prevalence in comparison to US adult women (8.55% score ≥ 10 using PHQ-9) [19]. However, comparison of prevalence data can be problematic owing to the differences in sampling framework, screening methods used, cutoff levels and in the few studies reporting data relating to women in midlife years.

Previous studies have shown that lower socioeconomic status was associated with higher rates of depression in women [20–24]. Although our study showed that depressive symptoms in midlife women were significantly associated with lower educational level, there was no association with lower household income or employment status. There may be several reasons for this perhaps 1) socioeconomic status play a minimal role in the occurrence of depressive symptoms in midlife or 2) socioeconomic inequalities may be buffered from household members income as 93% of women live with others and/or 3) socio-demographic parameters used in this study are not extensive or sensitive enough to detect individual social economic situations e.g. social relationships, financial strain, level of debt etc.

Previous studies have shown that stressful life events can precipitate the onset of depressive symptoms [25,26]. A similar community-based cross-sectional household survey conducted in Hong Kong show that midlife urban Chinese men who were single/divorced/separated/widowed, living alone and unemployed increased their vulnerability for clinically relevant depressive symptoms [27]. Whilst negative events such as "given up a hobby or activity" and "serious financial trouble" were independently associated with depressive symptoms in men; in our study of midlife women, living alone and employment status had no effect on depressive symptoms but "loss of a hobby or activity" and "separation from a close friend or relative" was more likely in women to have clinically relevant depressive symptoms. The effect of gender traditional roles [28] and women's tendency to "tend and befriend" [29]may explain these study findings. Traditional expectations of men to be the breadwinner may explain the negative effect of unemployment, financial trouble in men, whilst women's interpersonal and nurturing nature may explain the importance of close social support for women as a coping strategy. This is also consistent with the 'cost of caring' theory by Kessler and McRae [30] and Turner and Avison [31] who hypothesized that women tended to care more for others and thus were more vulnerable to events affecting close emotional ties rather than themselves. One study of couples with shared life events had suggested life events relating to children, housing or reproductive problems were specific in the onset of depression in women [32]. In our study of midlife women, these were not apparent and current worries regarding marriage, children, finance, job or health had no correlation with depressive symptoms. In midlife, changes such as the loss of hobby or activity in the past year and having poorer general health may highlight other physical or psychosocial pressures specifically facing those in midlife.

Hong Kong has a high life expectancy of 85.9 years, second to that of Japan [33] with midlife and elderly women making a substantial and increasing proportion of the population. The prevalence of depressive symptoms in the Chinese population appear to increase with age [34] and in the Chinese elderly age 70 years and above, significant depressive symptoms rise in both men and women [35,36], consistent with epidemiological studies which depict lower rates of depressive symptoms in midlife and elevated rates in the oldest old [37]. Differences in the prevalence of depressive symptoms in midlife and in older years may be attributable to the use of different assessment scales, patterns of health care utilization, acquisition of coping skills, cohort effect of those born at an earlier age, or period effect of different social environmental influences. Thus, there is a need for longitudinal cohort studies which can help us understand and identify those at risk of depression from the transition from midlife to elder years.

The association of poor physical health and comorbidity with depression is well documented [38,39], particularly in the older age community [35,36]. This association is also apparent in our study of midlife women, not surprisingly so, as this period is a vulnerable time for the onset of many chronic physical conditions.

Women that are married or in co-habiting partnerships in midlife appear to have less significant depressive symptoms. As midlife women play increasingly complex roles in their families and careers in urban societies, further studies exploring depressive symptoms and depression in midlife men and women are needed. The socio-demographics of Chinese midlife women in Hong Kong are changing with increasing numbers of women who have never married or are divorced or without children [13]. This is likely to impact the dynamic pattern of depressive symptoms in midlife women and close monitoring is required so that psychosocial interventions can be responsive and effective.

Limitations

This study was conducted in urban communities of Hong Kong. The demographic data of women in our sample compared to age-adjusted data of the census of the whole territory showed higher rates of low educational attainment to primary school level (44.5% vs. 34.1%) although comparative rates of employment (50.9% vs. 48.8%). Selection bias inherent in our study in selecting those of lower educational attainment may result in the overestimation of depressive symptoms and may not be representative of the whole region. In addition, the questionnaire was only conducted at one time point. It is unclear whether depressive symptoms are of new onset, persisting, recurrent or likely to resolve. The PHQ-9 was the screening tool used for detecting depressive symptoms in this study, and there are many other tools for this purpose which may yield a slight variation in prevalence results. The PHQ-9 and its shorter version PHQ-2, however is widely used clinically by health care professionals to screen for depression as a self administered tool or face to face interview and our study population would likely reflect the population that have detectable clinically relevant depressive symptoms in primary care.

Conclusion and Recommendation

The prevalence of clinically depressive symptoms in this study of urban midlife Chinese women was 11.0%. In midlife, being single/divorced/separated/widowed, having an educational level of primary school level or below, having multiple chronic diseases, loss of hobby or loss of close social support in the past 12 months were associated with clinically relevant depressive symptoms. Further studies of depressive symptoms in midlife are necessary to identify those at risk and to explore early psychosocial and community interventions to improve mental health for midlife women.

Author Contributions

Conceived and designed the experiments: JL MLC YHC LC KYW MSN MCSW CKMW. Analyzed the data: DCCC SYSW. Wrote the paper: CKMW.

References

1. Levav I, Rutz W (2002) The WHO World Health Report 2001 new understanding—new hope. Isr J Psychiatry Relat Sci 39(1): 50–56.
2. Blazer DG, Kessler RC, McGonagle KA, Swartz MS (1994) The prevalence and distribution of major depression in a national community sample: the National Comorbidity Survey. Am J Psychiatry 151(7): 979–986.
3. Kessler RC (1997) The effects of stressful life events on depression. Annu Rev Psychol: 48191–214.
4. Angst J, Merikangas K (1997) The depressive spectrum: diagnostic classification and course. J Affect Disord 45(1–2): 31–9; discussion 39–40.
5. Kessler RC, McGonagle KA, Nelson CB, Hughes M, Swartz M, et al. (1994) Sex and depression in the National Comorbidity Survey II: Cohort effects. J Affect Disord 30(1): 15–26.
6. Simpson HB, Nee JC, Endicott J (1997) First-episode major depression. Few sex differences in course. Arch Gen Psychiatry 54(7): 633–639.
7. Cohen LS, Soares CN, Vitonis AF, Otto MW, Harlow BL (2006) Risk for new onset of depression during the menopausal transition: the Harvard study of moods and cycles. Arch Gen Psychiatry 63(4): 385–390.
8. Freeman EW, Sammel MD, Lin H, Nelson DB (2006) Associations of hormones and menopausal status with depressed mood in women with no history of depression. Arch Gen Psychiatry 63(4): 375–382.
9. Bromberger JT, Matthews KA, Schott LL, Brockwell S, Avis NE, et al. (2007) Depressive symptoms during the menopausal transition: the Study of Women's Health Across the Nation (SWAN). J Affect Disord 103(1–3): 267–272.
10. Ho SC, Gaen Chan S, Bing Yip Y, Yee Chan S, Sham A (2003) Factors associated with menopausal symptom reporting in Chinese midlife women. Maturitas 44(2): 149-156.
11. Liu J, Eden J (2007) Experience and attitudes toward menopause in Chinese women living in Sydney—a cross sectional survey. Maturitas 58(4): 359–365.
12. Loh FH, Khin LW, Saw SM, Lee JJ, Gu K (2005) The age of menopause and the menopause transition in a multiracial population: a nation-wide Singapore study. Maturitas 52(3–4): 169–180.
13. Census and Statistics Department (2011) Census 2011. Hong Kong Special Adminstrative Region.
14. Lau EM, Egger P, Coggon D, Cooper C, Valenti L, et al. (1995) Low back pain in Hong Kong: prevalence and characteristics compared with Britain. J Epidemiol Community Health 49(5): 492–494.
15. Cheng CM, Cheng M (2007) To validate the Chinese version of the 2Q and PHQ-9 questionnaires in Hong Kong Chinese patients. The Hong Kong Practitioner 29: 381–390.
16. Kroenke K, Spitzer RL, Williams JB (2001) The PHQ-9: validity of a brief depression severity measure. J Gen Intern Med 16(9): 606–613.
17. Simonsick EM, Phillips CL, Skinner EA, Davis D, Kasper JD (1995) The Daily Lives of Disabled Older Women. In: Guralnik JM, Fried LM, Simonsick EM, et al., editors.The Women's Health and Aging Study: Health and Social Characteristics of Older Women with Disability.Bethesda Maryland: National Institute of Health, National Institute of Aging. Chapter 5. NIH Pub. No. 95-4009.
18. Shim RS, Baltrus P, Ye J, Rust G (2011) Prevalence, Treatment and control of Depressive symptoms in the United States: Results from the National Health and Nutrition Examination Survey (NHANES) 2005–1008. Journal Am Board Fam Med 24: 33–38
19. Bromberger JT, Harlow S, Avis N, Kravitz HM, Cordal A (2004) Racial/ethnic differences in the prevalence of depressive symptoms among middle-aged women: The Study of Women's Health Across the Nation (SWAN). Am J Public Health 94(8): 1378–1385.
20. Bracke P (2000) The three-year persistence of depressive symptoms in men and women. Soc Sci Med 51(1): 51–64.
21. Coiro MJ (2001) Depressive symptoms among women receiving welfare. Women Health 32(1–2): 1–23.
22. Eaton WW, Muntaner C, Bovasso G, Smith C (2001) Socioeconomic status and depressive syndrome: the role of inter- and intra-generational mobility, government assistance, and work environment. J Health Soc Behav 42(3): 277–294.
23. Elliott M (2001) Gender differences in causes of depression. Women Health 33(3–4): 163–177.
24. O'Campo P, Eaton WW, Muntaner C (2004) Labor market experience, work organization, gender inequalities and health status: results from a prospective analysis of US employed women. Soc Sci Med 58(3): 585–594.
25. Kendler KS, Karkowski LM, Prescott CA (1999) Causal relationship between stressful life events and the onset of major depression. Am J Psychiatry 156(6): 837–841.
26. Kendler KS, Kessler RC, Neale MC, Heath AC, Eaves LJ (1993) The prediction of major depression in women: an integrated etiologic model. Am J Psychiatry 150: 1139–1148.
27. Wong SY, Chan D, Leung PC (2006) Depressive symptoms in middle-aged men: results from a household survey in Hong Kong. J Affect Disord 92(2–3): 215–220.
28. Mirowsky J, Ross CE (1989) Social causes of psychological distress. New York: Aldine de Gruyter. 214 p.
29. Taylor SE, Klein LC, Lewis BP, Gruenewalk TL, Gurung RAR, et al. (2000) Biobehavioral responses to stress in females: tend-and-befriend, not fight-or-flight. Psychol Rev 107(3): 411–429.
30. Kessler RC, McRae JA (1981) Trends in the relationship between sex and psychological distress: 1957–1976. Am Sociol Rev 46(4): 443–452.
31. Turner RJ, Avison WR (1989) Gender and depression: assessing exposure and vulnerability to life events in a chronically strained population. J Nerv Ment Dis 177(8): 443–455.
32. Nazroo JY, Edwards AC, Brown GW (1997) Gender differences in the onset of depression following a shared life event: a study of couples. Psychol Med 27(1): 9–19.
33. Department of Health (2010) Annual report 2009/2010. Hong Kong Special Administrative Region.
34. Chou KL, Chi I (2005) Prevalence and correlates of depression in Chinese oldest-old. Int J Geriatr Psychiatry 20(1): 41–50.
35. Chi I, Yip PS, Chiu HF, Chou KL, Chan KS, et al. (2005) Prevalence of depression and its correlates in Hong Kong's Chinese older adults. Am J Geriatr Psychiatry 13(5): 409–416.
36. Woo J, Ho SC, Lau J, Yuen YK, Chiu H, et al. (1994) The prevalence of depressive symptoms and predisposing factors in an elderly Chinese population. Acta Psychiatr Scand 89(1): 8–13.
37. Krause N (1999) Mental disorder in late life: Exploring the influence of stress and socioeconomic status. In: Aneshensel CS, and Phelan JC, editors. Handbook of the sociology of mental health.New York: Kluwer Academic/Plenum Publishers. pp.183–208.
38. Buist-Bouwman MA, de Graaf R, Vollebergh WA, Ormel J (2005) Comorbidity of physical and mental disorders and the effect on work-loss days. Acta Psychiatr Scand 111(6): 436–443.
39. Scott KM, Bruffaerts R, Tsang A, Ormel J, Alonso J, et al. (2007) Depression-anxiety relationships with chronic physical conditions: results from the World Mental Health Surveys. J Affect Disord 103(1–3): 113–120.

8

Gastroesophageal Reflux Disease and Risk for Bipolar Disorder: A Nationwide Population-Based Study

Wan-Shan Lin[1¶], Li-Yu Hu[1,2,3¶], Chia-Jen Liu[2,3,4], Chih-Chao Hsu[1], Cheng-Che Shen[5], Yen-Po Wang[3,6,7], Yu-Wen Hu[3,8], Chia-Fen Tsai[3,9], Chiu-Mei Yeh[10], Pan-Ming Chen[11], Tung-Ping Su[3,9], Tzeng-Ji Chen[3,10], Ti Lu[1]*

1 Department of Psychiatry, Kaohsiung Veterans General Hospital, Kaohsiung, Taiwan, **2** Institute of Public Health, National Yang-Ming University, Taipei, Taiwan, **3** School of Medicine, National Yang-Ming University, Taipei, Taiwan, **4** Division of Hematology and Oncology, Department of Medicine, Taipei Veterans General Hospital, Taipei, Taiwan, **5** Department of Psychiatry, Chiayi Branch, Taichung Veterans General Hospital, Taipei, Taiwan, **6** Endoscopy Center of Diagnosis and Treatment, Taipei Veterans General Hospital, Taipei, Taiwan, **7** Division of Gastroenterology, Department of Medicine, Taipei Veterans General Hospital, Taipei, Taiwan, **8** Cancer Center, Taipei Veterans General Hospital, Taipei, Taiwan, **9** Department of Psychiatry, Taipei Veterans General Hospital, Taipei, Taiwan, **10** Department of Family Medicine, Taipei Veterans General Hospital, Taipei, Taiwan, **11** Department of Psychiatry, Su-Ao and Yuanshan Branch, Taipei Veterans General Hospital, Taipei, Taiwan

Abstract

Background: Studies have shown that chronic inflammation may play a vital role in the pathophysiology of both gastroesophageal reflux disease (GERD) and bipolar disorder. Among patients with GERD, the risk of bipolar disorder has not been well characterized.

Objective: We explored the relationship between GERD and the subsequent development of bipolar disorder, and examined the risk factors for bipolar disorder in patients with GERD.

Methods: We identified patients who were diagnosed with GERD in the Taiwan National Health Insurance Research Database. A comparison cohort without GERD was matched according to age, sex, and comorbidities. The occurrence of bipolar disorder was evaluated in both cohorts based on diagnosis and the prescription of medications.

Results: The GERD cohort consisted of 21,674 patients, and the comparison cohort consisted of 21,674 matched control patients without GERD. The incidence of bipolar disorder (incidence rate ratio [IRR] 2.29, 95% confidence interval [CI] 1.58–3.36, $P<.001$) was higher among GERD patients than among comparison cohort. Multivariate, matched regression models showed that the female sex (hazard ratio [HR] 1.78, 95% CI 1.76–2.74, $P=.008$), being younger than 60 years old (HR 2.35, 95% CI 1.33–4.16, $P=.003$), and alcohol use disorder (HR 4.89, 95% CI 3.06–7.84, $P=.004$) were independent risk factors for the development of bipolar disorder among GERD patients.

Conclusions: GERD may increase the risk of developing bipolar disorder. Based on our data, we suggest that attention should be focused on female patients younger than 60 years, and patients with alcohol use disorder, following a GERD diagnosis.

Editor: Melvin G. McInnis, University of Michigan, United States of America

Funding: This study is supported by a grant from Taipei Veterans General Hospital (V103B-022 and V103E10-001). The funders had no role in study design, data collection and analysis, decision to publish, or preparation of the manuscript.

Competing Interests: The authors have declared that no competing interests exist.

* Email: tlu@vghks.gov.tw

¶ These authors contributed equally to this work.

Introduction

Gastroesophageal reflux disease (GERD) is a condition which develops when the reflux of stomach contents causes troublesome symptoms and/or complications. It is one of the most common gastrointestinal disorder which presents as heartburn and regurgitation. It significantly affects quality of life and healthcare costs and rapidly increases in Asian countries. [1–3] However, the mechanisms involved in the pathogenesis of GERD symptoms have not been fully elucidated. Studies have shown that, in GERD patients, the esophageal mucosa produces significantly more amounts of various cytokines including interleukin-6 (IL-6), IL-8, IL-1 beta, interferon gamma (IFN-gamma), tumor necrosis factor alpha (TNF-alpha) compared with healthy people. [4] These inflammatory mediators activate immune cell recruitment and migration, and may play an important role in the generation of

GERD symptoms; in other words, GERD may be considered an inflammatory process. [4,5].

In clinical care, interest in the psychiatric aspects of gastroenterological diseases has grown. [6] Increasing numbers of gastroenterological diseases, including GERD, have been proved to be associated with psychiatric disorders, in particular, depression, anxiety, and sleep disturbance. [7–10] Evidence has showed that reflux symptoms are more common in patients with bipolar disorder. [11] However, the relationship between GERD and bipolar disorder has been less studied.

Studies have shown that cytokines circulating in the plasma may impair the function of the blood-brain barrier, [12] which may indicate that peripheral inflammation is associated with the upregulation of central nervous system (CNS) inflammation. [13] Several studies have shown that chronic inflammation plays a critical role in the pathophysiology of common mental disorders, [14] including depression and bipolar disorder. [15,16] Therefore, we hypothesized that a history of GERD increases the risk of the subsequent onset of bipolar disorder.

To prove our hypothesis, we designed a nationwide population-based study to investigate the incidence of bipolar disorder among patients with GERD.

Patients and Methods

Data Sources

The Taiwan's National Health Insurance (NHI) program offers a comprehensive, unified, universal health insurance program to all residents of Taiwan. The NHI program covers more than 96% of Taiwan residents, and has contracted with 99% of the hospitals and clinics in Taiwan. [17] The program provides coverage for outpatient, inpatient, emergency, and traditional Chinese medicine services, as well as for prescription drugs. Multiple NHI databases, including NHI enrollment files, claims data, and a prescription drug registry, are managed and publicly released by the National Health Research Institutes (NHRI) of Taiwan. The Bureau of NHI and NHRI regulations guarantee patient confidentiality, and data identifying patients is encrypted. Detailed information about the data source is provided on the NHRI website (http://nhird.nhri.org.tw) and any problems about the data request could be sent to e-mail address at the NHRI (e-mail: nhird@nhri.org.tw).

Ethics Statement

The Institutional Review Board of the Taipei Veterans General Hospital approved this study (2013-08-016BC). Written consent from study patients was not obtained because the NHI dataset consists of de-identified secondary data for research purposes, and the Institutional Review Board of Taipei Veterans General Hospital issued a formal written waiver for the need for consent.

Study Design and Participants

We conducted a retrospective cohort study of patients newly diagnosed with GERD between April 1, 2000 and December 1, 2009. We identified GERD cases in the Taiwan National Health Insurance Research Database (NHIRD) based on the International Classification of Diseases, 9th revision, Clinical Modification (ICD-9-CM) codes 530.11 and 530.81. To increase the validity of GERD diagnoses, we included only the patients who received proton pump inhibitor (PPI) and diagnosed as GERD. The Bureau of NHI requires that patients with GERD be diagnosed by performing either endoscopy or 24-hour pH-meter monitoring before a PPI can be prescribed for treatment. Patients with bipolar disorder were identified based on diagnoses of mood or behavior disturbances, related to a principal diagnosis of a bipolar disorder (ICD-9-CM codes 296.0X, 296.1X, 296.4X, 296.5X, 296.6X, 296.7X, 296.80, or 296.89). We also analyzed the use of drugs approved by the FDA (Food and Drug Administration) for treating one (or more) phases of bipolar disorder; the drugs were classified according to the World Health Organization (WHO) Anatomical Therapeutic Chemical (ATC) classification. In our study, only patients who were prescribed these drugs for at least one month were included in our study. In addition, patients with mood disorders resulting from a general medical condition (ICD-9-CM code 293.83) and patients with a history of mood disorders before the enrollment date were excluded from our study.

For each patient with GERD in the NHIRD, a patient without GERD matched for age, sex, comorbidities, [18] and enrollment date was included in the comparison cohort. Although there are many studies which have found several comorbidities to be risk factors for GERD, based on our inflammation hypothesis in this study, other inflammation-related comorbidities may be considered as potential confounders. Identical exclusion criteria were applied to the matched comparison cohort. Both the GERD and comparison patients were followed until the development of bipolar disorder, death, or the end of 2010.

Statistical Analysis

Diagnosis of bipolar disorder served as the primary dependent variable. We calculated bipolar disorder incidence rates (per 10,000 person-years) and incidence rate ratios (IRRs). The study groups were compared using the χ^2 test for categorical variables. The Kaplan-Meier method was used to estimate the cumulative incidence of bipolar disorder, and a Cox proportional hazards model was used to identify risk factors for bipolar disorder in patients with GERD. The qualifying criterion for inclusion in the multivariate analysis was a result in the univariate-analysis with a P value less than 0.1. The Perl programming language (version 5.12.2) was used to extract the data from the databases. Microsoft SQL Server 2005 (Microsoft Corp., Redmond, WA, USA) was used to execute data linkage, processing, and control sampling. SPSS software, version 19.0 for Windows (IBM, Armonk, NY, USA), and SAS software, version 9.2 (SAS Institute, Cary, NC, USA) were used to perform all statistical analyses. Comparison results with P values less than.05 were considered statistically significant.

Results

Participant Characteristics

Table 1 shows the demographic and comorbidity data of the GERD patients and comparison participants. The median age of the patients was 52 years. The majority of patients in both cohorts were men (54.2%). Hypertension, dyslipidemia, and chronic obstructive pulmonary disease were the most common comorbidities. There were no statistically significant differences in the baseline comorbidity data between the study groups.

Incidence of Bipolar Disorder

The cumulative incidences of bipolar disorder are shown in Figure 1. As shown in Table 2, the risk of developing bipolar disorder was significantly higher for patients with GERD than for the matched control patients (IRR 2.29, 95% confidence interval [CI] 1.58–3.36, $P<.001$). After stratifying patients according to age and sex, we observed that patients with GERD aged less than 60 years were associated with a higher risk of developing bipolar disorder (IRR 2.59, 95% CI 1.70–4.03, $P<.001$), but patients aged more than 60 years were not. This enhanced risk was

Table 1. Baseline characteristics of patients with gastroesophageal reflux disease (GERD) and matched cohort.

Demographic data	Patients with GERD (*n*=21,674)		Matched cohort *n*=21,674		*P* value
	n	%	*n*	%	
Age (years) (interquartile range)	52(40–65)		52(40–65)		
≥60	7,079	32.7	7,079	32.7	1.000
<60	14,595	67.3	14,595	67.3	
Sex					
Male	11,737	54.2	11,737	54.2	1.000
Female	9,937	45.8	9,937	45.8	
Comorbidities					
Alcohol use disorder	1,856	8.6	1,855	8.6	0.986
Autoimmune diseases	2,593	12.0	2,591	12.0	0.976
Chronic kidney disease	3,651	16.8	3,652	16.8	0.990
Cerebrovascular disease	4,333	20.0	4,331	20.0	0.981
Diabetes mellitus	5,974	27.6	5,976	27.6	0.983
Hypertension	9,289	42.9	9,289	42.9	1.000
Asthma	4,627	21.3	4,627	21.3	1.000
COPD	7,227	33.3	7,225	33.3	0.984
Malignancies	945	4.4	934	4.3	0.795
Cirrhosis	1,119	5.2	1,089	5.0	0.512
Dyslipidemia	8,444	39.0	8,443	39.0	0.992
Coronary artery disease	624	2.9	598	2.8	0.451
Obesity	483	2.2	469	2.2	0.646
Follow-up years (median)	3.03(1.86–4.39)		2.96(1.79–4.32)		<0.001

COPD, chronic obstructive pulmonary disease.

observed in both men and women. We also stratified patients according to follow-up duration, and observed that only patients with longer follow-up durations were associated with a higher risk of subsequent bipolar disorder (1–3 years and ≥3 years). Overall, our study showed that the incidence of the development of bipolar disorder after the diagnosis of GERD was 14.0 per 10,000 person-years.

Risks Factors for Bipolar Disorder in Patients with GERD

As demonstrated in the univariate and multivariate analyses, independent risk factors for the development of bipolar disorder among GERD patients were being younger than 60 years of age (HR 2.35, 95% CI 1.33–4.16, $P=.003$), female (HR 1.78, 95% CI 1.16–2.74, $P=.008$), and having an alcohol use disorder (HR 4.89, 95% CI 3.06–7.84, $P<.001$) (Table 3).

Discussion

This is the first population-based study to examine GERD as a risk factor for bipolar disorder by using a matched cohort design and a long-term follow-up period. This study observed a higher incidence of the development of subsequent bipolar disorder among patients with GERD. In addition, GERD patients who were female and aged less than 60 years had a greater risk of developing bipolar disorder than those who were male and aged more than 60 years. Alcohol use disorder was another risk factor for the development of bipolar disorder among patients with GERD.

In our study, patients with GERD were determined to be at higher risk for developing subsequent bipolar disorder. We hypothesize that this may be attributed to two possible mechanisms. First, the development of bipolar disorder after the onset of GERD may be the result of an inflammatory process activated by GERD. In patients with GERD, the esophageal mucosa produces higher amounts of various cytokines including IL-6, IL-8, IL-1 beta, IFN-gamma, TNF-alpha. [4] Even in non-erosive reflux disease (NERD), which the role of inflammation may be considered less obvious, enhanced expression of IL-8 and IL-1 beta has been found. [19,20] The chronic peripheral inflammatory process activated by GERD may increase the risk of subsequent bipolar disorder by upregulating CNS inflammation. [13] Studies have revealed that chronic, mild inflammation in the periphery and in the brain occurs in bipolar disorder. [21,22] Cytokines have been shown to access the brain and interact with pathophysiological domains relevant to bipolar disorder. Using animal models, it is shown that peripheral cytokines reach the brain through various mechanisms, including a leaky brain barrier, active transport, the activation of endothelial cells, and binding to cytokine receptors. [23] Levels of proinflammatory cytokines such as IL-2, IL-4, and IL-6 are elevated during mania, whereas IL-6 is elevated during depression. [24] Second, GERD and bipolar disorder share common risk factors, such as stress. Laboratory stress has been found to increase the perception of intraluminal acid stimuli and induced stress, anxiety, anger in GERD patients rather than normal control. [25] Stressful psychosocial factors can induce GERD, [26] and stress may also

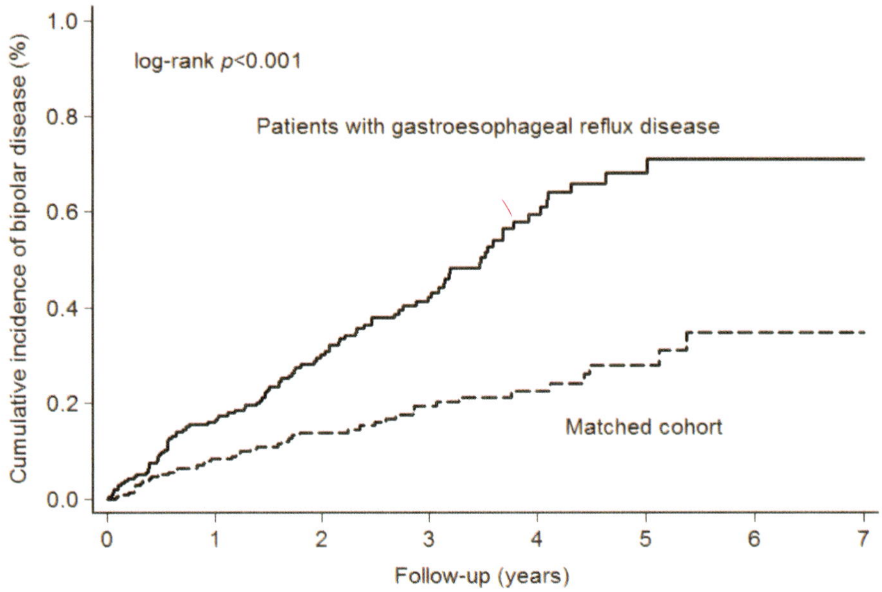

Figure 1. Cumulative incidence of bipolar disorder in patients with gastroesophageal reflux disease (GERD) and matched cohort.

induce bipolar disorder in patients genetically prone to developing bipolar disorder. [27,28] Psychological stress also may activate inflammatory responses in the brain. [29].

When stratifying according to follow-up duration, the risk of bipolar disorder among GERD patients was significantly higher after the first year following the GERD diagnosis, which is consistent with our hypothesis that inflammation is responsible for the association between GERD and bipolar disorder. We hypothesize that long periods of time are required for the chronic inflammatory process. Based on our results, detection bias was unlikely.

In our study, we observed that younger age was an independent risk factor for developing subsequent bipolar disorder among GERD patients. The incidence of bipolar disorder is determined to be relatively rare in people aged more than 60 years. [30] Our study confirmed this finding.

Epidemiological studies have shown that bipolar disorder is equally prevalent among men and women. However, in this study, we observed that women with GERD had a greater risk of developing a bipolar disorder than men did. One possible explanation is that women in our study group, with a median age of 52 years, were vulnerable to fluctuating estrogen levels, thereby increasing their risk of developing bipolar disorder. [31,32].

In our analysis of the risk factors associated with subsequent bipolar disorder in GERD patients, alcohol use disorder was an independent risk. Evidence has shown that alcohol use disorder

Table 2. Incidence of bipolar disorder in patients with gastroesophageal reflux disease (GERD) and matched cohort.

	Patients with GERD		Matched cohort		IRR (95% CI)	*P* value
	Bipolar No.	Per 10,000 person-year	Bipolar No.	Per 10,000 person-year		
Total	96	14.0	43	6.1	2.29(1.58–3.36)	<0.001
Age						
≥60	14	6.7	11	5.0	1.34(0.57–3.27)	0.473
<60	82	17.3	32	6.7	2.59(1.70–4.03)	<0.001
Sex						
Male	44	11.8	20	5.2	2.27(1.31–4.06)	0.002
Female	52	16.8	23	7.3	2.30(1.38–3.94)	0.001
Follow-up						
0–0.5 year	20	18.7	11	10.2	1.83(0.84–4.23)	0.105
0.5–1 year	15	14.3	7	6.6	2.18(0.84–6.32)	0.086
1–3 year	40	13.0	17	5.4	2.41(1.34–4.54)	0.002
≥3 year	21	12.8	8	4.7	2.73(1.16–7.12)	0.012

IRR, incidence rate ratio; CI, confidence interval.

Table 3. Analyses of risk factors for bipolar disorder in patients with gastroesophageal reflux disease (GERD).

Predictive variables	Univariate analysis		Multivariable analysis	
	HR (95% CI)	*P* value	HR (95% CI)	*P* value
Age <60	2.58(1.46–4.54)	0.001	2.35(1.33–4.16)	0.003
Sex(female)	1.42(0.95–2.12)	0.090	1.78(1.16–2.74)	0.008
Comorbidities				
Alcohol use disorder	4.38(2.81–6.84)	<0.001	4.89(3.06–7.84)	<0.001
Autoimmune diseases	1.63(0.96–2.75)	0.069	1.59(0.93–2.71)	0.088
Chronic kidney disease	1.16(0.69–1.96)	0.579		
Cerebrovascular disease	0.64(0.35–1.16)	0.141		
Diabetes mellitus	1.33(0.87–2.04)	0.196		
Hypertension	1.12(0.75–1.67)	0.593		
Asthma	1.31(0.82–2.08)	0.256		
COPD	1.33(0.88–2.01)	0.170		
Malignancies	0.59(0.15–2.41)	0.465		
Cirrhosis	1.61(0.75–3.48)	0.225		
Dyslipidemia	1.26(0.84–1.89)	0.259		
Coronary artery disease	2.08(0.85–5.12)	0.111		
Obesity	2.41(0.98–5.92)	0.056	1.96(0.79–4.86)	0.144

COPD, chronic obstructive pulmonary disease.

and bipolar disorder share certain common genetic characteristics, neuroimaging findings, and biochemical findings. [33,34].

This is the first retrospective study to examine GERD as a risk factor for the development of bipolar disorder. This study's strengths were its matched case-control design using a population-based cohort of GERD patients, and adequate controls for comorbidity. However, several limitations inherent to the use of claims databases must be considered. First, the results of endoscopies and patient's symptoms could not be obtained from the database. Consequently, the influence of GERD severity as a risk factor for developing subsequent bipolar disorder could not be determined. Second, the causal relationship between GERD and bipolar disorder was assessed mainly by determining the time of onset of these two conditions in particular patients. However, both conditions may need a long periods to seek treatment; thus, the possibility that bipolar disorder caused GERD cannot be completely ruled out. Finally, many demographic variables were unavailable in the database, such as socioeconomic status, lifestyle, and family medical history; analysis of these variables may have provided useful information regarding additional factors associated with GERD and bipolar disorder. [35–38].

In conclusion, the results of this study suggested that GERD increases the risk of developing bipolar disorder. Based on our data, we suggest that attention should be focused on female patients, patients aged less than 60 years, and patients with alcohol use disorders, following GERD diagnosis. Further prospective clinical studies on the relationship between GERD and bipolar disorder are warranted.

Acknowledgments

We thank Huei-Sing Chang, Cheng-Fang Hong, Chun-Hsin Hu, and Ai-Ling Hu for their technical assistance. The study is based in part on data from the National Health Insurance Research Database provided by the Bureau of National Health Insurance, Department of Health and managed by National Health Research Institutes. The interpretation and conclusions contained herein do not represent those of Bureau of National Health Insurance, Department of Health or National Health Research Institutes.

Author Contributions

Conceived and designed the experiments: WSL LYH CJL TL. Performed the experiments: CJL CCS YWH CFT CMY. Analyzed the data: WSL LYH CJL YPW CMY TL. Contributed reagents/materials/analysis tools: CJL PMC TPS TJC. Wrote the paper: WSL LYH CCH TL.

References

1. Sandler RS, Everhart JE, Donowitz M, Adams E, Cronin K, et al. (2002) The burden of selected digestive diseases in the United States. Gastroenterology 122: 1500–1511.
2. Jung HK (2011) Epidemiology of gastroesophageal reflux disease in Asia: a systematic review. J Neurogastroenterol Motil 17: 14–27.
3. Lu CL, Lang HC, Chang FY, Chen TJ, Chen CY, et al. (2005) Social and medical impact, sleep quality and the pharmaceutical costs of heartburn in Taiwan. Aliment Pharmacol Ther 22: 739–747.
4. Altomare A, Guarino MP, Cocca S, Emerenziani S, Cicala M (2013) Gastroesophageal reflux disease: Update on inflammation and symptom perception. World J Gastroenterol 19: 6523–6528.
5. Souza RF, Huo X, Mittal V, Schuler CM, Carmack SW, et al. (2009) Gastroesophageal reflux might cause esophagitis through a cytokine-mediated mechanism rather than caustic acid injury. Gastroenterology 137: 1776–1784.
6. Mikocka-Walus A, Turnbull D, Andrews JM, Moulding N, Wilson I, et al. (2009) Psychogastroenterology: a call for psychological input in Australian gastroenterology clinics. Intern Med J 39: 127–130.
7. Chou PH, Lin CC, Lin CH, Tsai CJ, Cheng C, et al. (2013) Prevalence of Gastroesophageal Reflux Disease in Major Depressive Disorder: A Population-Based Study. Psychosomatics.
8. Jansson C, Nordenstedt H, Wallander MA, Johansson S, Johnsen R, et al. (2007) Severe gastro-oesophageal reflux symptoms in relation to anxiety, depression and coping in a population-based study. Aliment Pharmacol Ther 26: 683–691.
9. Kim JY, Kim N, Seo PJ, Lee JW, Kim MS, et al. (2013) Association of sleep dysfunction and emotional status with gastroesophageal reflux disease in Korea. J Neurogastroenterol Motil 19: 344–354.

10. Jansson C, Nordenstedt H, Wallander MA, Johansson S, Johnsen R, et al. (2009) A population-based study showing an association between gastroesophageal reflux disease and sleep problems. Clin Gastroenterol Hepatol 7: 960–965.
11. Avidan B, Sonnenberg A, Giblovich H, Sontag SJ (2001) Reflux symptoms are associated with psychiatric disease. 2001 15: 1907–1912.
12. Abbott NJ, Ronnback L, Hansson E (2006) Astrocyte-endothelial interactions at the blood-brain barrier. Nat Rev Neurosci 7: 41–53.
13. Lampa J, Westman M, Kadetoff D, Agreus AN, Le Maitre E, et al. (2012) Peripheral inflammatory disease associated with centrally activated IL-1 system in humans and mice. Proc Natl Acad Sci U S A 109: 12728–12733.
14. Kivimaki M, Shipley MJ, Batty GD, Hamer M, Akbaraly TN, et al. (2013) Long-term inflammation increases risk of common mental disorder: a cohort study. Mol Psychiatry.
15. Berk M, Williams LJ, Jacka FN, O'Neil A, Pasco JA, et al. (2013) So depression is an inflammatory disease, but where does the inflammation come from? BMC Med 11: 200.
16. Stertz L, Magalhaes PV, Kapczinski F (2013) Is bipolar disorder an inflammatory condition? The relevance of microglial activation. Curr Opin Psychiatry 26: 19–26.
17. Wu CY, Chen YJ, Ho HJ, Hsu YC, Kuo KN, et al. (2012) Association between nucleoside analogues and risk of hepatitis B virus-related hepatocellular carcinoma recurrence following liver resection. JAMA 308: 1906–1914.
18. Khan NF, Perera R, Harper S, Rose PW (2010) Adaptation and validation of the Charlson Index for Read/OXMIS coded databases. BMC Fam Pract 11: 1.
19. Isomoto H, Saenko VA, Kanazawa Y, Nishi Y, Ohtsuru A, et al. (2004) Enhanced expression of interleukin-8 and activation of nuclear factor kappa-B in endoscopy-negative gastroesophageal reflux disease. Am J Gastroenterol 99: 589–597.
20. Monkemuller K, Wex T, Kuester D, Fry LC, Peitz U, et al. (2009) Interleukin-1beta and interleukin-8 expression correlate with the histomorphological changes in esophageal mucosa of patients with erosive and non-erosive reflux disease. Digestion 79: 186–195.
21. Goldstein BI, Kemp DE, Soczynska JK, McIntyre RS (2009) Inflammation and the phenomenology, pathophysiology, comorbidity, and treatment of bipolar disorder: a systematic review of the literature. J Clin Psychiatry 70: 1078–1090.
22. Hamdani N, Tamouza R, Leboyer M (2012) Immuno- inflammatory markers of bipolar disorder: a review of evidence. Front Biosci (Elite Ed) 4: 2170–2182.
23. Miller AH, Maletic V, Raison CL (2009) Inflammation and its discontents: the role of cytokines in the pathophysiology of major depression. Biol Psychiatry 65: 732–741.
24. Brietzke E, Stertz L, Fernandes BS, Kauer-Sant'anna M, Mascarenhas M, et al. (2009) Comparison of cytokine levels in depressed, manic and euthymic patients with bipolar disorder. J Affect Disord 116: 214–217.
25. Fass R, Naliboff BD, Fass SS, Peleg N, Wendel C, et al. (2008) The effect of auditory stress on perception of intraesophageal acid in patients with gastroesophageal reflux disease. Gastroenterology 134: 696–705.
26. Jansson C, Wallander MA, Johansson S, Johnsen R, Hveem K (2010) Stressful psychosocial factors and symptoms of gastroesophageal reflux disease: a population-based study in Norway. Scand J Gastroenterol 45: 21–29.
27. Proudfoot J, Whitton A, Parker G, Doran J, Manicavasagar V, et al. (2012) Triggers of mania and depression in young adults with bipolar disorder. J Affect Disord 143: 196–202.
28. Etain B, Henry C, Bellivier F, Mathieu F, Leboyer M (2008) Beyond genetics: childhood affective trauma in bipolar disorder. Bipolar Disord 10: 867–876.
29. Wager-Smith K, Markou A (2011) Depression: a repair response to stress-induced neuronal microdamage that can grade into a chronic neuroinflammatory condition? Neurosci Biobehav Rev 35: 742–764.
30. Kroon JS, Wohlfarth TD, Dieleman J, Sutterland AL, Storosum JG, et al. (2013) Incidence rates and risk factors of bipolar disorder in the general population: a population-based cohort study. Bipolar Disord 15: 306–313.
31. Graae L, Karlsson R, Paddock S (2012) Significant association of estrogen receptor binding site variation with bipolar disorder in females. PLoS One 7: e32304.
32. Frey BN, Dias RS (2013) Sex hormones and biomarkers of neuroprotection and neurodegeneration: implications for female reproductive events in bipolar disorder. Bipolar Disord.
33. Farren CK, Hill KP, Weiss RD (2012) Bipolar disorder and alcohol use disorder: a review. Curr Psychiatry Rep 14: 659–666.
34. Pettinati HM, O'Brien CP, Dundon WD (2013) Current status of co-occurring mood and substance use disorders: a new therapeutic target. Am J Psychiatry 170: 23–30.
35. Minatsuki C, Yamamichi N, Shimamoto T, Kakimoto H, Takahashi Y, et al. (2013) Background factors of reflux esophagitis and non-erosive reflux disease: a cross-sectional study of 10,837 subjects in Japan. PLoS One 8: e69891.
36. Waxmonsky JA, Thomas MR, Miklowitz DJ, Allen MH, Wisniewski SR, et al. (2005) Prevalence and correlates of tobacco use in bipolar disorder: data from the first 2000 participants in the Systematic Treatment Enhancement Program. Gen Hosp Psychiatry 27: 321–328.
37. Moshkowitz M, Horowitz N, Halpern Z, Santo E (2011) Gastroesophageal reflux disease symptoms: prevalence, sociodemographics and treatment patterns in the adult Israeli population. World J Gastroenterol 17: 1332–1335.
38. Schoeyen HK, Birkenaes AB, Vaaler AE, Auestad BH, Malt UF, et al. (2011) Bipolar disorder patients have similar levels of education but lower socio-economic status than the general population. J Affect Disord 129: 68–74.

9

A Study of Remitted and Treatment-Resistant Depression Using MMPI and Including Pessimism and Optimism Scales

Masatoshi Suzuki[1], Michio Takahashi[1], Katsumasa Muneoka[1], Koichi Sato[1], Kenji Hashimoto[2], Yukihiko Shirayama[1]*

1 Department of Psychiatry, Teikyo University Chiba Medical Center, Ichihara, Japan, **2** Division of Clinical Neuroscience, Chiba University Center for Forensic Mental Health, Chiba, Japan

Abstract

Background: The psychological aspects of treatment-resistant and remitted depression are not well documented.

Methods: We administered the Minnesota Multiphasic Personality Inventory (MMPI) to patients with treatment-resistant depression (n = 34), remitted depression (n = 25), acute depression (n = 21), and healthy controls (n = 64). Pessimism and optimism were also evaluated by MMPI.

Results: ANOVA and post-hoc tests demonstrated that patients with treatment-resistant and acute depression showed similarly high scores for frequent scale (F), hypochondriasis, depression, conversion hysteria, psychopathic device, paranoia, psychasthenia and schizophrenia on the MMPI compared with normal controls. Patients with treatment-resistant depression, but not acute depression registered high on the scale for cannot say answer. Using Student's t-test, patients with remitted depression registered higher on depression and social introversion scales, compared with normal controls. For pessimism and optimism, patients with treatment-resistant depression demonstrated similar changes to acutely depressed patients. Remitted depression patients showed lower optimism than normal controls by Student's t-test, even though these patients were deemed recovered from depression using HAM-D.

Conclusions: The patients with remitted depression and treatment-resistant depression showed subtle alterations on the MMPI, which may explain the hidden psychological features in these cohorts.

Editor: Robert Stewart, Institute of Psychiatry, United Kingdom

Funding: Funding for this study was provided by Teikyo University Chiba Medical Center, Ichihara, Japan. The funders had no role in study design, data collection and analysis, decision to publish, or preparation of the manuscript.

* Email: shirayama@rapid.ocn.ne.jp

Introduction

Approximately 80 to 90 percent of depressed patients respond to antidepressant treatment, while the remaining 5 to 15 percent are deemed non-responders. Treatment-resistant depression is defined as a non-response to at least two types of antidepressant medication [1,2]. A response is defined as a reduction in depressive symptoms to less than 50 percent while remission means a full recovery.

The Minnesota Multiphasic Personality Inventory (MMPI) is a screening instrument for the differentiation of various forms of psychopathology [3]. Personality is considered to be a modifier for depression. It is not surprising that high depression scores are found to be modestly accurate in predicting depression [4–6], as it is well known that a high score on the MMPI depression scale is not specific to depression [7]. A previous study showed that the MMPI profile for patients with unipolar depression was characterized by an elevation on the depression scale and a secondary elevation on the schizophrenia scale, while the MMPI profile for the bipolar depression group showed comparable elevations on both depression and schizophrenia scales [8]. Another study showed small but significant differences between dysthymia and major depression, but the presence of a personality disorder increased the neurotic triad, namely the hypochondriasis, depression and hysteria scales [9]. Similarly, comorbidity of a personality disorder with major depression increased schizophrenia scores, while major depression without a personality disorder increased psychasthenia scores on the MMPI [10]. Furthermore, when scoring depressed patients on the MMPI, the high scoring scales excluding depression, were hysteria, psychopathic deviation, schizophrenia and psychasthenia [11]. Therefore, on the MMPI, combinations of scores excluding depression may be useful for detecting the psychological mechanisms involved in remitted and treatment-resistant depression.

Interestingly, a previous study demonstrated that scores on the MMPI were useful for evaluating pessimism and optimism [12]. This scale was developed on the basis of a working hypothesis. The hypothesis states that the manner in which people attempt to understand the causes of a stressful or adverse life event can significantly undermine their psychological and physiological function or adversely affect the course of a disease [13,14]. Peterson and Seligman put forward that a pessimistic explanatory style could predict an escalation in depressive symptoms [13]. A recent study reported pessimistic personality traits increased all-cause mortality [15].

The present study attempts to explore the psychological features underlying both treatment-resistant and remitted depression (single episode) using the MMPI. We administered the MMPI to patients with treatment-resistant depression, remitted depression and acute depression, and compared them with normal healthy controls. In addition, we evaluated the pessimism or optimism scores in these same cohorts of patients using the MMPI.

Methods

Ethics Statement

The study was approved by the ethics committee of Teikyo University Chiba Medical Center (study number 09–30), and performed in accordance with the Declaration of Helsinki. Written informed consent was obtained from all participants after a full explanation of all procedures.

Participants

Sixty four healthy subjects, 25 remitted depressed patients, 21 acutely depressed patients and 34 antidepressant treatment-resistant depressed patients were enrolled in this study (**Table 1**). All patients met the DSM-IV criteria for major depressive disorder (first episode) [16]. All patients were recruited from the outpatient clinics of Teikyo University Chiba Medical Center. Two senior-level psychiatrists assessed the psychopathology of patients with treatment-resistant depression. Participants were physically healthy and free from alcohol or drug abuse. Inclusion criteria for treatment-resistant depression required symptoms of moderate depression after treatment with at least two antidepressants, for eight weeks. Patients with treatment-resistant depression had typically received at least two antidepressants, whereas acutely depressed patients were medication-free or receiving their first antidepressant trials. The remitted group received one or two antidepressants trials (Table 1). The depression scores of patients with acute depression and treatment-resistant depression were 14 or more on the 17-item Hamilton Rating Scale for Depression (HAM-D), on which, the definition of remission (recovery) was defined as 7 or less in patients with remitted depression [1,2] (Table 1). Only patients who had suffered a single depressive episode were included in the study. The controls were healthy volunteers recruited from hospital staff, their associates and friends. Those who had a current or past history of psychiatric treatment or drug dependence were not enrolled in this study. All controls were employed men or women.

Personality evaluated by MMPI

MMPI is used worldwide to assess patient personality types [3]. For the purpose of shortening procedural times, we used the short version of the MMPI, which consists of 383 questions and 13 domains (4 validity scales and 9 clinical scales). MMPI data provides a standardized and quantitative measure of personality traits. Validity scales involve the cannot say answer scale (?), the lie scale (L), the frequent scale (F), and correction scale (K). The clinical scales detect the presence of psychopathological features, namely, hypochondriasis (scale 1), depression (scale 2), hysteria (scale 3), psychopathic device (scale 4), paranoia (scale 6), psychasthenia (scale 7), schizophrenia (scale 8), hypomania (scale 9) and social introversion (scale 0). Scale 5 (masculinity-femininity) was not used since the participants included both males and females.

A raw score on the can not say answer scale greater than 30 was considered grounds for declaring a profile invalid. A total of six MMPIs data were discarded for this reason.

MMPI for pessimism and optimism

Briefly, the habit of voicing pessimistic or optimistic explanations for the cause of a stressful or adverse life event can undermine their psychological functioning [13] or adversely affect the course of a disease [14]. Pessimism and optimism were evaluated using the methods of a previous study [12]. Half of the MMPI items described good or bad, both of which mirrored various life experiences. Thus, this scale is capable of assessing a patient's beliefs around the cause of good and bad events, based on the pattern of item endorsement.

Since the short version of MMPI is used to reduce clinical procedural time, we checked coefficients between the 550 original and 383 short versions of the MMPI in the same participants, using Pearson coefficient ($n = 20$). The coefficients of pessimism and optimism were 0.9919 and 0.9488, respectively (both P values were less than 0.0001), validating the short version of MMPI for pessimism and optimism.

Statistical Analysis

Data from 13 domains (4 validity scales and 9 clinical scales) of the MMPI were first analyzed using multiple analysis of variance (MANOVA) to confirm the ability to determine the simultaneous, significant differences. Statistical differences among the four groups were determined by a one-way factorial analysis of variance (ANOVA), followed by multiple comparison testing (Scheffe's test). Statistical evaluation between the two groups was performed using two-tailed Student's t-test or Chi-square test. Differences were considered to be significant when p values were less than 0.05.

Results

MANOVA for all scales (validity and clinical scales) indicated a significant effect for group ($F = 7.154$, $P < 0.0001$).

MMPI for validity

MANOVA for validity scales indicated a significant effect for group ($F = 8.320$, $P < 0.0001$). Subsequent one-way ANOVA demonstrated statistical significance on the cannot say answer scale ($F = 16.926$, $P < 0.0001$), F ($F = 11.164$, $P < 0.0001$), K ($F = 3.874$, $P = 0.0107$), but not the L scale ($F = 1.493$, $P = 0.2193$). Post hoc testing (Scheffe's test) demonstrated that patients with treatment-resistant depression and those with acute depression showed significantly altered scores on the MMPI, relative to patients with remitted depression and healthy controls (**Figure 1**). Patients with treatment-resistant depression showed significantly higher scores in the cannot say answer scale compared with normal controls and patients with acute depression ($P < 0.0001$).

MMPI for clinical features

MANOVA for clinical scales indicated a significant effect for group ($F = 7.236$, $P < 0.0001$). One-way ANOVA demonstrated

Table 1. Demographic information for subjects.

	Healthy Control	Remitted Depression	Acute Depression	Treatment-resistant Depression	P values
	n = 64	n = 25	n = 21	n = 34	
Current age (years)	37.47±8.46 (24–53)	40.08±9.92 (22–58)	40.19±10.79 (23–58)	39.03±9.48 (22–53)	0.526
Sex (male/female)	54/10	18/7	16/5	24/10	0.370
Age at onset (years)		36.56±9.65 (22–54)	39.81±10.93 (23–55)	36.15±8.99 (17–50)	0.369
Duration of depressive state (months)		23.70±20.67 (4–68)	2.24±3.07^{a} (1–7)	37.15±21.24^{a,b} (9–98)	<0.001
Duration of treatment (months)		26.88±26.68 (6–54)	0.14±0.64^{a} (0–1)	30.65±21.30^{a,b} (4–97)	<0.001
HAM-D		4.36±1.73 (3–7)	20.62±4.27^{a} (16–30)	18.35±4.04^{a} (14–28)	<0.001
Trial numbers of antidepressants		1.28±0.45 (1–2)	0.05±0.21^{a} (0–1)	2.50±1.26^{a,b} (2–9)	<0.001

Data are shown as mean ± SD.
HAM-D: Hamilton Rating Scale for Depression
^{a}P<0.001 as compared to the remitted group.
^{b}p<0.01 as compared to the acute depression group.
Parenthesis denotes the range.

statistical significances for hypochondriasis (F = 14.570, P< 0.0001), depression (F = 77.949, P<0.0001), hysteria (F = 12.875, P<0.0001), psychopathic deviate (F = 9.668, P<0.0001), paranoia (F = 13.027, P<0.0001), psychasthenia (F = 37.567, P<0.0001), schizophrenia (F = 22.698, P<0.0001), and social introversion (F = 27.778, P<0.0001), but not hypomania (F = 2.078, P = 0.1059).

Patients with treatment-resistant depression and acute depression showed significantly altered scores on the MMPI relative to patients with remitted depression and healthy controls (**Figure 1**). However, we found a significant difference only in the cannot say answer scale between treatment-resistant depression and acute depression patients. We found no significant differences in any scales between remitted depression patients and healthy controls.

Comparisons between the two groups

Since ANOVA and post hoc testing showed a trend for significance between patients with treatment-resistant depression and those with acute depression in some scales (paranoia, P = 0.0670; mania, P = 0.1074), we used Student's t-test to detect small differences between the two groups. We found statistically significant differences between treatment-resistant depression and acute depression on the paranoia (t = 2.141, P = 0.0369), and mania scales (t = 2.088, P = 0.0416) (**Figure 1**).

Similarly, since ANOVA and post hoc testing showed a trend for significance between patients with remitted depression and normal controls in some scales (depression, P = 0.1397; social introversion, P = 0.0744), we used Student's t-test to detect small differences between the two groups. We found a significant difference between remitted depression and normal controls on the depression (t = 2.577, P = 0.0117), and social introversion scales (t = 2.837, P = 0.0057) (**Figure 1**).

Pessimism and optimism by MMPI

MANOVA for pessimism and optimism scales demonstrated a significant effect for group (F = 17.472, P<0.0001). One-way ANOVA highlighted statistically significant differences on pessimism (F = 26.958, P<0.0001) and optimism (F = 35.357, P< 0.0001). Patients with treatment-resistant depression and acute depression showed significantly altered scores on the MMPI, compared with patients suffering remitted depression, or healthy controls (**Figure 2**).

Although post hoc testing failed to show significant changes between patients with remitted depression and normal controls on the optimism scale (P = 0.2572), we used Student's t-test to detect small differences between the two groups, and found a significant difference between remitted depression and normal controls in this trait (t = 2.116, P = 0.0372) (**Figure 2**).

Discussion

This study found that patients with treatment-resistant depression or remitted depression exhibited psychological features in their MMPI profile, different to those in acutely depressed patients or normal controls. These data are supported by a previous study which showed that unipolar depression patients had a higher elevation in the depression scale, predominant over disturbances in the hypocondriasis, depression, hysteria, psychopathic deviate, paranoia, paychasthenia, schizophrenia and social introversion scales on the MMPI [8]. Another study showed that disturbances in unipolar depression, psychopathic deviation, paranoia, psychasthenia and schizophrenia predominanted over disturbances in hypochondriasis, hysteria and social introversion on the MMPI [17]. A more recent study recorded mean scores for hypochondriasis, depression, hysteria, psychotic deviate, paranoia, psychasthenia and schizophrenia as greater than 65 T in major depression using MMPI-2 [18].

A review by Gross et al., showed that many studies used the depression scale with cut-off scores over 65 or 70 T in MMPI, suggesting that the depression scale in the MMPI is moderately accurate for predicting depression [6]. Clinically, 65 T is 1.5 standard deviations over the mean. The percentage of depression scores above 65 or 70 T is 95 and 81 percent in acutely depressed patients, 94 and 88 percent in patients with treatment-resistant disease, 32 and 4 percent in remitted depression, and 8 and 5 percent in normal controls, respectively. Between the two groups, we found a significant difference between patients with remitted depression and normal controls in the depression scale over 65 T (Chi-square 8.432, p = 0.0037), but not over 70 T. Furthermore, depressed patients in remission showed a significant elevation in the depression scale when evaluated by Student's t-test, but not by ANOVA or post-hoc testing (Figure 1). Therefore, it is likely that

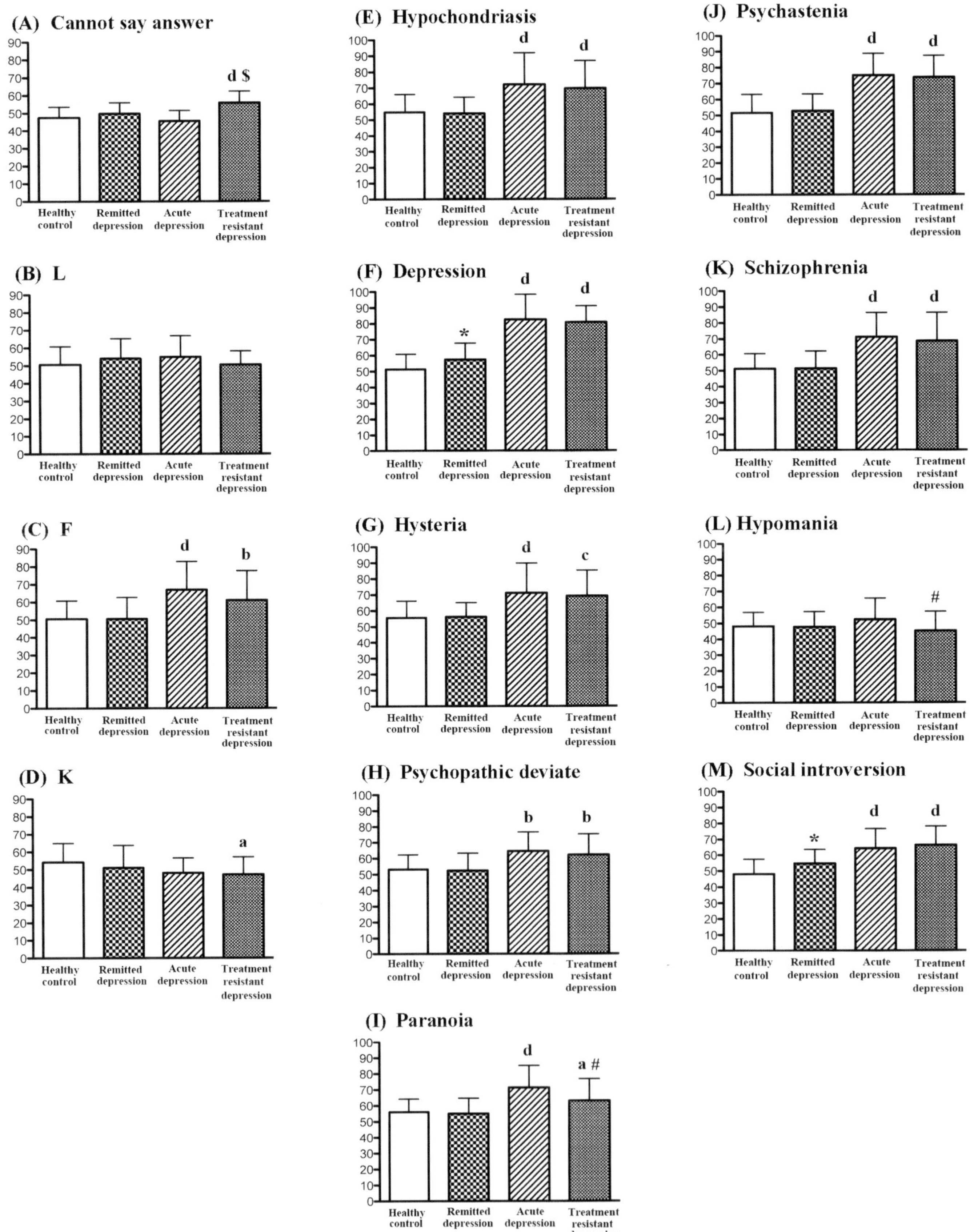
(A) Cannot say answer
d $
(B) L
(C) F
d
b
(D) K
a
(E) Hypochondriasis
d
d
(F) Depression
*
d
d
(G) Hysteria
d
c
(H) Psychopathic deviate
b
b
(I) Paranoia
d
a #
(J) Psychastenia
d
d
(K) Schizophrenia
d
d
(L) Hypomania
#
(M) Social introversion
*
d
d
0
10
20
30
40
50
60
70
80
90
100
Healthy control
Remitted depression
Acute depression
Treatment resistant depression

Figure 1. MMPI scales. Data are shown as mean ± SD. [a]p<0.05, [b]p<0.01, [c]p<0.001, [d]p<0.0001, as compared to the normal control group (ANOVA and post-hoc test). [$] p<0.0001 as compared to the acute depression group (ANOVA and post-hoc test). [#] P<0.05 as compared to the acute depression group (Student's t-test). * P<0.05 as compared to the normal control group (Student's t-test).

small depressive traits are present but masked in remitted depression patients, even though they scored less than 7 on HAM-D. This is supported by a recent study which found depressed outpatients who were deemed to be in remission according to HAM-D [19].

Our study demonstrated that when using the MMPI, criteria other than the depression scale were useful to understand the psychological status of depressed patients. The MMPI profile of depression is characterized by elevations on the depression, psychasthenia and schizophrenia scales [5,17]. The psychasthenia scale assesses ruminative worry and is called the anxious personality scale, indicating generalized feelings of anxiety and discomfort. The schizophrenia scale assesses cognitive confusion or bizarreness. A previous study using two-high scales proposed seven MMPI personality profiles in depressed inpatients, namely, depression plus schizophrenia, depression plus psychasthenia, depression plus psychopathic deviate, depression plus hysteria, schizophrenia plus psychopathic deviate, schizophrenia plus psychasthenia and schizophrenia plus hypomania [11], indicating

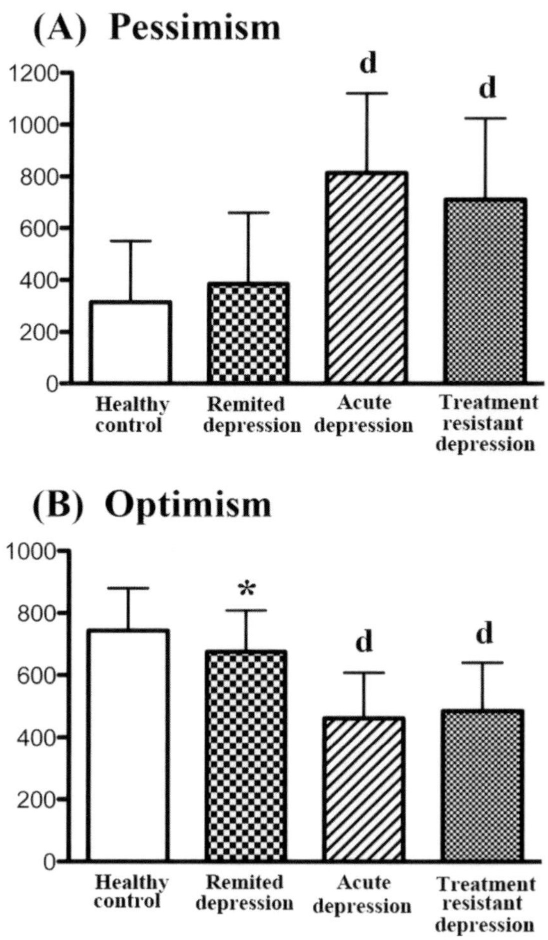

Figure 2. Pessimism and Optimism on the MMPI. Data are shown as mean ± SD. [d] p<0.0001 as compared to the normal control group (ANOVA and post-hoc test). * P<0.05 as compared to the normal control group (Student's t-test).

that depression and schizophrenia scales predominante psychopathic deviate or psychasthenia scales, and to a lesser extent, hysteria and hypomania scales, on the MMPI. Another study reported that psychopathic deviate plus schizophrenia scales were frequently found in depressed patients with personality disorders [10]. However, in our results, the depression scale took precedence over schizophrenia or psychasthenia, and to a lesser extent, hypochondriasis and hysteria in patients with acute and treatment-resistant depression (Figure 1).

Influence of neurotic based mechanisms was indicated by high scores in all three neurosis related MMPI profiles (hypochondriasis, depression and hysteria). Hypochondriasis assesses somatic complaints, while hysteria assesses a state of repression, low coping skills and excessive response to strong trauma. Hysteria correlates with a high body resistance. Patients with somatization disorder showed high hypochondriasis and hysteria compared with primary depression [20]. Another study reported differences between dysthymia and major depression for scales in hypochondriasis and hysteria, and to a lesser extent, depression, in the MMPI profile [9]. The theorized presence of neurotic mechanisms in patients with treatment-resistant depression seems to be justified, since these patients often feel frustrated with the difficulty of adhering to regular work or social schedules. This study demonstrated that the percentage of the neurotic triad evaluating all three items over 65 or 70 T was 71 and 47 percent in acutely depressed patients and 44 and 38 percent in patients with treatment-resistant depression, respectively. We found a statistically significant difference between patients with treatment-resistant depression and those with acute depression over 65 T (Chi-square 3.905, p = 0.0481), but not over 70 T. In contrast to our expectation, patients with treatment-resistant depression suffered equally or lower levels of neurotic pathophysiology, compared with those suffering acute depression.

A previous study demonstrated that psychopathic deviate plus paranoia, or psychopathic deviate plus hypomania at a T-score above 70 in the MMPI, met the criteria for personality dysfunction [21]. The psychopathic deviate scale indicates anti-social behavior, hostility or conflict. Here, the percentage of patients with a psychopathic deviate plus paranoia pattern over 65 or 70 T, was 42 and 33 percent in acutely depressed patients and 29 and 30 percent in patients with treatment-resistant depression respectively. The percentage of a psychopathic deviate plus hypomania pattern over 65 or 70 T was 6 percent in acutely depressed patients and 10 percent in patients with treatment-resistant depression, in both groups. These were no statistical differences between any of the two examined groups by Chi-square method.

The patients with treatment-resistant depression showed weak alterations on paranoia and hypomania scales compared to those with acute depression by Student's t-test (Figure 1). Since the paranoia scale assesses sensitivity to personal communication, low paranoia levels, although still above normal controls, indicate impaired sensitivity in personal communication. Low hypomania scores point to low activity. It is likely that patients with treatment-resistant depression exhibit low social activity, compared with acutely depressed patients.

For validity scales scores, ANOVA and post-hoc testing demonstrated that the cannot say answer scale was significantly increased in treatment-resistant depression patients, relative to acutely depressed patients (Figure 1). This seems to reflect enhanced difficulty in decisions making in this cohort, compared with other groups. Additionally, the K scale was significantly decreased in patients, but only in those with treatment-resistant depression (Figure 1). Since low K scores denote a tendency for self-criticism, patients with treatment-resistant depression appear to be introversive. However, F scales were significantly increased in both treatment-resistant and acute depression patients, compared with normal controls (Figure 1). The F scale is an atypical response and is thought to reflect an exaggeration of complaints, poor thinking ability or inattention. On this scale, patients with treatment-resistant depression are similar with those with acute depression.

Recently we reported on the psychological profiles of patients with treatment-resistant depression, namely, low scores for reward dependence and cooperativeness on the (Temperament and Character Inventory) TCI and low scores for openness on the NEO Personality Inventory, in contrast with depressed patients [22,23]. It is conceivable that these alterations share some relationship with our current results.

Patients in remitted depression showed significantly higher rises in depression or social introversion scores on the MMPI, compared with normal controls when evaluated by Student's t test, and a trend for significance by ANOVA and post-hoc testing (Figure 1). High social introversion assesses introversive tendencies or withdrawal. This is a unique characteristic of patients in remitted depression.

Looking at pessimism and optimism, patients with treatment-resistant and acute depression demonstrated higher pessimism and lower optimism than normal controls (Figure 2). Although the explanatory styles for pessimism and optimism in the two groups are different from normal controls, the degrees of alteration were not significantly different between the two groups, indicating similar levels in patients with treatment-resistant and acute disease. Therefore, these characteristics are not unique to patients with treatment-resistant depression.

Patients with remitted depression showed lower optimism compared with normal controls when evaluated by Student's t-test (Figure 2). The exact cause of this marginally lower optimism is unknown, but seems noteworthy. Our recent study revealed that patients in remitted depression who had suffered a single depressive episode, had higher scores of harm avoidance on the TCI, compared with healthy controls [22]. This lower optimism on the MMPI and higher harm avoidance on the TCI may well be interrelated pathological mechanisms in these patients.

Self-directedness on the TCI increased during remission from major depression [24]. Previous studies showed that patients with remitted depression exhibited low self-directedness as well as high harm avoidance on the TCI [25–27]. However, it is conceivable that these traits are related to the recurrence of depressive episodes since the remitted depression patients in these studies were characterized by recurrent episodes. Other studies on remitted depression with patients suffering single episodes, failed to show any changes using the Maudsley Personality Inventory [28] or the NEO [23]. Studies therefore should distinguish whether their remitted depression patients suffered single or recurrent episodes of depression. Considering these differences, the characteristics identified in this study using remitted patients after a single episode of depression, are unique and useful for future studies.

This study has a number of limitations. First, the study is of a cross-sectional design, making it difficult to accurately determine the degree to which a participant's depressed state influences their responses. In addition the recruits were volunteers with potentially limited generalisability. Also, there was no adjustment for potential confounding factors, such as gender difference, duration of treatment, duration of depressive state and education. This means that the independence of associations cannot be assumed, and that negative associations need to be viewed with caution because of the relatively small sample size. Finally, the remission and control groups differed in that the former groups had suffered, and received treatment for depression. It is therefore possible that the remitted group could still be experiencing sub-case symptomatology, since their depression scores fell between 3 and 7 on the HAM-D (Table 1).

In conclusion, there are subtle but important alterations on the MMPI, which may underpin the hidden psychological features of patients with both remitted and treatment-resistant depression.

Acknowledgments

The authors would like to thank Mrs. Minako Nagayo for her technical support.

Author Contributions

Conceived and designed the experiments: YS. Performed the experiments: MS MT KM KS YS. Analyzed the data: MS MT KM YS. Contributed reagents/materials/analysis tools: MT KS KH YS. Wrote the paper: KS KH YS.

References

1. Thase ME, Rush AJ (1995) Treatment-resistant depression. In F. E. . Bloom and D. J . Kupfer (EDs.), Psychopharmacology: the fourth generation of progress. New York: Raven Press. 1081–1097.
2. Souery D, Oswald P, Massat I, Bailer U, Bollen J, et al. (2007) Clinical factors associated with treatment resistance in major depressive disorder: results from a European multicenter study. J Clinical Psychiatry 68:1062–1070.
3. Hathaway SR, McKinley JC (1940) A multiphasic personality schdule (Minnesota): 1. Construction of the schedule. J Psychology 10:249–254.
4. Plutchik R, van Praag HM (1987) Interconvertability of five self-report measures of depression. Psychiatry Res 22:243–256.
5. Wetzler S, Kahn R, Strauman TJ, Dubro A (1989) Diagnosis of major depression by self-report. J Pers Asses 53:22–30.
6. Gross K, Keyes MD, Greene RL 2000) Assessing depression with the MMPI and MMPI-2. J Pers Assess 75:464–477.
7. Ganellen RJ (1996) Comparing the diagnostic efficiency of the MMPI, MMPI-II, and Rorschach: a review. J Pers Assess 67:219–243.
8. Wetzler S, Khadivi A, Oppenheim S (1995) The psychological assessment of depression: unipolars vesus bipolars. J Pers Asses 65:557–566.
9. Klonsky ED, Bertelson AD (2000) MMPI-2 clinical scale differences between dysthymia and major depression. Assessment 7:143–149.
10. Brems C (1991) Depression and personality disorder: differential diagnosis with the MMPI. J Clin Psychol 47:669–675.
11. Wetzler S, Marlowe DB, Sanderson WC (1994) Assessment of depression: using the MMPI, Millon, and Millon-II. Psychol Rep 75:755–768.
12. Colligan RC, Offord KP, Malinchoc M, Schulman P, Seligman MEP (1994) Caveing the MMPI for an optimism-pessimism scale: Seligman's attributional model and the assessment for explanatory style. J Clin Psychol 50 (1): 71–95.
13. Peterson C, Seligman ME (1984) Causal explanation as a risk factor depression: theory and evidence. Psychol Rev 91: 347–374.
14. Levenson JL, Bemis C (1991) The role of psychological factors in cancer onset and progression. Psychosomatics 32:124–132.
15. Grosssardt BR, Bower JH, Geda YE, Colligan RC, Rocca WA (2009) Pessimistic, anxious, and depressive personality traits predict all-cause mortality: the Mayo clinic cohort study of personality and aging. Psychosomatic Medicine 71:491–500.
16. American Psychiatric Association (1994) Diagnostic and Statistical Manual of Mental Disorders (4th ed., text rev): Washington, DC: American Psychiatric Press.
17. Moldin SO, Gottesman II, Erlenmeyer-Kimling L (1987) Psychometric validation of psychiatric diagnoses in the New York high-risk study. Psychiat Res 22:159–177.
18. Bagby RM, Marshall MB, Basso MR, Nicholson RA, Bacchiochi J, et al. (2005) Distinguishing bipolar depression, major depression, and schizophrenia with the MMPI-2 clinical and content scales. J Pers Assess 84:89–95.
19. Zimmerman M, Martinez JA, Attiullah N, Friedman M, Toba C, et al. (2012) Why do some depressed outpatients who are in remission according to the Hamilton depression rating scale not consider themselves to be in remission? J Clin Psychiatry 73:790–795.

20. Wetzel R, Brim J, Guze SB, CloningerRB, Martin RL, et al. (1999) MMPI screening scales for somatization disorder. Psychol Reports 85:341–348.
21. Norman WH, Keitner GI, Miller IW (1985) MMPI, personality dysfunction and the dexamethasone suppression test in major depression. J Affect Disord 9:97–101.
22. Takahashi M, Shirayama Y, Muneoka K, Suzuki M, Sato K, et al. (2013) Personality traits as possible risk factors for treatment-resistant depression. Plos One 8: e63756.
23. Takahashi M, Shirayama Y, Muneoka K, Suzuki M, Sato K, et al. (2013) Low openness on the NEO and its relationship with low reward dependence and cooperativeness on the TCI in the patients with treatment-resistant depression. Plos One 9: e71964.
24. Goekoop JG, De Winter RFP, Goekoop R (2011) An increase of the character of self-directedness is centrally involved in symptom reduction during remission from major depression. Depression Research and Treatment: 749640.
25. Richter J, Eisemann M, Richter G (2000) Temperament and character during the course of unipolar depression among inpatients. Eur Arch Psychiatry Clin Neurosci 250:40–47.
26. Smith DJ, Duffy L, Stewart ME, Muir WJ, Blackwood DH (2005) High harm avoidance and low self-directedness in euthymic young adults with recurrent, early-onset depression. J Affect Disord 87:83–89.
27. Nery FG, Hatch JP, Nicoletti MA, Monkul ES, Najt P, et al. (2009) Temperament and character traits in major depressive disorder: influence of mood state and recurrence of episodes. Depress Anxiety 26:382–388.
28. Shea MT, Leon AC, Mueller TI, Solomon DA, Warshaw MG, et al. (1996) Dose major depression result in lasting personality change? Am J Psychiatry 153:1404–1410.

10

Embryonic $GABA_B$ Receptor Blockade Alters Cell Migration, Adult Hypothalamic Structure, and Anxiety- and Depression-Like Behaviors Sex Specifically in Mice

Matthew S. Stratton[1], Michelle Staros[1], Tomaz Budefeld[2], Brian T. Searcy[1], Connor Nash[1], Chad Eitel[1], David Carbone[3], Robert J. Handa[3], Gregor Majdic[2], Stuart A. Tobet[1,4]*

1 Department of Biomedical Sciences, Colorado State University, Fort Collins, Colorado, United States of America, **2** Center for Animal Genomics, Veterinary Faculty, University of Ljubljana, Ljubljana, Slovenia, **3** Department of Basic Medical Sciences, University of Arizona College of Medicine, Phoenix, Arizona, United States of America, **4** School of Biomedical Engineering, Colorado State University, Fort Collins, Colorado, United States of America

Abstract

Neurons of the paraventricular nucleus of the hypothalamus (PVN) regulate the hypothalamic- pituitary-adrenal (HPA) axis and the autonomic nervous system. Females lacking functional $GABA_B$ receptors because of a genetic disruption of the R1 subunit have altered cellular characteristics in and around the PVN at birth. The genetic disruption precluded appropriate assessments of physiology or behavior in adulthood. The current study was conducted to test the long term impact of a temporally restricting pharmacological blockade of the $GABA_B$ receptor to a 7-day critical period (E11–E17) during embryonic development. Experiments tested the role of $GABA_B$ receptor signaling in fetal development of the PVN and later adult capacities for adult stress related behaviors and physiology. In organotypic slices containing fetal PVN, there was a female specific, 52% increase in cell movement speeds with $GABA_B$ receptor antagonist treatment that was consistent with a sex-dependent lateral displacement of cells *in vivo* following 7 days of fetal exposure to $GABA_B$ receptor antagonist. Anxiety-like and depression-like behaviors, open-field activity, and HPA mediated responses to restraint stress were measured in adult offspring of mothers treated with $GABA_B$ receptor antagonist. Embryonic exposure to $GABA_B$ receptor antagonist resulted in reduced HPA axis activation following restraint stress and reduced depression-like behaviors. There was also increased anxiety-like behavior selectively in females and hyperactivity in males. A sex dependent response to disruptions of $GABA_B$ receptor signaling was identified for PVN formation and key aspects of physiology and behavior. These changes correspond to sex specific prevalence in similar human disorders, namely anxiety disorders and hyperactivity.

Editor: Christine Jasoni, University of Otago, New Zealand

Funding: This work was funded by ORWH-NIMH P50 MH082679. The funders had no role in study design, data collection and analysis, decision to publish, or preparation of the manuscript.

Competing Interests: The authors have declared that no competing interests exist.

* Email: stuart.tobet@colostate.edu

Introduction

The formation of functional circuits in the developing brain depends on the orchestrated regulation of cellular developmental processes including cell division, signal induced cell death, cell migration, specification, axon outgrowth and connectivity. These processes are dependent on a combination of genetic programming and responses to external cues [1]. In the hypothalamus, the paraventricular nucleus (PVN) is the final common neuronal pathway for regulation of the hypothalamic - pituitary - adrenal (HPA) axis, which provides a key hormonal component of stress responses [2]. The neurons of the PVN also help regulate the autonomic nervous system and thereby, cardiovascular functions [3]. Dysregulation of the HPA axis has been implicated in human anxiety and depression related disorders, both of which display significant sex dependence [4].

In the fetal mouse brain, the developing PVN is surrounded by cellular elements containing high levels of the GABA synthesizing enzymes, glutamic acid decarboxylase (GAD) 65 and 67 (also referred to as GAD2 and 1, respectively in humans), as well as GABA itself. At the same time, cells within the developing PVN contain abundant amounts of GABA receptors [5]. The receptor expression pattern provides a basis for the hypothesis that GABA directs key developmental steps in this brain region. Previous work showed that disruption of the gene encoding the $GABA_B$ receptor led to altered protein expression and cell placement in and around the neonatal PVN [5,6]. In addition, embryonic treatment with a $GABA_A$ receptor antagonist (bicuculline) decreased the number of cells containing immunoreactive estrogen receptors (ER-alpha specifically) within the PVN, again in neonates [5]. The current study was designed to determine the role of $GABA_B$ receptor signaling on the formation of the PVN and potential adult consequences of blocking $GABA_B$ receptor signaling during embryonic development. The evidence for altered GABA signaling contributing to depression and anxiety disorders is growing (reviewed; [7–10]). There are decreased GABA concentrations in plasma [11], CSF and brain [12–14], and fewer GABA neurons in the orbitofrontal cortex of individuals with various forms of depression [15]. There are links for polymorphisms of the GAD 65 gene with anxiety behaviors in children [16] and of the GAD 67 gene with depression in women [17]. Also, GAD 67 is less abundant in the brains of patients with mood disorders relative to controls [18]. In animal models, disrupting GAD genes [19,20], $GABA_A$, or $GABA_B$ receptors [21–23] all cause anxiety-like phenotypes and some have been reported to cause changes in depression-like behavior. In these cases, even though the given mutations and chemical imbalances are present throughout development, results have been interpreted from the perspective of GABA acting in adults to regulate neuronal excitability without investigation of developmental processes.

Understanding fetal antecedents to adult diseases may provide key tools for diagnosis and treatment of many debilitating conditions [24]. The current work tested the effect of $GABA_B$ receptor blockade on acute cell movements in the embryonic PVN *ex vivo* and subsequent behavioral and physiological consequences of similar treatments that resulted in altered cell placements in and around the PVN. Pharmacological blockade was chosen for these studies to restrict the treatment to a critical fetal period and compare to prior work with a genetic disruption that is present throughout the lifespan.

Materials and Methods

Animals

B6.Cg-Tg (Thy1-YFP)16Jrs/J transgenic mice [25] were used for fluorescence video microscopy as described previously. The Thy-1 promoter drives YFP neuronal expression in the brain and allows for tracking of individual immature neurons in specific regions of the developing hypothalamus [26], including the PVN in the current study (e.g., figure 1A, C).

To block $GABA_B$ receptor activation during PVN development, time mated pregnant dams (C57BL/6J) were injected (s.c.) with 0.1 mg/kg CGP 55845 [27] (Tocris Biosciences) or vehicle (1% DMSO, 0.25% EtOH, PBS) daily from E11 through E17. Five pregnant dams were treated with CGP 55845 and five pregnant dams were treated with vehicle. Offspring were weaned at postnatal day (P) 19, assigned random numbers and marked by ear punch. At 11 weeks of age animals started behavior testing and restraint stress HPA axis activation testing. At the conclusion of testing animals were perfused through the heart with 4% paraformaldehyde and immunohistochemical analyses were conducted.

Ethics Statement

All experiments were carried out in accordance with the NIH Guide for the Care and Use of Laboratory Animals and approval of the Colorado State University Institutional Animal Care and Use Committee.

Fluorescence Video Microscopy

Fetal mice were taken at embryonic day (E) 13, a developmental age when the majority of cells destined to become part of the PVN have had their last mitotic event but have not yet completed their migration. Live slice preparations followed previously published methods [26,28]. Briefly, dissections were limited to a maximum of two hours to minimize cellular damage. Following each dissection, brains were embedded in 8% agarose and cut in a coronal plane at 250 μm in Krebs buffer using a vibrating microtome (Leica VT1000S). Slices that contained regions of the hypothalamus that included the PVN were chosen for video microscopy and were transferred to culture media (Hybernate-E; GIBCO-Invitrogen Corporation, Carlsbad, CA), with 2% pen-strep, and incubated at 36°C with 5% CO_2 for 30 minutes. Following the 30-minute

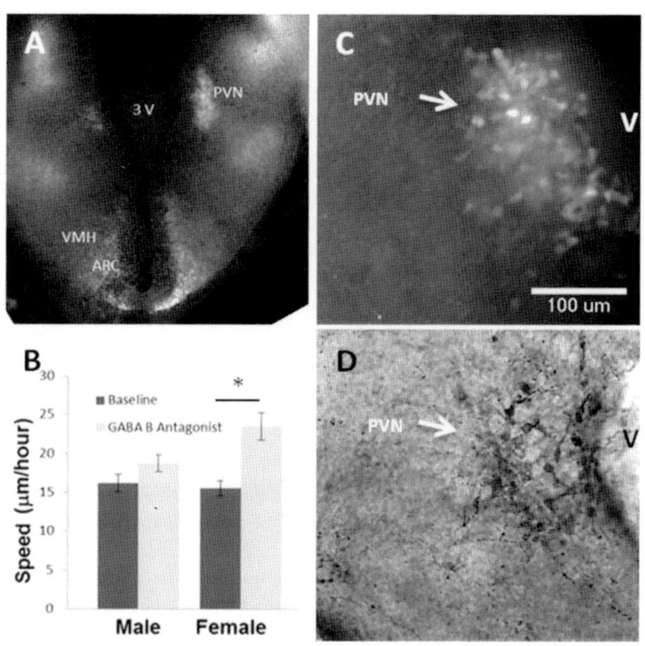

Figure 1. Effects of $GABA_B$ receptor antagonists 2 Hydroxy Saclofen and CGP 55845 on cell movements in *ex vivo* brain slice cultures. $GABA_B$ receptor antagonists caused cells in slices from female embryos, but not male embryos, to increase their speed of movement. Panel A shows a low magnification image of fluorescence in the hypothalamus of Thy1 YFP mice. Labeled neurons are also seen in the arcuate (ARC) and ventromedial nuclei (VMH). The data is summarized by sex and treatment in panel B, illustrating a significant effect of antagonists on rate of motion only for cells from slices taken from female embryos (statistically significant sex × treatment interaction, $p<0.05$). (C) Representative image of fluorescently labeled neurons in the developing PVN. A subset of slices was processed for CRH immunohistochemistry (D) to verify that video recordings were taken from developing PVN. (female n = 50 cells from 14 slices; male n = 34 cells from 16 slices).

incubation period, each slice was plated onto glass bottom dishes pre-coated by the manufacturer with poly-d-lysine (MatTek; P35G-0-20-C) and coated with an additional 1:1 dilution of Purecol (Advanced Biomatrix, San Diego, CA) and water. The slices were put back into the 36°C incubator for up to 30 minutes to promote adhesion. To prevent slice movement during video observation, 40 μL of a collagen solution (1 mL Purecol, 125 μL 10XMEM, 23 μL penicillin/streptomycin, and 33 μL 1 M sodium bicarbonate) was placed over each slice. The slices were then placed in the 36°C incubator for up to 1 hour to allow the Purcol to polymerize. 1 mL of Neurobasal media (10% L-glutamine, 2% B-27, 1.1% glucose, 2% pen-strep, 2% glutamine) was pipetted into each dish. The slices were maintained at 36°C and 5% CO_2 until use for video microscopy - as early as the following morning and as late as 2 days post plating.

In preparation for video microscopy, slices were washed with warm Neurobasal media (GIBCO-Invitrogen), and placed on a heated stage maintained at 37°C with 5% CO_2 with fresh Neurobasal medium. Data were collected using an inverted Nikon TE2000-U (Nikon USA, Melville, NY) microscope with a 20x plan Apo phase objective (0.75 na) or an upright Olympus BX61W (Olympus America, Center Valley, PA) microscope with an XLUM PLAN FLN-W 20x objective (1.0 na). Cells expressing yellow fluorescent protein (YFP) were imaged using Metamorph software (Molecular Devices Inc., Sunnyvale, CA). At least 1.5 hours of baseline video microscopy was taken before the addition of $GABA_B$ receptor antagonists, 2-hydroxy saclofen ([29]; Sigma-Aldrich, St. Louis, MO) or CGP 55845 ([30]; Tocris Biosciences, Bristol, UK). Then an additional 1.5 hours of video was taken to compare baseline to treatments. Vehicle was used to serve as an additional control. E13 embryos have only 1 or 2, sections that contain developing PVN when sectioned at 250 μm.

Immunohistochemistry

Immunohistochemistry was performed as previously reported [6]. Briefly, fixed tissue was embedded in 5% agarose and cut into coronal 50 μm thick sections using a vibrating microtome (Leica VT1000S). Alternating sections were collected in 0.05 M phosphate buffered saline (PBS), pH 7.5. Excess unreacted aldehyde was neutralized using a 30-minute incubation in 0.1 M glycine and 15 minutes in 0.5% sodium borohydride in PBS. After washing the tissue sections in PBS the sections were incubated in a PBS blocking solution containing 5% normal goat serum, 0.3% Triton-X 100 (Tx) and 1% hydrogen peroxide for 60 minutes at 4°C. Tissue was then incubated in primary antisera containing 1% bovine serum albumin (BSA) and 0.3%Tx over 2 nights at 4°C. Primary antisera were used at a 1:10,000 dilution (rabbit anti-ERα; C1355, Upstate Biotechnology, Charlottesville, VA) or a 1:5,000 dilution (rabbit anti-cFOS; sc-52, Santa Cruz Biotechnology, Santa Cruz, CA). Anti-rabbit secondary antiserum was diluted to 1:2500 (Rabbit IgG-fab fragment; Jackson Immunoresearch, West Grove, PA). Sections were washed at room temperature in PBS containing 1% normal goat serum and 0.02% Tx then incubated at room temperature in secondary antisera buffer containing 1% normal goat serum and 0.32% Tx with a biotin conjugated anti-rabbit secondary diluted to 1:2500 (Rabbit IgG-fab fragment; Jackson Immunoresearch, West Grove, PA). Sections were developed using a Vectastain ABC Elite kit (Vector Laboratories; Burlingame, CA) for 1 hour at room temperature and then exposed for 5 minutes to a solution containing 0.025% diaminobenzidine with 0.02% nickel ammonium sulfate and 0.02% H_2O_2 diluted in tris-buffered saline (pH 7.5).

Radioimmunoassay (RIA)

Blood was collected via the tail vain at the start of restraint stress (placement in a 50 ml plastic conical tube) and after 30 minutes of restraint stress. Plasma corticosterone concentrations were measured by RIA. Plasma samples were diluted 1:25 in 0.01 M PBS, and corticosterone binding globulin was denatured by incubating the samples at 65°C for one hour. All samples and standards were then incubated overnight at 4°C in the presence of antiserum (MP Biomedicals, Solon OH) and [3H] corticosterone (Perkin- Elmer, Boston, MA) in 0.1% gelatin dissolved in 0.01 M PBS. Unbound corticosterone was removed by adding dextran-coated charcoal, which was then separated by centrifugation. Bound corticosterone was decanted into new vials, mixed with scintillation fluid, and counted using a Beckman Coulter LS6500 Multipurpose Scintillation Counter (Brea, CA). Plasma corticosterone concentrations were determined by comparison to a standard curve (5–700 ng/ml). The intra-assay variance was 3.26%, and was determined by an internal control that was measured at regular intervals throughout the assay.

Analysis

Images of the PVN were carefully matched by an investigator blinded to treatment condition to ensure that the same section (relative to rostral-caudal location) was used in analyses for each animal. Images of sections containing immunoreactive ERα were normalized for optimal contrast in Adobe Photoshop (version CS for Macintosh) and immunoreactive area above threshold (not densitometry) was quantified in IP Lab Imaging software (Scanalytics Inc., part of BD Biosciences, Rockville, MD) as reported previously [5]. Eight 100 μm (width) × 500 μm (height) columns were placed over the images starting 100 μm lateral from the edge of the ventricle (to eliminate impact of an immunoreactive edge artifact) and 200 μm above the top of the ventricle. Cells containing immunoreactive ERα were selected for in vivo cell placement analysis due to their sensitivity to displacement in previous studies and because their clearly identifiable cell bodies/nuclei were amenable to quantification. Other immunoreactive components of the PVN (i.e. vasopressin or corticotropin releasing factor) were not selected for cell placement analysis due complications of immunoreactive content in axons and dendrites relative to the placement of cell bodies. For FOS analysis, an investigator manually counted FOS immunoreactive cell nuclei in the PVN (both left and right sides) from two sections per animal in the mid-region of the PVN.

For analysis of the distribution of ERα immunoreactive cells, significance was determined by three way ANOVA analyzing Sex × Treatment × Location (columns as a repeated measure) with SPSS software (SPSS Inc., Chicago, IL). See results section for additional detail on posthoc analyses.

For all behavior testing and HPA axis activation assessment, sex differences in response to CGP 55845 were determined by analyzing the Sex × Treatment interaction in two-way ANOVAs along with examining the main effects of sex and treatment. Once an overall significance was established via ANOVA, posthoc group differences were based on non-overlapping 95% confidence intervals. All data are expressed as mean±SEM.

Behavior Testing

Behavior testing (details in supplemental material) started when mice were approximately 11 weeks of age. Females were tested while in estrus as determined by primarily cornified epithelial cells in the vaginal cytology. Animals were handled for two weeks prior to the start of testing and for two days before each individual test. The testing order was Elevated Plus Maze, Open Field, Tail

Suspension, Forced Swim (Figure S1 in file S1), Sucrose Preference, and Restraint Stress for each animal. Except for the sucrose preference test, the testing order was least stressful to most stressful. Sucrose preference test was assessed after forced swim testing because animals must be housed individually to measure individual fluid intake. The intention was to avoid confounding effects of social isolation and/or re-socialization for the rest of the behavior tests. Restraint stress was assessed last so that FOS activation could be quantified via immunohistochemistry at an acute time point following restraint stress. Tests were conducted during the same 4-hour window each day (11:00 am–3:00 pm) in the light phase of the animal's daily cycle. Tests were spaced at least 4 days apart for each animal. During each testing day the order of animal testing (i.e. sex and treatment) was randomized. Analysis was blinded through a random animal numbering system. Thirty-six animals were behavior tested and each group consisted of offspring from at least three different nulliparous dams. Specific numbers of animals that were included in each analysis are reported in the appropriate figure legends.

Results

Ex Vivo cell movement with $GABA_B$ receptor blockade

To determine the effect of $GABA_B$ receptor antagonists on cell movement in the developing PVN, mouse embryos were harvested on E13 and organotypic slices containing fluorescently labeled neurons in the developing PVN (Figure 1A, 1C) were maintained in vitro. Blockade of $GABA_B$ receptors in these brain slices resulted in increased rates of cell movement in the developing PVN in a sex specific manner (Figure 1B). Cells in organotypic slices from female but not male embryos increased their speed (μm/h) of migration by 52% following $GABA_B$ receptor antagonist treatment compared to baseline movement (female baseline = 15.6±0.93 female antagonist = 23.5±1.7, Sex × Treatment ANOVA $F(1,82) = 5.56$, $p<0.05$) (male baseline = 16.21±1.16, male antagonist = 18.7±1.08) (Figure 1B). Immunoreactive vasopressin and corticotropin releasing hormone (CRH) provided posthoc evidence that sections chosen for video microscopy contained authentic PVN (e.g., Figure 1D). The speed of cell movements were affected similarly regardless of which $GABA_B$ receptor antagonist was used (no significant difference between 1 μM CGP55845 and 20 μM 2-hydroxy saclofen). Vehicle treatment did not alter cell movement speeds (Supplemental table S1 in file S1).

In Vivo cell placement following fetal $GABA_B$ receptor blockade

Cells containing immunoreactive ERα were present in the PVN in a pattern extending laterally from the third ventricle to juxtaparaventricular and perifornical areas [31,32]. A pilot experiment examined the placement of cells containing immunoreactive ERα at birth following embryonic treatment with CGP 55845 (data not shown). The results provided a positive basis to continue raising the cohort of mice that were tested for behavior and ultimately analyzed for immunoreactive ERα in adulthood (see below).

Fetal treatment with the $GABA_B$ receptor antagonist CGP 55845 reproduced in adults the phenotype seen previously in the neonatal $GABA_B$ R1 subunit knockout mouse [5]. In female offspring from mothers treated with CGP 55845 there was a lateral shift in the distribution of cells containing immunoreactive ERα toward juxtaparaventricular and perifornical areas (Figure 2D–F). There was no difference in the positions of cells in males from the same litters (figure 2A–C). In the most medial column quantified, females treated with CGP 55845 had 71% less immunoreactivity compared to controls while in the two most lateral columns quantified, females treated with CGP 55845 had 60% more immunoreactivity compared to vehicle treated animals (Sex × Treatment × Location as a repeated measure; $F(7,154) = 3.20$, $p<0.05$). To determine to what extent the significant 3-way interaction was due selectively to females versus males, orthogonal contrasts were run for each sex individually in a Treatment × Location as repeated measure posthoc analysis. There was statistical significance in females ($F(7,154) = 5.28$, $p<0.01$), but not males ($F(7,154) = 0.46$, $p = 0.86$).

Increased anxiety-like behavior in female offspring of mothers treated with $GABA_B$ receptor antagonist

Adult offspring of dams treated with CGP 55845 or vehicle were subjected to the elevated plus maze test to assess anxiety-like behavior [33]. Female offspring of CGP 55845 treated mothers showed significantly increased anxiety-like behavior. This was indicated by decreased time in the open arms of an elevated plus maze (ratio of time spent in open arm divided by time spent in any arm; Figure 3A, vehicle = 0.31±0.04, CGP 55845 = 0.158±0.04; Figure 3A). Male offspring of fetal CGP 55845 treated mothers showed increased time in the open arms (Figure 3A, vehicle = 0.11±0.02; CGP 55845 = 0.23±0.04), which may be indicative of decreased anxiety-like behavior. The sex difference in the effect of exposure to fetal CGP exposure was established by a statistically significant Sex × Treatment interaction ($F(1,31) = 12.50$, $p<0.05$).

To interpret a finding of increased time in open arms as less "anxiety-like" behavior one must control for total activity of the animals. The increased time in the open arms in male offspring of CGP treated mothers was accompanied by a trend toward an increased total number of arm entries. This suggested increased activity (entries vehicle = 12.4±0.86; CGP 55845 = 15.6±1.2), although there was no significant main effect of treatment or Sex × Treatment interaction. Male open arm ratios and male total arm entries were significantly correlated ($R = 0.688$, $p<0.005$). Overall, females were more active than males in the EPM as indicated by more arm entries (female vehicle = 16.0±1.2; male vehicle = 12.4±0.86; $F(1,31) = 4.4$, $p<0.05$).

Increased activity in adult male offspring of mothers treated with $GABA_B$ receptor antagonist

The apparent male hyperactivity indicated by arm entries in the elevated plus maze with embryonic $GABA_B$ receptor blockade was confirmed by analyzing animal mobility in an open field (Figure 3C, D). Total time spent mobile, latency to immobility (Figure S2 in file S1) and number of immobile episodes were quantified using Anymaze software (Stoelting Co.). There was a 45% decrease in time spent immobile in male offspring of CGP 55845 treated mothers relative to controls (Figure 3C, immobile time male vehicle = 98.9±10.7; male CGP 55845 = 53.9±16.6) without significant main effects of treatment or sex due to variability within the females. However, when males were analyzed alone in a two tailed T test, statistical significance was attained when comparing vehicle and CGP 55845 treatment ($p<0.05$). Also, male offspring from mothers treated with CGP 55845 showed significantly increased latency to immobility (latency in seconds: male vehicle = 45.1±12.8; male CGP 55845 = 125.9±29.2; Sex × Treatment ANOVA $F(1,32) = 7.57$, $p<0.05$) and significantly decreased immobile episodes relative to controls (Figure 3D, male vehicle = 23.7±2.5, male CGP 55845 = 11.7±2.8; Sex × Treatment ANOVA $F(1,32) = 12.4$,

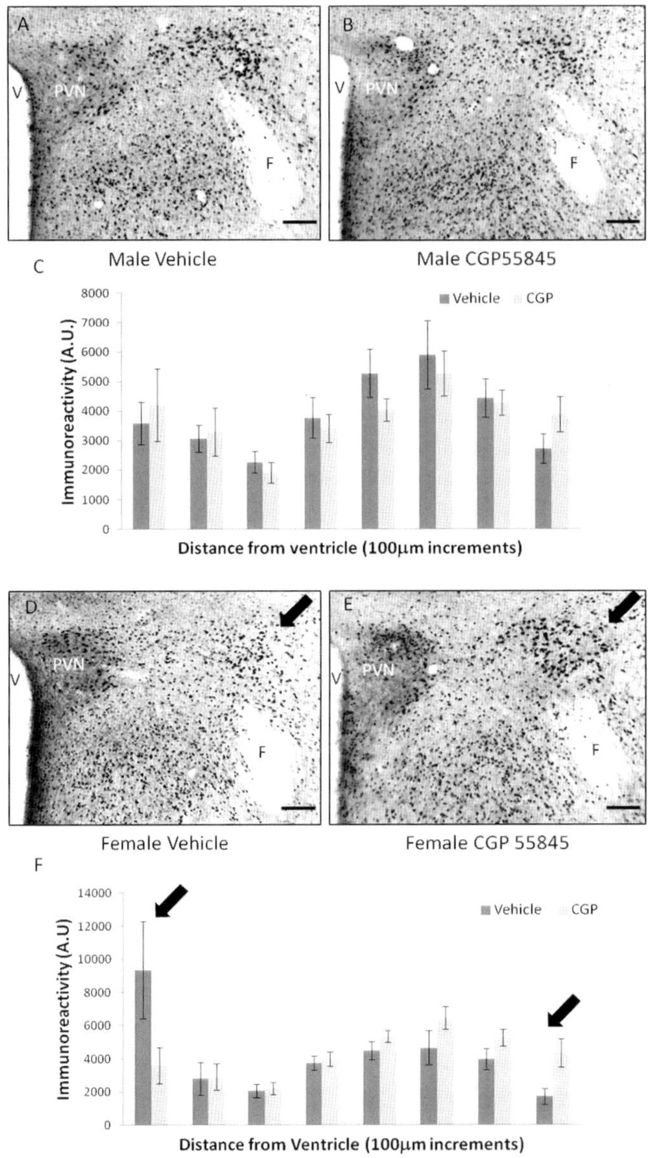

Figure 2. Distribution of cells containing immunoreactive ERα in the region of the PVN. When mothers were treated with CGP 55845, male offspring (Panels A–C) had no difference in the position of immunoreactive ERα containing cells (B) relative to vehicle treated controls (A). The distribution of immunoreactive cells relative to distance from the third ventricle is shown quantitatively in panel C. In female offspring of mothers treated with vehicle (Panels D,F) a large number of immunoreactive cells were concentrated close to the third ventricle (V). By contrast, when mothers were treated with CGP 55845, female offspring (Panel E,F) had fewer cells noted in medal positions and more cells were located in positions lateral to the paraventricular nucleus (PVN) and closer to the perifornical area (black arrows). Post hoc analysis revealed that CGP 55845 selectively shifted this immunoreactivity in females (medial to lateral indicated by black arrows panel F) ($p<0.05$). F in panels A, B, D, E = fornix, scale bars represent 200 μm. ($n=6$ vehicle male, $n=7$ CGP 55845 male, $n=6$ vehicle female, $n=7$ CGP 55845 female).

$p<0.05$). This suggests that fetal $GABA_B$ receptor blockade resulted in the male offspring growing up to be hyperactive. There was no indication of an effect of fetal CGP treatment on female activity. As detailed in the supplemental material and methods section, the dimensions of the open box used for activity assessment was smaller than that needed for an appropriate anxiety-like behavior assessment by analysis of time spent on the box's interior vs time spent on the perimeter. Consequently, anxiety-like behavior was not assessed in this open field test.

Less depression-like behavior adult offspring of mothers treated with $GABA_B$ receptor antagonist

To assess the impact of developmental inhibition of $GABA_B$ receptors on adult depression-like behavior, a tail suspension test was used. This test quantifies an animal's "efforts" to fight/struggle out of what for most is an inescapable situation [33]. Mice are suspended by their tail for a period of five minutes and the time spent struggling and time spent motionless is counted. Male and female offspring of mothers treated with CGP 55845 displayed less depression-like behavior as indicated by shorter immobile times and increased struggling (Figure 4A). In females, time spent immobile was 66% less (female vehicle = 123.0±9.7;

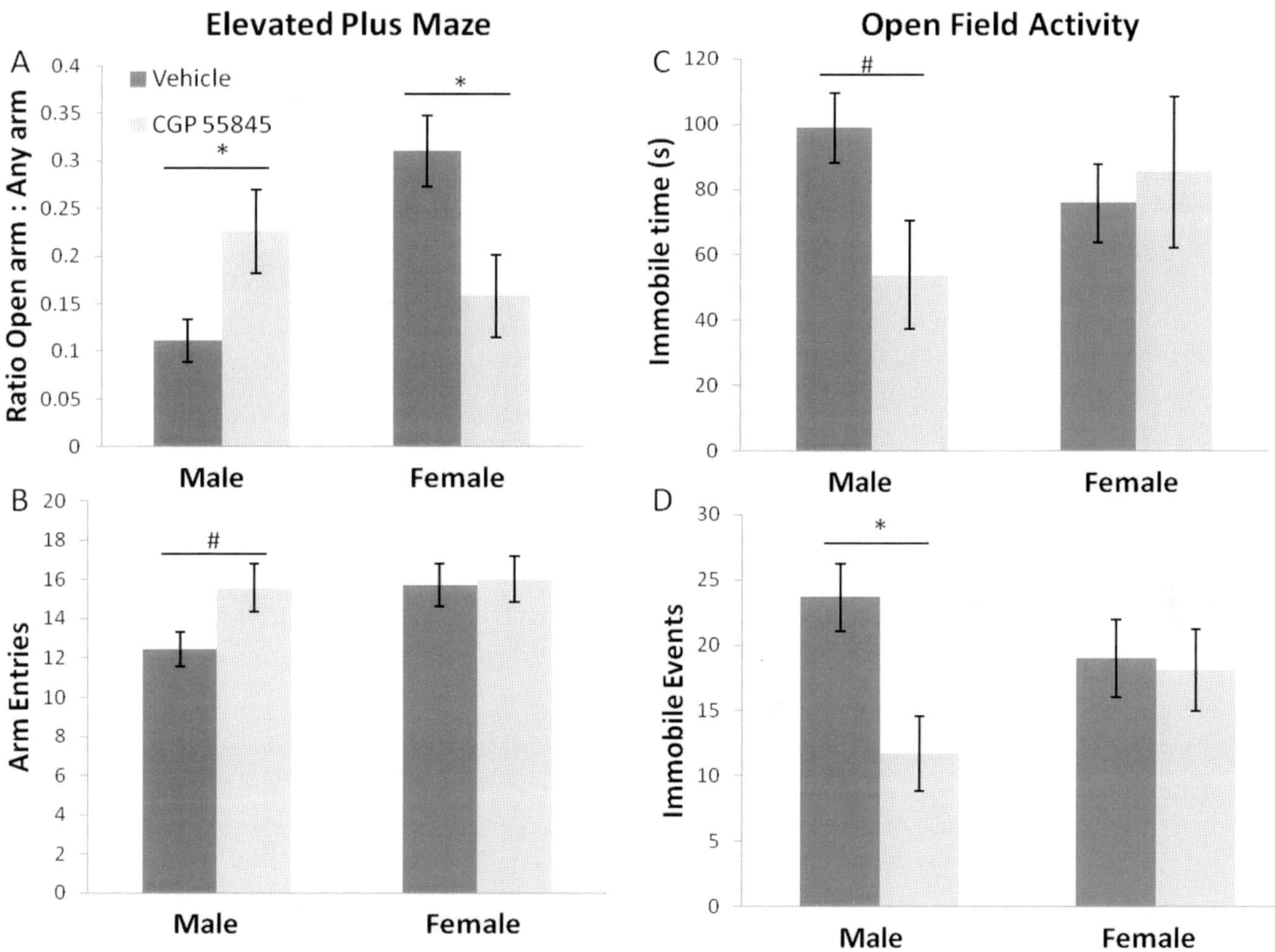

Figure 3. Anxiety- and hyperactivity-like behaviors: Elevated Plus Maze and activity in an Open Field. Panel A depicts the open arm ratio of the Elevated Plus Maze test (time in open arms divided by time spent in any of the four arms), while panel B depicts the total number of arm entries for the elevated plus maze test. Female offspring of mothers treated with CGP 55845 spent less time in the open arm compared to vehicle controls. Male offspring of mothers treated with CGP 55845 showed increased open arm ratio and an increased trend in number of arm entries (n = 9 vehicle male, n = 7 CGP 55845 male, n = 11 vehicle female, n = 9 CGP 55845 female). As measures of activity in an 'open-field', time spent immobile (C) and number of immobile events (D) were quantified. Male offspring from mothers treated with CGP 55845 during pregnancy displayed a hyperactivity-like phenotype that was most obvious for the number of immobile events (D). Males also showed decreased latency to immobility with embryonic exposure to the $GABA_B$ receptor antagonist (see text) and a trend toward decreased time spent immobile. There were no obvious treatment effects on the activity of females (n = 9 vehicle male, n = 7 CGP 55845 male, n = 11 vehicle female, n = 9 CGP 55845 female). (*indicates non-overlapping 95% confidence interval following significant treatment effect or significant Sex × Treatment interaction).

female CGP 55845 = 73.9±10.9) with fetal exposure to CGP 55845 while in males immobile time was 14% less (male vehicle = 147.7±11.2; male CGP 55845 = 129.2±13.4). There was a significant main effect of fetal treatment ($F(1,27) = 8.67$, $p < 0.05$) and a significant main effect of sex ($F(1,27) = 12.17$, $p < 0.05$). The Sex × Treatment interaction was not statistically significant, suggesting that male and female offspring were similarly affected by fetal treatment with CGP 55845. Nonetheless, the effect in females was almost 5 times larger than the effect in males and male 95% confidence intervals did overlap. Three males and two females "climbed their tails" and were excluded from this analysis on that basis. Interestingly, tail climbing was found only in the vehicle treated group.

Less anhedonic/more hedonic-like behavior in adult offspring of mothers treated with $GABA_B$ receptor antagonist

Depression- and anhedonic-like behavior was assessed using a sucrose preference test (Figure 4B). This test measures an animal's pleasure seeking behavior by measuring its consumption of plain water compared to water sweetened with sucrose. Typically, when the constellation of depression-like behavior is increased, animals show no or reduced preference for sucrose over plain water which is interpreted as animals not going out of their way to seek pleasure [33]. Fetal exposure of males and females to CGP 55845 resulted in increased preference for 1% sucrose solution versus water (Treatment effect $F(1,31) = 6.9$, $p < 0.05$, with no Treatment × Sex interaction). The ratio of sucrose consumption to water consumption increased 70% from 1.84 for offspring of vehicle treated mothers to 3.18 for offspring of CGP 55845 treated mothers.

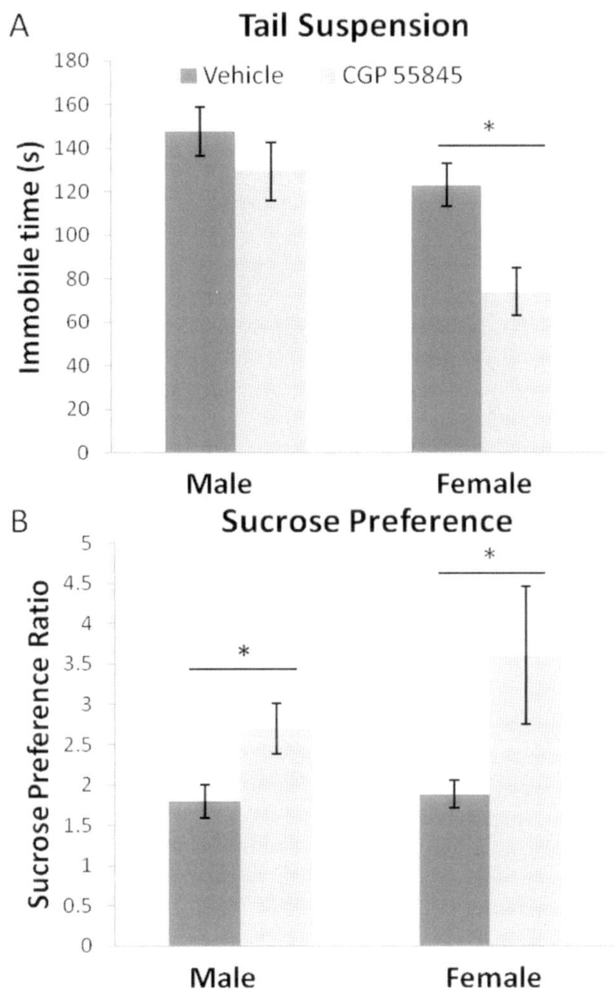

Figure 4. Measures of depression-like behavior: tail suspension and sucrose preference tests. Panel A shows that CGP 55845 treatment during pregnancy caused decreased immobility in the tail suspension test. However, only in females did the 95% confidence intervals not overlap (n = 6 vehicle male, n = 7 CGP 55845 male, n = 9 vehicle female, n = 9 CGP 55845 female). Panel B shows that male and female offspring exposed to fetal CGP 55845 had increased sucrose preference (n = 9 vehicle male, n = 7 CGP 55845 male, n = 11 vehicle female, n = 9 CGP 55845 female). (*indicates non overlapping 95% confidence intervals following significant main effect of treatment).

Decreased adult HPA axis activation in adult offspring of mothers treated with $GABA_B$ receptor antagonist

The neuronal responses in the HPA axis to stress were assessed using short-term physical restraint. One hour after release from restraint stress, neuronal activation in the PVN as indicated by immunoreactive Fos was markedly attenuated (31%) in offspring of mothers that were treated with $GABA_B$ receptor antagonist relative to vehicle controls (Figure 5C; main effect of treatment $F(1,12) = 8.5$, $p<0.05$). This occurred similarly in males and females as there was no statistically significant Treatment × Sex interaction.

Plasma corticosterone was measured after restraint stress to assess neuroendocrine output of the HPA axis (Figure 5D). At the start of restraint stress (time 0), female corticosterone values were significantly higher than in males (male = 10.3±3.5, female = 24.6±3.4) based on the main effect of sex ($F(1,29) = 8.46$, $p<0.05$) without a Sex × Treatment interaction. After 30 minutes of restraint stress, offspring of dams treated with CGP 55845 displayed a blunted stress response as indicated by decreased plasma corticosterone levels relative to vehicle treated controls (vehicle = 163.0±13.1, CGP 55845 = 121.9±15.0). There was a significant main effect of treatment ($F(1,31) = 4.3$, $p<0.05$) without a Sex × Treatment interaction.

Discussion

In the current study, treatment of pregnant mice with a $GABA_B$ receptor antagonist for a restricted period resulted in offspring that had altered cell positions within and around the PVN. The same animals displayed a general pattern of increased anxiety-like behavior in females and increased hyperactivity in males along with decreased stress response and decreased depression-like behavior in both sexes (although tending toward greater effects in females). Genetic and environmental influences combine in the developing fetus to contribute to an individual's ability to respond to stressors as an adult and the likelihood of developing pathology as a result of stress [24]. The results of the current study suggest that 1) GABA can act through $GABA_B$ receptors to impact cell migration in the PVN of females selectively, and 2) that time-restricted maternal treatment with $GABA_B$ receptor antagonist can alter the behaviors of adult offspring in ways that are directly related to animal models for human psychiatric disorders.

Direct application of $GABA_B$ receptor antagonists caused neurons in the PVNs of organotypic slices from females ex vivo to increase their speed of movement. An *in vivo* correlate was seen as a lateral shift in the location of cells containing immunoreactive ERα from within the PVN to the perifornical area in adult female offspring of mothers treated with $GABA_B$ receptor antagonist. The shift following fetal CGP treatment created a neuroanatomical phenocopy of a $GABA_B$ R1 subunit knockout mouse in terms of changing the distribution of cells containing immunoreactive ERα in the PVN and juxtaparaventricular and perifornical areas [5]. The in vitro results are consistent with the in vivo results being a function of direct $GABA_B$ antagonism in the fetus as opposed to an influence of $GABA_B$ antagonism in the mother that then secondarily impacts the fetus. Taken together this provides additional evidence consistent with a hypothesis that GABA restricts cell migration for some neurons so that they remain within the PVN during fetal development. It is also an interesting complementary finding to studies in which prenatal stress has been shown to alter the migration of GABAergic neurons in the developing cerebral cortex [34]. Thus GABA may influence migration of other cells on the one hand in some places (e.g., PVN this study; [35,36]) and GABAergic cells may be influenced by other fetal factors in other places (e.g., cerebral cortex, [34,37]).

The perifornical region is part of the hypothalamic area controlling emotional responses (HACER) in the primate [38] and is involved in the regulation of cardiovascular responses to emotions [39]. This region has also been implicated in aggressive behaviors and autonomic cardiovascular responses [40,41]. Estradiol can enhance the sensitivity of PVN CRH neurons in the HPA response to stress [42]. The lateral population of cells containing immunoreactive ERα is comprised of approximately 70% GABAergic neurons with projections to the PVN in the adult rat. Estradiol can block glucocorticoid dependent negative feedback on the PVN via ERα signaling in the perifornical region [43]. This lateral population of ERα containing cells may be part of the limbic inputs that exert an inhibitory tone on the PVN [44]. Changing the position or levels of ERα could change the ability of estrogens to modulate the HPA axis.

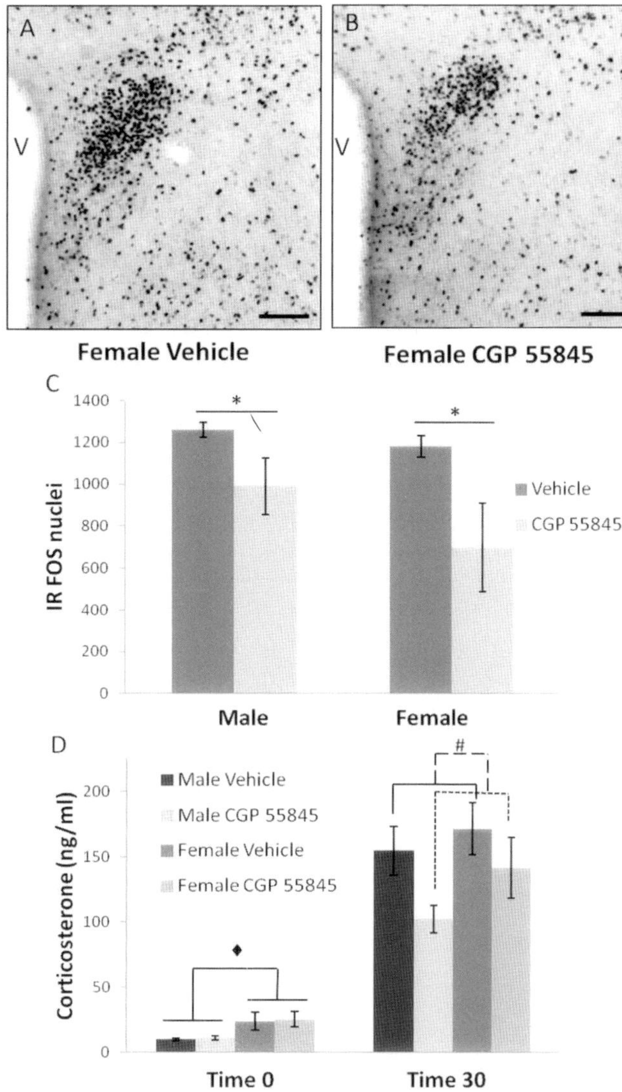

Figure 5. HPA axis output following acute stress. Immunoreactive Fos in the PVN one hour after release from restraint, vehicle treated (A) and CGP 55845 treated (B) female mice. Adult offspring of mothers treated with CGP 55845 during pregnancy had less immunoreactive Fos in the PVN one hour after release from restraint stress compared to controls in both males and females (C; n = 4 vehicle male, n = 4 CGP 55845 male, n = 4 vehicle female, n = 4 CGP 55845 female). At baseline, females had increased plasma corticosterone relative to males. After 30 minutes of restraint stress, offspring from mothers treated with CGP 55845 had blunted stress responses indicated by a smaller increase in corticosterone concentration relative to vehicle treated controls (D) (*indicates non overlapping 95% confidence intervals following significant main effect of treatment; ♦ indicates significant main effect of sex; # indicates significant main effect of treatment; V = 3rd ventricle, scale bars represent 200 μm).

Why the developing PVN appears to be more dependent on $GABA_B$ signaling in females than in males remains an open question. The simplest explanation would be that there are sex differences in the GABA concentration seen by the developing PVN or in the distribution of $GABA_B$ receptors in the developing PVN. A preliminary survey of $GABA_B$ R1 subunit immunoreactivity in embryonic mice suggested no difference in $GABA_B$ R1 protein expression between the sexes in the PVN (Stratton and Tobet, unpublished observations). While sex differences in concentrations of GABA have been reported, the studies have either been in adult or early postnatal animals, and PVN was contained in tissue blocks that also contained other hypothalamic nuclei [45,46].

Adult offspring of mothers treated with CGP 55845 displayed more anxiety-like behavior and less depressive-like behaviors if they were female. In male offspring from the same litters, there was a hyperactivity-like phenotype and less depressive-like behavior. These findings suggest that the same insult (maternal exposure to $GABA_B$ receptor antagonist) may result in the phenotype of a female predominant disorder in females (anxiety) and the phenotype of a male predominant disorder in males (hyperactivity). Previous studies using $GABA_B$ receptor knockout mice that could be raised to adulthood also reported increased anxiety and antidepressant-like behavior, but without any sex dependence [47]. Importantly, these studies taken together indicate that the behavioral phenotypes seen in mice lacking functional $GABA_B$ receptors (throughout the life span) may be explained at least in part by brain patterning effects of GABA during embryonic development.

Cells of the PVN provide the ultimate output regulation for the HPA axis modulating the hormonal response to stress. Anxiety- and depressive-like behaviors in animal models can be manifested as a result of manipulating the HPA axis and increasing circulating levels of CRH [48]. The importance of the PVN and the HPA axis as it relates to anxiety-related disorders has also been suggested in human studies [49–51]. In the current study, maternal treatment with a $GABA_B$ receptor antagonist resulted in offspring with altered cytoarchitecture in the region of the PVN and this altered cytoarchitecture correlated with altered anxiety- and depression-like behaviors. Unfortunately, a direct cause and effect relationship cannot be drawn as the entire developing embryo was exposed to the CGP 55845 compound. Many brain regions contribute to anxiety- and depression-like behaviors [52] and it was not feasible to assay each of them to determine if CGP 55845 administration altered their cellular or chemoarchitecture.

Despite the blunted stress response in both sexes, females showed increased anxiety-like behavior in the elevated plus maze. This apparent disparity may be related to the timing and relative stressful nature of the tests. For instance the stress response was measured with corticosterone concentrations after 30 minutes of stress (similar longer term measurement for Fos) while the elevated plus maze was conducted over 5 minutes and did not involve an acute stressor other than minor handling and the presence of open and elevated platforms. This highlights the complexities of the ontogeny of diseases like anxiety and depression and the shortcomings of current rodent behavior models in capturing realistic correlates of human disease. Of course other brain regions also likely impact rodent performance in elevate plus mazes [53]. Nonetheless, the increased anxiety-like behavior and decreased depression-like behavior replicated phenotypes seen in $GABA_B$ receptor knockout mice [8]. The importance lies in the suggestion that the loss of $GABA_B$ signaling may be most critical during a restricted fetal period rather than throughout life.

In summary, the results of the current study are consistent with the hypothesis that GABA acts through $GABA_B$ receptors to direct cell migration in the developing female PVN and that altered $GABA_B$ receptor signaling during development has life long, and possibly sex specific consequences for physiology and behavior [54]. Identifying and understanding fetal antecedents to adult psychiatric disorders will greatly enhance the ability to develop prevention and treatment strategies specific to sex, genotype and known environmental conditions (e.g., fetal and maternal stress, infection, medications; [55]).

Acknowledgments

We would like to thank Drs. Klemens Kaupmann and Stephan Urwyler for advice regarding $GABA_B$ receptor antagonists. We thank Dr. Jill Goldstein for comments during the course of the project.

Author Contributions

Conceived and designed the experiments: MSS SAT DC GM RJH BTS. Performed the experiments: MSS GM SAT CN MS DC TB BTS. Analyzed the data: MSS GM SAT CN MS DC TB. Contributed reagents/materials/analysis tools: CE GM RJH. Wrote the paper: MSS SAT.

References

1. Dodd J, Kolodkin AL (2005) Development: Edging towards circuitry, behavior and disease. Curr Opin Neurobiol. 15: 1–6.
2. Pyner S (2009) Neurochemistry of the paraventricular nucleus of the hypothalamus: implications for cardiovascular regulation. J Chem Neuroanat 38: 197–208.
3. Ferguson AV, Latchford KJ, Samson WK (2008) The paraventricular nucleus of the hypothalamus - a potential target for integrative treatment of autonomic dysfunction. Expert Opin Ther Targets. 12(6): 717–27.
4. Kessler RC, McGonagle KA, Swartz M, Blazer DG, Nelson CB (1993) Sex and depression in the National Comorbidity Survey. I: Lifetime prevalence, chronicity and recurrence. J Affect Disord 29: 85–96.
5. McClellan KM, Stratton MS, Tobet SA (2010) Roles for gamma-aminobutyric acid in the development of the paraventricular nucleus of the hypothalamus. J Comp Neurol 518: 2710–2728.
6. Stratton MS, Searcy BT, Tobet SA (2011) GABA regulates corticotropin releasing hormone levels in the paraventricular nucleus of the hypothalamus in newborn mice. Physiol Behav 104: 327–333.
7. Kalueff AV, Nutt DJ (2007) Role of GABA in anxiety and depression. Depress Anxiety 24: 495–517.
8. Cryan JF, Slattery DA (2010) GABAB Receptors and Depression: Current status. Advances in Pharmacology 58: 427–51.
9. Luscher B, Shen Q, Sahir N (2011) The GABAergic deficit hypothesis of major depressive disorder. Mol Psychiatry. 16: 383–406.
10. Ghose S, Winter MK, McCarson KE, Tamminga CA, Enna SJ (2011) The GABAB receptor as a target for antidepressant drug action. Br J Pharmacol. 162: 1–17.
11. Prosser J, Hughes CW, Sheikha S, Kowatch RA, Kramer GL, et al. (1997) Plasma GABA in children and adolescents with mood, behavior, and comorbid mood and behavior disorders: a preliminary study. J Child Adolesc Psychopharmacol. 7: 181–99.
12. Sundman-Eriksson I, Allard P (2002) [(3)H]Tiagabine binding to GABA transporter-1 (GAT-1) in suicidal depression. J Affect Disord 71: 29–33.
13. Kugaya A, Sanacora G, Verhoeff NP, Fujita M, Mason GF, et al. (2003) Cerebral benzodiazepine receptors in depressed patients measured with [123I]iomazenil SPECT. Biol Psychiatry 54: 792–799.
14. Epperson CN, Gueorguieva R, Czarkowski KA, Stiklus S, Sellers E, et al. (2006) Preliminary evidence of reduced occipital GABA concentrations in puerperal women: a 1H-MRS study. Psychopharmacology (Berl) 186: 425–433.
15. Rajkowska G, O'Dwyer G, Teleki Z, Stockmeier CA, Miguel-Hidalgo JJ (2007) GABAergic neurons immunoreactive for calcium binding proteins are reduced in the prefrontalcortex in major depression. Neuropsychopharmacology. 32(2): 471–82.
16. Smoller JW, Rosenbaum JF, Biederman J, Susswein LS, Kennedy J, et al. (2001) Genetic association analysis of behavioral inhibition using candidate loci from mouse models. Am J Med Genet 105: 226–235.
17. Utge S, Soronen P, Partonen T, Loukola A, Kronholm E, et al. (2010) A population-based association study of candidate genes for depression and sleep disturbance. Am J Med Genet B Neuropsychiatr Genet. 153B: 468–76.
18. Thompson M, Weickert CS, Wyatt E, Webster MJ (2009) Decreased glutamic acid decarboxylase(67) mRNA expression in multiple brain areas of patients with schizophrenia and mood disorders. J Psychiatr Res 43: 970–7.
19. Kash SF, Tecott LH, Hodge C, Baekkeskov S (1999) Increased anxiety and altered responses to anxiolytics in mice deficient in the 65-kDa isoform of glutamic acid decarboxylase. Proc Natl Acad Sci USA 96: 1698–1703.
20. Stork O, Ji FY, Kaneko K, Stork S, Yoshinobu Y, et al. (2000) Postnatal development of a GABA deficit and disturbance of neural functions in mice lacking GAD65. Brain Res 865: 45–58.
21. Crestani F, Lorez M, Baer K, Essrich C, Benke D, et al. (1999) Decreased GABAA-receptor clustering results in enhanced anxiety and a bias for threat cues. Nat Neurosci 2: 833–839.
22. Mombereau C, Kaupmann K, Froestl W, Sansig G, van der Putten H, et al. (2004) Genetic and pharmacological evidence of a role for GABA(B) receptors in the modulation of anxiety- and antidepressant-like behavior. Neuropsychopharmacology 29: 1050–1062.
23. Gassmann M, Shaban H, Vigot R, Sansig G, Haller C, et al. (2004) Redistribution of GABAB(1) protein and atypical GABAB responses in GABAB(2)-deficient mice. J Neurosci 24: 6086–6097.
24. Viveros MP, Mendrek A, Paus T, López-Rodríguez AB, Marco EM, et al. (2012) A comparative, developmental, and clinical perspective of neurobehavioral sexual dimorphisms. Front Neurosci. 6: 84.
25. Feng G, Mellor RH, Bernstein M, Keller-Peck C, Nguyen QT, et al. (2000) Imaging neuronal subsets in transgenic mice expressing multiple spectral variants of GFP. Neuron. 28: 41–51.
26. Tobet SA, Walker HJ, Seney ML, Yu KW (2003) Viewing cell movements in the developing neuroendocrine brain. Integr Comp Biol 43: 794–801.
27. LaSarge CL, Bañuelos C, Mayse JD, Bizon JL (2009) Blockade of GABA(B) receptors completely reverses age-related learning impairment. Neuroscience. 164: 941–7.

28. McClellan KM, Calver AR, Tobet SA (2008) GABAB receptors role in cell migration and positioning within the ventromedial nucleus of the hypothalamus. Neuroscience 151: 1119–1131.
29. Kerr DI, Ong J, Johnston GA, Abbenante J, Prager RH (1988) 2-Hydroxy-saclofen: an improved antagonist at central and peripheral GABAB receptors. Neurosci Lett 92: 92–96.
30. Mann EO, Kohl MM, Paulsen O (2009) Distinct roles of GABA(A) and GABA(B) receptors in balancing and terminating persistent cortical activity. J Neurosci 29: 7513–7518.
31. Hahn JD, Swanson LW (2010) Distinct patterns of neuronal inputs and outputs of the juxtaparaventricular and suprafornical regions of the lateral hypothalamic area in the male rat. Brain Res Rev 64: 14–103.
32. Carbone DL, Zuloaga DG, Lacagnina AF, Handa RJ (2012) Prepro-thyrotropin releasing hormone expressing neurons in the juxtaparaventricular region of the lateral hypothalamus are activated by leptin and altered by prenatal glucocorticoid exposure. Brain Res 1477: 19–26.
33. Crawley JN (2007) What's Wrong With My Mouse? Behavioral Phenotyping of Transgenic and Knockout Mice. John Wiley & Sons, Inc., Hoboken, New Jersey, Second Edition.
34. Stevens HE, Su T, Yanagawa Y, Vaccarino FM (2013) Prenatal stress delays inhibitory neuron progenitor migration in the developing neocortex. Psychoneuroendocrinology. 38(4): 509–21.
35. Behar TN, Smith SV, Kennedy RT, McKenzie JM, Maric I, et al. (2001) GABA(B) receptors mediate motility signals for migrating embryonic cortical cells. Cereb Cortex. 11(8): 744–53.
36. Inada H, Watanabe M, Uchida T, Ishibashi H, Wake H, et al. (2011) GABA regulates the multidirectional tangential migration of GABAergic interneurons in living neonatal mice. PLoS One. 6(12): e27048.
37. Crandall JE, McCarthy DM, Araki KY, Sims JR, Ren JQ, et al. (2007) Dopamine receptor activation modulates GABA neuron migration from the basal forebrain to the cerebral cortex. J Neurosci. 27(14): 3813–22.
38. Smith OA, DeVito JL, Astley CA (1990) Neurons controlling cardiovascular responses to emotion are located in lateral hypothalamus-perifornical region. Am J Physiol. 259(5 Pt 2): R943–54.
39. Risold PY, Canteras NS, Swanson LW (1994) Organization of projections from the anterior hypothalamic nucleus: a Phaseolus vulgaris-leucoagglutinin study in the rat. J Comp Neurol. 1994 Oct 1;348(1): 1–40.
40. Peyron C, Tighe DK, van den Pol AN, de Lecea L, Heller HC, et al. (1998) Neurons containing hypocretin (orexin) project to multiple neuronal systems. J Neurosci. 18(23): 9996–10015.
41. Steininger TL, Kilduff TS, Behan M, Benca RM, Landry CF (2004) Comparison of hypocretin/orexin and melanin-concentrating hormone neurons and axonal projections in the embryonic and postnatal rat brain. J Chem Neuroanat. 27(3): 165–81.
42. Lund TD, Hinds LR, Handa RJ (2006) The androgen 5alpha-dihydrotestosterone and its metabolite 5alpha-androstan-3beta, 17beta-diol inhibit the hypothalamo-pituitary-adrenal response to stress by acting through estrogen receptor beta-expressing neurons in the hypothalamus. J Neurosci. 26(5): 1448–56.
43. Weiser MJ, Handa RJ (2009) Estrogen impairs glucocorticoid dependent negative feedback on the hypothalamic-pituitary-adrenal axis via estrogen receptor alpha within the hypothalamus. Neuroscience. 159(2): 883–95.
44. Herman JP, Ostrander MM, Mueller NK, Figueiredo H (2005) Limbic system mechanisms of stress regulation: hypothalamo-pituitary-adrenocortical axis. Prog Neuropsychopharmacol Biol Psychiatry. 29(8): 1201–13.
45. Flugge G, Wuttke W, Fuchs E (1986) Postnatal development of transmitter systems: sexual differentiation of the GABAergic system and effects of muscimol. Int J Dev Neurosci. 1986;4: 319–26.
46. Frankfurt M, Fuchs E, Wuttke W (1984) Sex differences in gamma-aminobutyric acid and glutamate concentrations in discrete rat brain nuclei. Neurosci Lett 50: 245–50.
47. Mombereau C, Kaupmann K, Gassmann M, Bettler B, van der Putten H, et al. (2005) Altered anxiety and depression-related behaviour in mice lacking GABAB(2) receptor subunits. Neuroreport. 16(3): 307–10.
48. Kasckow JW, Baker D, Geracioti TD Jr (2001) Corticotropin-releasing hormone in depression and post-traumatic stress disorder. Peptides 22: 845–851.
49. Bao AM, Meynen G, Swaab DF (2008) The stress system in depression and neurodegeneration: focus on the human hypothalamus. Brain Res Rev 57: 531–553.
50. Bao AM, Swaab DF (2007) Gender difference in age-related number of corticotropin-releasing hormone-expressing neurons in the human hypothalamic paraventricular nucleus and the role of sex hormones. Neuroendocrinology 85: 27–36.
51. Wang SS, Kamphuis W, Huitinga I, Zhou JN, Swaab DF (2008) Gene expression analysis in the human hypothalamus in depression by laser microdissection and real-time PCR: the presence of multiple receptor imbalances. Mol Psychiatry 13: 786–799, 741.
52. Holsen LM, Spaeth SB, Lee JH, Ogden LA, Klibanski A, et al. (2011) Stress response circuitry hypoactivation related to hormonal dysfunction in women with major depression. J Affect Disord 131: 379–87.
53. Heldt SA, Mou L, Ressler KJ (2012) In vivo knockdown of GAD67 in the amygdala disrupts fear extinction and the anxiolytic-like effect of diazepam in mice. Transl Psychiatry. 2: e181.
54. Tobet SA, Handa RJ, Goldstein JM (2013) Sex-dependent pathophysiology as predictors of comorbidity of major depressive disorder and cardiovascular disease. Pflugers Arch. 465: 585–94.
55. Goldstein JM, Handa RJ, Tobet SA (2014)Disruption of fetal hormonal programming (prenatal stress) implicates shared risk for sex differences in depression and cardiovascular disease. Front Neuroendocrinol 35: 140–58.

11

Striatal Dopamine $D_{2/3}$ Receptor Availability in Treatment Resistant Depression

Bart P. de Kwaasteniet[1,2*¶], Chedwa Pinto[3¶], Eric H. G. Ruhé[1,2,6], Guido A. van Wingen[1,2], Jan Booij[2,4], Damiaan Denys[1,2,5]

1 Department of Psychiatry, Academic Medical Center, Amsterdam, the Netherlands, **2** Brain Imaging Center, Academic Medical Center, Amsterdam, the Netherlands, **3** Department of Psychiatry, MC groep, Lelystad, the Netherlands, **4** Department of Nuclear Medicine, Academic Medical Center, Amsterdam, the Netherlands, **5** The Institute for Neuroscience, an institute of the Royal Netherlands Academy of Arts and Sciences, Amsterdam, the Netherlands, **6** University of Groningen, University Medical Center Groningen, Mood and Anxiety Disorders, Department of Psychiatry, Groningen, the Netherlands

Abstract

Several studies demonstrated improvement of depressive symptoms in treatment resistant depression (TRD) after administering dopamine agonists which suggest abnormal dopaminergic neurotransmission in TRD. However, the role of dopaminergic signaling through measurement of striatal dopamine $D_{2/3}$ receptor (D2/3R) binding has not been investigated in TRD subjects. We used [^{123}I]IBZM single photon emission computed tomography (SPECT) to investigate striatal D2/3R binding in TRD. We included 6 severe TRD patients, 11 severe TRD patients on antipsychotics (TRD AP group) and 15 matched healthy controls. Results showed no significant difference ($p = 0.75$) in striatal D2/3R availability was found between TRD patients and healthy controls. In the TRD AP group D2/3R availability was significantly decreased (reflecting occupancy of D2/3Rs by antipsychotics) relative to TRD patients and healthy controls ($p<0.001$) but there were no differences in clinical symptoms between TRD AP and TRD patients. This preliminary study therefore does not provide evidence for large differences in D2/3 availability in severe TRD patients and suggests this TRD subgroup is not characterized by altered dopaminergic transmission. Atypical antipsychotics appear to have no clinical benefit in severe TRD patients who remain depressed, despite their strong occupancy of D2/3Rs.

Editor: Huaibin Cai, National Institute of Health, United States of America

Funding: Dr. H.G. Ruhé is supported by a NWO/ZonMW VENI-Grant #016.126.059. The funders had no role in study design, data collection and analysis, decision to publish, or preparation of the manuscript.

Competing Interests: One of the authors (Chedwa Pinto) is employed at a commercial MC groep.

* Email: b.p.dekwaasteniet@amc.nl

¶ These authors contributed equally to this work.

Introduction

About one third of patients with major depressive disorder (MDD) do not respond to two or more trials with different classes of antidepressants and are considered treatment resistant [1,2]. Treatment resistant depression (TRD) is associated with an overall worse prognosis and high medical costs [3]. At present, little is known about the pathophysiology of TRD, however several studies in TRD subjects demonstrated improvement of depressive symptoms after treatment with dopamine agonists [4–6]. These findings therefore suggest that abnormal dopaminergic neurotransmission is implicated in the pathophysiology of TRD [7].

In addition, aberrant dopaminergic neurotransmission is also associated with dysfunctional reward/motivational systems and anhedonia; the absolute or relative inability to experience pleasure. Anhedonia is one of the two key symptoms required for the diagnosis of MDD [8]. In TRD, anhedonia is often more profound and long-lasting and associated with a deficiency of the reward/motivational systems in the brain. Reward and motivation are mediated by the mesolimbic system, which is one of the major brain dopaminergic tracts [7]. This mesolimbic tract arises from the ventral tegmental area (VTA) and projects to the ventral striatum (including the nucleus accumbens), hippocampus and amygdala.

Relatively few neuroimaging studies examined the dopaminergic system in MDD with either positron emission tomography (PET) or single photon emission computed tomography (SPECT), and reported inconsistent findings [9,10]. Studies investigating dopamine $D_{2/3}$ receptor (D2/3R) availability reported increased striatal D2/3R availability in MDD patients compared to controls [11,12], as well as increased striatal D2/3R availability in a subgroup of MDD patients with psychomotor retardation [13,14]. Increased D2/3R availability may reflect either an up-regulation of $D_{2/3}$ receptors, increased affinity of the receptor for the radioligand or a decreased synaptic dopamine concentration [7]. Therefore, the evidence of altered dopaminergic function in MDD is equivocal, also, as other studies demonstrated no differences between MDD and healthy controls [15,16]. An explanation for these inconsistent findings may be that these studies included MDD patients with heterogeneous clinical characteristics which might underlie different clinical subgroups. Interestingly, it has been suggested that TRD is characterized by a more profound dysfunction of mood regulating networks relative to non-treatment resistant depression [17,18], which suggests that TRD patients are at the worst end of a continuous depression spectrum. Furthermore, as TRD patients are often more severely anhedonic and psychomotorically retarded, and most of the time did not respond to serotonergic or noradrenergic drugs, abnormalities in TRD patients may be related to reduced dopaminergic signaling. To date, striatal D2/3R binding has not been investigated in TRD patients.

Therefore, the aim of the present study was to investigate striatal D2/3R binding in severe TRD patients to test the hypothesis whether TRD patients are characterized by diminished dopaminergic transmission, reflected by increased D2/3R binding. We performed in vivo measurements of striatal D2/3 binding in 6 TRD patients compared to 15 healthy controls. We additionally investigated the effect of antipsychotics on striatal D2/3R availability in 11 TRD patients and whether these drugs were associated with improvement of symptomatology.

Methods

Subjects

We included 6 TRD patients, 11 TRD patients on antipsychotics (TRD AP group) and 15 healthy control subjects matched for age and gender. TRD patients were recruited at the department of Psychiatry of the Academic Medical Center (AMC) in Amsterdam and St. Elisabeth Hospital in Tilburg. The study was approved by the Medical Ethical Committee of the AMC of the University of Amsterdam (METC AMC), and the Medical Ethical Committee of the St. Elizabeth Hospital (METC St. Elisabeth). All subjects provided written informed consent. Inclusion criteria for TRD and TRD AP subjects were: (i) age between 18 and 65 years; (ii) total Hamilton Depression Rating Scale (HAM-D) ≥18; (iii) primary diagnosis of MDD according to the Diagnostic and Statistical Manual of Mental Disorders (DSM-IV) criteria and assessed by The Structured Clinical Interview for DSM-IV (SCID) [19]. To capture the most severely TRD patients, we included only patients with an illness duration of >2 years, who did not respond to (i) at least two adequate treatments of two different modern antidepressants (selective serotonin reuptake inhibitors, serotonin–norepinephrine reuptake inhibitors, or noradrenergic and specific serotonergic antidepressants), and (ii) a tricyclic antidepressant, and (iii) an irreversible monoamine oxidase (MAO) inhibitor, and (iv) at least 6 sessions of bilateral electroconvulsive therapy (ECT). Exclusion criteria were: (i) Parkinson's disease, dementia or epilepsy; (ii) bipolar disorder; (iii) schizophrenia or a history of psychosis unrelated to MDD; (iv) alcohol or substance abuse during last 6 months; and (v) antisocial personality disorder. Healthy controls were screened by the structured clinical interview for DSM-IV disorders in order to confirm the absence of psychiatric or neurological illness [19]. None of the healthy participants reported a family history of psychiatric illness. We used the HAM-D [20] and Montgomery Asberg Depression Rating Scale (MADRS) [21] to quantify depression severity. The Maudsley Staging Method (MSM) was used to quantify the level of treatment resistance [22,23]. The MSM score includes various clinical parameters; duration of the current depressive episode, symptom severity, and level of functioning as measured by the Global Assessment of Functioning (GAF) score. For a complete list of these clinical variables we refer to Fekadu et al [22].

Single Photon Emission Computed Tomography protocol

SPECT scanning was performed using a 12-detector single-slice brain-dedicated scanner (Neurofocus, Inc., Medfield, MA, USA). Subjects underwent a measurement of the striatal D2/3R binding potential (BP_{ND}) using the selective D2/3R antagonist [^{123}I]iodobenzamide ([^{123}I]IBZM). We applied a bolus/constant infusion technique, which has been described in detail previously [24,25]. SPECT data were acquired for 60 minutes, starting 120 minutes after infusion of the radioligand. At the day of scanning subjects were not allowed to use alcohol, coffee and cigarettes since this has been associated with altered striatal dopamine release [26,27].

Image reconstruction and analysis

SPECT data were reconstructed in 3-D mode and attenuation correction of all images was performed as described earlier [28]. For quantification, a region of interest (ROI) analysis was performed. Fixed ROIs were positioned for the striatum and, as a reference, the occipital cortex [25]. Mean striatal and mean occipital binding were averaged from right and left ROIs. Then, BP_{ND} was calculated as the ratio of specific to non-specific binding ((total activity in striatum - activity in occipital cortex)/activity in the occipital cortex). All scans were analyzed by one investigator (CP) who was blind to the clinical data. To measure the inter-rater agreement, two authors (CP and BdK) independently analysed BP_{ND} in ten subjects. The intraclass correlation coefficient (ICC) was 0.94 for left- and 0.95 for right striatum which indicates an excellent agreement between both raters.

Statistical analysis

Differences in age, HAM-D and MADRS scores were evaluated with a one way analysis of variance (ANOVA), and gender differences using a chi-square test. Comparison of striatal D2/3R availability between TRD, TRD AP and healthy control subjects was performed with an ANOVA as well. Using a Least Significant Difference (LSD) ANOVA post-hoc test, differences in D2/3R availability were investigated between TRD patients and healthy controls, between TRD AP patients and healthy controls and between TRD AP and TRD patients. Since D2/3R availability is influenced by age [29] and gender [30], we additionally included these variables as covariates in the group analyses using a one way analysis of covariance (ANCOVA). A two tailed probability value of 0.05 was selected as significance level.

Results

Patient characteristics

TRD, TRD AP and control subjects were comparable for age and gender (Table 1). HAM-D and MADRS scores did not differ between TRD and TRD AP patients which indicates no difference in severity of depression between both groups. Mean MSM scores of TRD patients were 11.8 (±1.0) and for TRD AP patients 11.8 (±0.5) which indicates a high level of treatment resistance in both groups. An overview of medication use of each TRD and TRD AP patient is reported in Table 2.

SPECT imaging

There were no significant differences in mean striatal D2/3R availability between TRD patients and healthy controls ($p = 0.75$) suggesting that dopaminergic neurotransmission was not significantly altered in TRD patients (Table 1, Figure 1 and 2). The standardized effect size was 0.21. Furthermore, the mean D2/3R availability of the TRD AP group was significantly lower compared to both the TRD ($p = 0.001$) and healthy control group ($p<0.001$). Since the antipsychotics used by the TRD AP patients

Table 1. Demographic and clinical measures of TRD, TRD AP and healthy control subjects.

Characteristic	TRD (n = 6)	TRD AP (n = 11)	HCs (n = 15)	p-value
Age (years±SEM)	48.7±3.7	55.9±2.0	54.5±2.0	0.17[1]
Gender (female/male)	3/3	7/4	10/5	0.63[2]
HAM-D (SEM)	20.2±1.3	22.2±1.5	n.a.	0.38
MADRS (SEM)	33.4±3.4	34.8±1.5	n.a.	0.66
Duration of current episode in months (SEM)	82±20.0	73±14.9	n.a.	0.73
Age of onset (SEM)	25.2±5.2	32.1±4.7	n.a.	0.36
MSM scores (SEM)	11.8±1.0	11.8±0.5	n.a.	0.98
Psychomotor retardation Item 8 HAM-D (SEM)	1±0.3	2±0.2	n.a.	0.02
Striatal D2/3R availability (BP_{ND}) (±SEM)	0.84±0.06	0.50±0.06	0.81±0.05	<0.001[1] TRD>HC: 0.75 TRD AP>HC: <0.001 TRD AP>TRD: 0.001

Abbreviations: TRD; Treatment resistant depression, TRD AP; Treatment resistant depression patients using antipsychotics, HCs; Healthy Controls, SEM; standard error of the mean MADRS; Montgomery Asberg Depression Rating Scale, HAM-D; Hamilton Depression Rating Scale, MSM; Maudsley Staging Method, BP_{ND}; Binding Potential non-displaceable (reflects striatal D2/3R availability)
[1]One way ANOVA.
[2]Chi square test.

were all dopamine receptor antagonists, this demonstrates strong occupancy of striatal D2/3Rs (Table 1, Figure 2; occupancy of 50%±20%). Correction for age and gender did not significantly affect these results.

Discussion

This preliminary study is, to the best of our knowledge, the first to investigate striatal D2/3R availability in TRD. We included a unique group of severe TRD patients which were eligible for deep brain stimulation, with an illness duration of more than 2 years defined as non-response to at least four adequate treatments of different antidepressants and at least 6 sessions of bilateral ECT. We showed no significant differences in striatal D2/3R availability in TRD patients relative to healthy controls which suggests that dopaminergic neurotransmission is not significantly altered in TRD. Furthermore, the TRD AP subjects showed significantly decreased striatal D2/3R availability relative to both TRD and healthy control subjects, which reflects a significant occupancy of D2/3Rs (estimated to be approximately 50%) by these atypical antipsychotics. Interestingly, despite these large differences in receptor occupancy depressive symptoms were not improved in the TRD AP subjects.

Previously, it was suggested that particularly TRD is associated with dopaminergic dysfunction [7]. Since TRD is characterized by a more profound dysfunction of mood regulating networks [17,18], we expected them to show more severe dopaminergic dysfunction and as such an increased D2/3R availability compared to controls. Nevertheless, we observed no significant difference in striatal D2/3R availability in TRD patients compared to controls. We propose several explanations for this finding. First, other studies reported differences in D2/3R availability in psychomotor retarded patients [13,14]. In our sample we used item 8 (range 0 to 4) of the HAM-D scores to measure psychomotor retardation which showed these TRD patients suffered only moderately from psychomotor retardation. Unfortunately, our study lacks more sensitive tests to measure motor retardation such as a finger tapping task [14]. We therefore

Table 2. Psychopharmacological drugs used in TRD and TRD AP patients.

Subject	TRD AP patients (n = 11)	TRD patients (n = 6)
1.	Olanzapine 5 mg Zoplicon 15 mg	None
2.	Lithiumcarbonate 600 mg Quetiapine 300 mg Lorazepam 3 mg	Tranylcypromine 10 mg Zopiclon 7.5 mg
3.	Quetiapine 500 mg Lorazepam 1 mg	None
4.	Tranylcypromine 90 mg Quetiapine 100 mg Aripiprazol 30 mg	Lithiumcarbonate 800 mg Zolpidem 20 mg
5.	Olanzapine 12.5 mg Flurazepam 15 mg Lorazepam 6 mg	None
6.	Quetiapine 600 mg Venlafaxine 75 mg	Mirtazapine 400 mg
7.	Dipiperon 80 mg Lorazepam 5.5 mg Zoplicon 7.5 mg	
8.	Quetiapine 700 mg Oxazepam 10 mg Zolpidem 20 mg	
9.	Tranylcypromine 20 mg Dipiperon 80 mg	
10.	Imipramine 25 mg Olanzapine 10 mg	
11.	Quetiapine 900 mg	

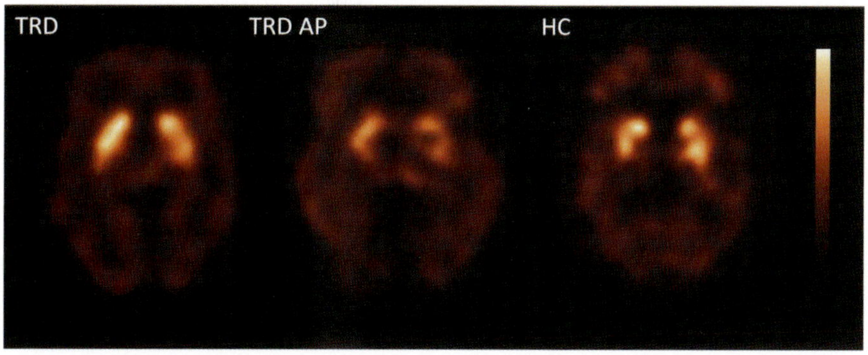

Figure 1. Transversal images of D2/3R availability. Transversal [123I]IBZM SPECT slices at the level of the striatum showing D2/3 receptor availability in a TRD patient, a TRD patient on antipsychotics (TRD AP), and a healthy control subject.

cannot exclude the option that our patients were less psychomotorically retarded than in previous studies [13,14]. Second, in the present sample TRD patients were only included after a non-response to MAO-inhibitors. As MAO-inhibitors increase dopamine concentrations, it could be hypothesized that especially in a subgroup of patients with a good response to MAO-inhibitors a hypodopaminergic state might exist. This could explain why in the current sample of non-responders to MAO-inhibitors no differences in striatal D2/3R availability were found. However, this hypothesis has not been investigated yet. Third, the present sample might be too small to detect differences in striatal D2/3R availability between TRD and control subjects. Importantly, however, the standardized effect size was small ($d = 0.21$). This implies that at least 343 patients should be included to demonstrate a significant group difference (at a statistical power of 0.8). Therefore the chance that future larger studies will find increased D2/3R availability in this subgroup of TRD-patients appears to be low. Furthermore, our present findings are consistent with several MDD studies which also reported no differences in striatal D2/3R availability relative to healthy controls [15,16]. However these studies included different clinical groups with mostly treatment sensitive patients and a shorter duration of illness which therefore hampers direct comparisons.

As expected, the TRD AP subjects showed significantly decreased striatal D2/3R availability relative to TRD subjects (which reflects occupancy of D2/3Rs by the antipsychotics). The present D2/3R occupancy (approximately 50%) in the TRD AP group is comparable with that of atypical antipsychotics in schizophrenia patients [31,32]. Since we showed no significant differences in depressive symptoms between these groups at

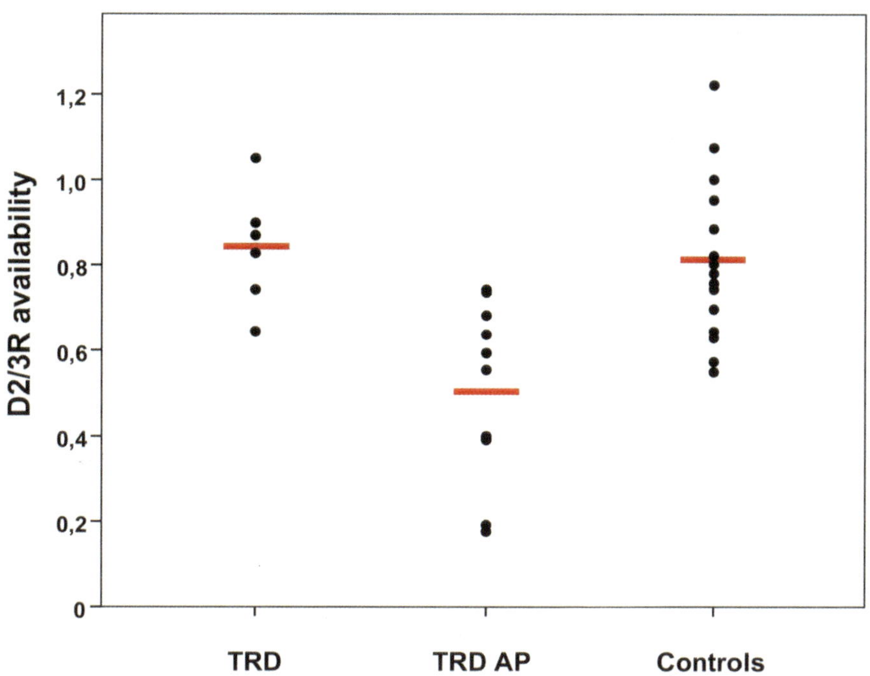

Figure 2. Striatal D2/3R availability for TRD, TRD AP and healthy control subjects. Striatal D2/3 receptor (D2/3R) availability of TRD patients, TRD patients with antipsychotics (TRD AP) and healthy control subjects. The black dots represents the striatal D2/3R availability of each subject. The horizontal lines indicate the mean D2/3R availability of each group which is 0.84 for the TRD, 0.50 for the TRD AP and 0.81 for the healthy control subjects.

adequate occupancy levels, this suggests that either monotherapy or augmentation with atypical antipsychotics does not provide clinical benefits in this specific TRD group, suggesting that these antipsychotics could be tapered in these patients. Importantly, all antipsychotic drugs used by the TRD AP patients have appreciable 5-HT_{2A} receptor occupancy which has been shown to improve depressive symptoms [33]. The 5-HT_{2A} receptor occupancy in these patients therefore cannot explain the lack of clinical improvement in this group. An explanation for the non-response might be that these atypical antipsychotics are all dopamine receptor antagonists. Interestingly, several studies showed that adjunctive dopamine agonists like pramipexole are effective in TRD patients [6,34,35] which suggests that dopamine agonist augmentation therapy might also be effective in the present severe TRD patients. We speculate that direct stimulation of dopamine D2/3 receptors may be helpful to increase motivational processes in the brain [36].

Despite the frequent use of atypical antipsychotic drugs in psychotic depression [37,38], low-dose augmentation of these drugs in (non-psychotic) TRD patients has been proven to be effective [39,40]. However, in these augmentation studies TRD was mostly defined as a non-response to only two trials of antidepressants. The present TRD patients additionally did not respond to more classes of antidepressants such as tricyclic antidepressants and MAO-inhibitors which may further explain the non-response to atypical antipsychotics, which might have no clinical benefit in more severe TRD patients. However, a randomized controlled trial would be necessary to definitely conclude whether antipsychotic augmentation in severe TRD is clinically useful.

We acknowledge several limitations of the present study. First, several studies showed that the striatum contains not only D2/3 receptors but also dopamine D1 receptors which operate via different intracellular pathways [41]. The dopamine D1 receptor is part of a D1-like subfamily which also comprises the dopamine D5 receptor [41]. Striatal D1 receptors are part of the direct nigrostriatal output pathway whereas D2 receptors are more prevalent in the indirect pathway [42]. Despite these functional differences, an animal study demonstrated that concurrent activation of D1 and D2 receptors in the shell of the nucleus accumbens produces a cooperative effect on the regulation of motivation, i.e. dopamine mediated reward processes [43]. Since depression has been associated with a dysfunctional reward/ motivational system [44,45], these findings suggest that altered expression of D1 receptors might lead to disturbances in the motivational system in MDD patients. However, as far as we know no human study has investigated striatal D1 availability in MDD nor in TRD. The Positron Emission Tomography (PET) radioligand [^{11}C] SCH23390 binds to dopamine D1-like receptors [46], and to a lesser extent to D5 receptors. Since the expression of the D5 receptors in the striatum is lower, [^{11}C] SCH23390 binding will predominantly reflect D1 receptor availability. [^{11}C] SCH23390, but also other ligands like [^{11}C]NNC 756 [47] or [^{11}C]SKF 82957 [48] could therefore be used to investigate striatal dopamine D1 receptor availability in MDD and TRD patients.

Second, three out six TRD patients used psychotropic medication which might have influenced striatal D2/3R availability. One of these patients used a MAO-inhibitor which increases the synaptic dopamine concentration in the striatum [49]. Therefore, use of this drug could have reduced striatal D2/ 3R availability in this patient by increased competition with the radioligand. However, exclusion of this patient did not change results. In fact, large increases in dopamine concentrations are needed to reduce the [^{123}I]IBZM binding in vivo. Another TRD patient used mirtazapine which is a noradrenergic and specific serotonergic antidepressant (NaSSA). Although mirtazapine has no affinity for dopamine receptors it does increase dopamine release in the prefrontal and occipital cortex by activation of the 5-HT_{1A} receptor and blockade of the α2-adrenergic receptors [50,51]. However, there is no evidence that mirtazapine increases striatal dopamine release which suggests striatal D2/3R binding is not altered by mirtazapine use. Third, with [^{123}I]IBZM we are able to measure striatal D2/3Rs in vivo. However, consequently we cannot exclude differences in extra-striatal D2/3Rs in TRD, which cannot be quantified. Finally, we did not select TRD-patients based on symptomatology like psychomotor retardation and/or anhedonia which might represent a subgroup with decreased D2/3R availability.

In conclusion, the present study did not detect differences in striatal D2/3R receptor availability in severely treatment resistant MDD patients relative to healthy controls. This contradicts the hypothesis that TRD is characterized by altered dopaminergic transmission. Furthermore, the results showed that additional treatment with antipsychotics decreased striatal D2/3R receptor availability (due to occupancy of D2/3R by the antipsychotics) in TRD. Importantly, because depressive symptoms were not reduced in these TRD AP patients, this suggest that in patients who have been administered different antidepressant drugs and remain depressed, atypical antipsychotics do not have a clinical advantage.

Acknowledgments

We gratefully acknowledge Elsmarieke van de Giessen and Evelien Zoons for providing healthy controls, and both patients and healthy controls for participating in SPECT-scanning. Provided healthy controls: EvdG, EZ.

Author Contributions

Conceived and designed the experiments: BDK CP JB ER. Performed the experiments: BDK CP. Analyzed the data: BDK CP. Contributed reagents/materials/analysis tools: BDK CP JB. Wrote the paper: BDK CP JB ER GVW DD.

References

1. Greden JF (2001) The burden of disease for treatment-resistant depression. *J Clin Psychiatry* 62 Suppl 16:26–31.
2. Rush AJ, Trivedi MH, Wisniewski SR, Nierenberg AA, Stewart JW, et al. (2006) Acute and longer-term outcomes in depressed outpatients requiring one or several treatment steps: a STAR*D report. *Am J Psychiatry* 163:1905–1917.
3. Ustun TB, Kessler RC (2002) Global burden of depressive disorders: the issue of duration. *Br J Psychiatry* 181:181–183.
4. Cusin C, Iovieno N, Iosifescu DV, Nierenberg AA, Fava M, et al. (2013) A randomized, double-blind, placebo-controlled trial of pramipexole augmentation in treatment-resistant major depressive disorder. *J Clin Psychiatry* 74:e636–e641.
5. Inoue T, Kitaichi Y, Masui T, Nakagawa S, Boku S, et al. (2010) Pramipexole for stage 2 treatment-resistant major depression: an open study. *Prog Neuropsychopharmacol Biol Psychiatry* 34:1446–1449.
6. Lattanzi L, Dell'Osso L, Cassano P, Pini S, Rucci P, et al. (2002) Pramipexole in treatment-resistant depression: a 16-week naturalistic study. *Bipolar Disord* 4:307–314.
7. Dunlop BW, Nemeroff CB (2007) The role of dopamine in the pathophysiology of depression. *Arch Gen Psychiatry* 64:327–337.
8. American Psychiatric Association (1994) Diagnostic and Statistical Manual of Mental Disorders, 4th ed: American Psychiatric Press.
9. Dunlop BW, Nemeroff CB (2007) The role of dopamine in the pathophysiology of depression. *Arch Gen Psychiatry* 64:327–337.
10. Ruhe HG, Visser KD, Frokjaer VG, Haarman CM, Klein C, et al. (2014) Molecular imaging of depressive disorders *PET and SPECT in Psychiatry*, den Boer,J.A.; ed: Springer Verlag, pp 93–172.

11. D'haenen HA, Bossuyt A (1994) Dopamine D2 receptors in depression measured with single photon emission computed tomography. *Biol Psychiatry* 35:128–132.
12. Shah PJ, Ogilvie AD, Goodwin GM, Ebmeier KP (1997) Clinical and psychometric correlates of dopamine D2 binding in depression. *Psychol Med* 27:1247–1256.
13. Ebert D, Feistel H, Loew T, Pirner A (1996) Dopamine and depression–striatal dopamine D2 receptor SPECT before and after antidepressant therapy. *Psychopharmacology (Berl)* 126:91–94.
14. Meyer JH, McNeely HE, Sagrati S, Boovariwala A, Martin K, et al. (2006) Elevated putamen D(2) receptor binding potential in major depression with motor retardation: an [11C]raclopride positron emission tomography study. *Am J Psychiatry* 163:1594–1602.
15. Parsey RV, Oquendo MA, Zea-Ponce Y, Rodenhiser J, Kegeles LS, et al. (2001) Dopamine D(2) receptor availability and amphetamine-induced dopamine release in unipolar depression. *Biol Psychiatry* 50:313–322.
16. Yang YK, Yeh TL, Yao WJ, Lee IH, Chen PS, et al. (2008) Greater availability of dopamine transporters in patients with major depression–a dual-isotope SPECT study. *Psychiatry Res* 162:230–235.
17. Konarski JZ, Kennedy SH, McIntyre RS, Rafi-Tari S, Soczynska JK, et al. (2007) Relationship between regional brain metabolism, illness severity and age in depressed subjects. *Psychiatry Res* 155:203–210.
18. Paillere Martinot ML, Martinot JL, Ringuenet D, Galinowski A, Gallarda T, et al. (2011) Baseline brain metabolism in resistant depression and response to transcranial magnetic stimulation. *Neuropsychopharmacology* 36:2710–2719.
19. First MB (2012) Structured Clinical Interview for DSM-IV-TR Axis I Disorders, Research Version, Patient Edition: New York State Psychiatric Institute.
20. Hamilton M (1960) A rating scale for depression. *J Neurol Neurosurg Psychiatry* 23:56–62.
21. Montgomery SA, Asberg M (1979) A new depression scale designed to be sensitive to change. *Br J Psychiatry* 134:382–389.
22. Fekadu A, Wooderson S, Donaldson C, Markopoulou K, Masterson B, et al. (2009) A multidimensional tool to quantify treatment resistance in depression: the Maudsley staging method. *J Clin Psychiatry* 70:177–184.
23. Ruhe HG, van RG, Spijker J, Peeters FP, Schene AH (2012) Staging methods for treatment resistant depression. A systematic review. *J Affect Disord* 137:35–45.
24. Booij J, Korn P, Linszen DH, van Royen EA, et al. (1997) Assessment of endogenous dopamine release by methylphenidate challenge using iodine-123 iodobenzamide single-photon emission tomography. *Eur J Nucl Med* 24:674–677.
25. Boot E, Booij J, Zinkstok JR, Linszen DH, Baas F, et al. (2010) Striatal D(2) receptor binding in 22q11 deletion syndrome: an [123I]IBZM SPECT study. *J Psychopharmacol* 24:1525–1531.
26. Kaasinen V, Aalto S, Nagren K, Rinne JO (2004) Dopaminergic effects of caffeine in the human striatum and thalamus. *Neuroreport* 15:281–285.
27. Nevo I, Hamon M (1995) Neurotransmitter and neuromodulatory mechanisms involved in alcohol abuse and alcoholism. *Neurochem Int* 26:305–336.
28. Booij J, Tissingh G, Boer GJ, Speelman JD, Stoof JC, et al. (1997) [123I]FP-CIT SPECT shows a pronounced decline of striatal dopamine transporter labelling in early and advanced Parkinson's disease. *J Neurol Neurosurg Psychiatry* 62:133–140.
29. Rinne JO, Hietala J, Ruotsalainen U, Sako E, Laihinen A, et al. (1993) Decrease in human striatal dopamine D2 receptor density with age: a PET study with [11C]raclopride. *J Cereb Blood Flow Metab* 13:310–314.
30. Trainor BC (2011) Stress responses and the mesolimbic dopamine system: social contexts and sex differences. *Horm Behav* 60:457–469.
31. Kapur S, Zipursky RB, Remington G (1999) Clinical and theoretical implications of 5-HT2 and D2 receptor occupancy of clozapine, risperidone, and olanzapine in schizophrenia. *Am J Psychiatry* 156:286–293.
32. Tauscher J, Hussain T, Agid O, Verhoeff NP, Wilson AA, et al. (2004) Equivalent occupancy of dopamine D1 and D2 receptors with clozapine: differentiation from other atypical antipsychotics. *Am J Psychiatry* 161:1620–1625.
33. Celada P, Puig M, Amargos-Bosch M, Adell A, Artigas F (2004) The therapeutic role of 5-HT1A and 5-HT2A receptors in depression. *J Psychiatry Neurosci* 29:252–265.
34. Hori H, Kunugi H (2012) The efficacy of pramipexole, a dopamine receptor agonist, as an adjunctive treatment in treatment-resistant depression: an open-label trial. *ScientificWorldJournal* 2012:372474.
35. Izumi T, Inoue T, Kitagawa N, Nishi N, Shimanaka S, et al. (2000) Open pergolide treatment of tricyclic and heterocyclic antidepressant-resistant depression. *J Affect Disord* 61:127–132.
36. Leentjens AF, Koester J, Fruh B, Shephard DT, Barone P, et al. (2009) The effect of pramipexole on mood and motivational symptoms in Parkinson's disease: a meta-analysis of placebo-controlled studies. *Clin Ther* 31:89–98.
37. Farahani A, Correll CU (2012) Are antipsychotics or antidepressants needed for psychotic depression? A systematic review and meta-analysis of trials comparing antidepressant or antipsychotic monotherapy with combination treatment. *J Clin Psychiatry* 73:486–496.
38. Wijkstra J, Lijmer J, Burger H, Geddes J, Nolen WA (2013) Pharmacological treatment for psychotic depression. *Cochrane Database Syst Rev* 11:CD004044.
39. Corya SA, Williamson D, Sanger TM, Briggs SD, Case M, et al. (2006) A randomized, double-blind comparison of olanzapine/fluoxetine combination, olanzapine, fluoxetine, and venlafaxine in treatment-resistant depression. *Depress Anxiety* 23:364–372.
40. Nelson JC, Papakostas GI (2009) Atypical antipsychotic augmentation in major depressive disorder: a meta-analysis of placebo-controlled randomized trials. *Am J Psychiatry* 166:980–991.
41. Vallone D, Picetti R, Borrelli E (2000) Structure and function of dopamine receptors. *Neurosci Biobehav Rev* 24:125–132.
42. Gerfen CR, Engber TM, Mahan LC, Susel Z, Chase TN (1990) D1 and D2 dopamine receptor-regulated gene expression of striatonigral and striatopallidal neurons. *Science* 250:1429–1432.
43. Ikemoto S, Glazier BS, Murphy JM, McBride WJ (1997) Role of dopamine D1 and D2 receptors in the nucleus accumbens in mediating reward. *J Neurosci* 17:8580–8587.
44. Pizzagalli DA, Holmes AJ, Dillon DG, Goetz EL, Birk JL, et al. (2009) Reduced caudate and nucleus accumbens response to rewards in unmedicated individuals with major depressive disorder. *Am J Psychiatry* 166:702–710.
45. Smoski MJ, Felder J, Bizzell J, Green SR, Ernst M, et al. (2009) fMRI of alterations in reward selection, anticipation, and feedback in major depressive disorder. *J Affect Disord* 118:69–78.
46. Plaven-Sigray P, Gustavsson P, Farde L, Borg J, Stenkrona P, et al. (2014) Dopamine D1 receptor availability is related to social behavior: A positron emission tomography study. *Neuroimage* 102P2:590–595.
47. Abi-Dargham A, Simpson N, Kegeles L, Parsey R, Hwang DR, et al. (1999) PET studies of binding competition between endogenous dopamine and the D1 radiotracer [11C]NNC 756. *Synapse* 32:93–109.
48. Palner M, McCormick P, Parkes J, Knudsen GM, Wilson AA, et al. (2010) Systemic catechol-O-methyl transferase inhibition enables the D1 agonist radiotracer R-[11C]SKF 82957. *Nucl Med Biol* 37:837–843.
49. Yamada M, Yasuhara H (2004) Clinical pharmacology of MAO inhibitors: safety and future. *Neurotoxicology* 25:215–221.
50. Devoto P, Flore G, Pira L, Longu G, Gessa GL (2004) Mirtazapine-induced corelease of dopamine and noradrenaline from noradrenergic neurons in the medial prefrontal and occipital cortex. *Eur J Pharmacol* 487:105–111.
51. Nakayama K, Sakurai T, Katsu H (2004) Mirtazapine increases dopamine release in prefrontal cortex by 5-HT1A receptor activation. *Brain Res Bull* 63:237–241.

12

Characteristics of Effective Collaborative Care for Treatment of Depression

Peter A. Coventry[1]*, Joanna L. Hudson[2], Evangelos Kontopantelis[3], Janine Archer[4], David A. Richards[5], Simon Gilbody[6], Karina Lovell[4], Chris Dickens[5], Linda Gask[1], Waquas Waheed[7], Peter Bower[3]

1 Collaboration for Leadership in Applied Health Research and Care, Centre for Primary Care and Manchester Academic Health Science Centre, University of Manchester, Manchester, United Kingdom, **2** Health Psychology Section, Psychology Department, Institute of Psychiatry, King's College London, London, United Kingdom, **3** NIHR School for Primary Care Research, Centre for Primary Care and Manchester Academic Health Science Centre, University of Manchester, Manchester, United Kingdom, **4** School of Nursing, Midwifery & Social Work, University of Manchester, Manchester, United Kingdom, **5** Institute of Health Service Research, University of Exeter Medical School, University of Exeter, Exeter, United Kingdom, **6** Mental Health Research Group, Department of Health Sciences and Hull York Medical School, University of York, York, United Kingdom, **7** Lancashire Care NHS Foundation Trust, Preston, United Kingdom

Abstract

Background: Collaborative care is a complex intervention based on chronic disease management models and is effective in the management of depression. However, there is still uncertainty about which components of collaborative care are effective. We used meta-regression to identify factors in collaborative care associated with improvement in patient outcomes (depressive symptoms) and the process of care (use of anti-depressant medication).

Methods and Findings: Systematic review with meta-regression. The Cochrane Collaboration Depression, Anxiety and Neurosis Group trials registers were searched from inception to 9th February 2012. An update was run in the CENTRAL trials database on 29th December 2013. Inclusion criteria were: randomised controlled trials of collaborative care for adults ≥18 years with a primary diagnosis of depression or mixed anxiety and depressive disorder. Random effects meta-regression was used to estimate regression coefficients with 95% confidence intervals (CIs) between study level covariates and depressive symptoms and relative risk (95% CI) and anti-depressant use. The association between anti-depressant use and improvement in depression was also explored. Seventy four trials were identified (85 comparisons, across 21,345 participants). Collaborative care that included psychological interventions predicted improvement in depression (β coefficient −0.11, 95% CI −0.20 to −0.01, p = 0.03). Systematic identification of patients (relative risk 1.43, 95% CI 1.12 to 1.81, p = 0.004) and the presence of a chronic physical condition (relative risk 1.32, 95% CI 1.05 to 1.65, p = 0.02) predicted use of anti-depressant medication.

Conclusion: Trials of collaborative care that included psychological treatment, with or without anti-depressant medication, appeared to improve depression more than those without psychological treatment. Trials that used systematic methods to identify patients with depression and also trials that included patients with a chronic physical condition reported improved use of anti-depressant medication. However, these findings are limited by the observational nature of meta-regression, incomplete data reporting, and the use of study aggregates.

Editor: Phillipa J. Hay, University of Western Sydney, Australia

Funding: This study was funded by a Research and Capability Funding grant awarded by the NIHR Collaboration for Leadership in Applied Health Research and Care for Greater Manchester (ref:RCF_R10_PC). The funders had no role in study design, data collection and analysis, decision to publish, or preparation of the manuscript.

Competing Interests: The authors have been/are involved in the conduct of trials of collaborative care in the United Kingdom funded by the Medical Research Council and the National Institute for Health Research.

* Email: peter.a.coventry@manchester.ac.uk

Introduction

Major depressive disorder accounted for 8.2% of years living with disability in 2010, making it the second leading direct cause of global disease burden [1]. People with depression and a chronic physical disease have worse health status than people with depression alone or people with any combination of chronic physical disease without depression [2].

Significant advances have occurred in primary care in recent years to improve the management of chronic disease, principally by introducing structured disease management programmes that draw on the Chronic Care Model [3]. The chronic care model promotes a more proactive, planned and population-based approach to disease management and has been instrumental in transforming ambulatory care in primary care [4]. The concept and components of the chronic care model are fully specified here: http://www.improvingchroniccare.org/. Depression shares with other chronic diseases many features that can be addressed by the chronic care model, such as multiple recurrent episodes [5], where successful management hinges on regular monitoring, care coordination, enhancing providers' expertise, and supporting patients to self-manage. Interventions that include at least one component of the chronic care model have been shown to improve clinical outcomes and the process of care for people with chronic disease, including depression [6].

'Collaborative care' is the most promising chronic care model-based strategy for improving care of depression. While the make-up of collaborative care interventions for treatment of depression vary, they typically include a multi-professional approach to patient care, structured management, scheduled patient follow-ups, and enhanced inter-professional communication [7]. A recent Cochrane review that included 79 randomised controlled trials (RCTs) and 24,308 participants conclusively showed that collaborative care is more effective than usual care for both depression and anxiety after treatment, and up to two years later [8]. There is also ample evidence that these benefits are cost effective [9].

However, while some authors suggest that there is now sufficient evidence about effectiveness and that research should now shift to implementation [10], collaborative care is a complex intervention and there is significant variation in the exact nature of the intervention between trials, as well as differences in patient populations, contexts, comparators, and design. A number of these factors have already been shown to be related to estimates of effect: setting (i.e. country), recruitment of patients using systematic or population health approaches (e.g. disease registers), using case managers with a mental health background, and regular clinical supervision of case managers [11]. There has since been considerable international expansion of collaborative care outside of the United States and extension of this care model to populations with depression and chronic physical disease. We have therefore used meta-regression with a comprehensive and updated data set of randomised controlled trials of collaborative care to identify factors associated with improvement in patient outcome (i.e. depressive symptoms) and/or the process of care (i.e. anti-depressant use). The results will be used to distinguish which features of collaborative care effectively improve patient outcomes and/or the process of care and which do not.

Methods

This systematic review and meta-regression is reported in accordance with the Preferred Reporting Items for Systematic Reviews and Meta-Analyses Statement (see Figure 1 and Checklist S1) [12].

Information sources

The Cochrane Collaboration Depression, Anxiety and Neurosis Group (CC-DAN) trials registers (including both the references register and the studies register) were searched from inception to 9th February 2012. The CC-DAN registers include Randomised Controlled Trials indexed in MEDLINE, EMBASE, PsycINFO, CENTRAL, World Health Organisation's trials portal (ICTRP), Clinicaltrials.gov, and CINAHL. Details of the search strategy used can be found in Archer et al [8]. The CENTRAL search used in the Cochrane review by Archer et al [8] was updated on 29th December 2013 (see Methods S1 for search strategy). For the purposes of an update the comprehensive coverage of the CENTRAL database makes exhaustive searching of individual bibliographic databases unnecessary [13]. All reference lists of included studies and previously published reviews were checked.

Characteristics of collaborative care and conceptual model to be tested

For the purposes of this review we used a definition of collaborative care derived from a systematic review of complex interventions for managing depression in primary care [7]. Collaborative care consists of four key criteria: multi-professional approach to patient care, structured management, scheduled patient follow-ups, and enhanced inter-professional communication (Table 1).

A key innovation arising from collaborative care is the introduction of a non-medical case or care manager who works with a medical practitioner and under the supervision of a mental health specialist to deliver and coordinate psychological treatment, and to monitor progress with psychological and/or pharmacological treatment [14]. While chronic disease management interventions that include one or more features of patient or provider education, feedback, and reminders can lead to improved disease control and adherence to guidelines [15] enhanced roles in primary care for case managers are seen as central to the provision of effective and integrated interventions for depression [16]. Based on current understanding about how the intervention might work and based on previous knowledge about mechanisms of change and active ingredients of collaborative care we tested 10 factors (study covariates) that could potentially moderate patient and process outcomes (Table 2).

Eligibility criteria

Studies were included in this meta-analysis and meta-regression if they:

1) Were RCTs or clustered RCTs of collaborative care delivered in primary care settings or community settings. Primary care was defined as a person's first and ongoing contact point for health care [17].
2) Included adults over the age of 18 with a primary diagnosis of depression or mixed anxiety and depressive disorder according to clinical diagnosis or research assessment (observer interview or validated self-report measure). No restrictions on severity or chronicity of depression were made.
3) Compared the effectiveness of collaborative care with standard or enhanced usual care.

Standard usual care was defined as care routinely provided by primary care providers to patients with depression or mixed anxiety and depressive disorder. This could include onward referral to mental health teams or feedback on participants' depressive status if specified in the protocol.

Enhanced usual care was defined as care where any one or more of the following were present:

i. The patient received additional resources (i.e. educational leaflets, lists of locally available resources, letter from research team with self-help advice) OR the patient had access to enhanced care systems (i.e. consultation-liaison, enhanced referral systems to psychology services, case reviews between health professionals, equal contact time with a health professional, medication management, patient-primary care provider electronic messaging system, person-

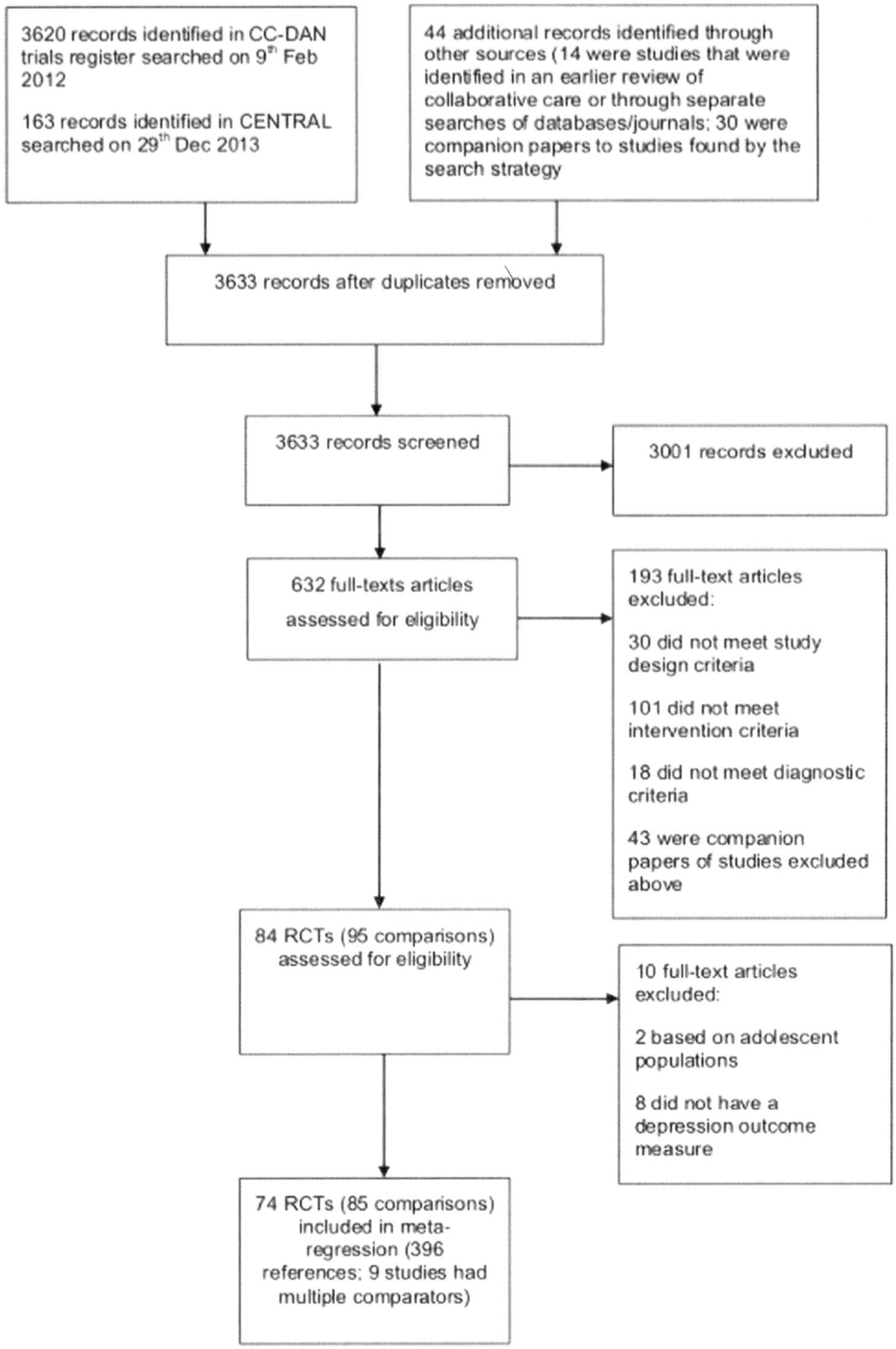

Figure 1. PRISMA Flow Diagram.

alised patient treatment plans from the principal investigator).

ii. Didactic training for the primary care provider.

iii. Primary care providers were supplied with manualised treatment algorithms or evidence based guidelines.

iv. Primary care providers received educational materials other than evidence based guidelines (e.g. educational DVD).

4) Measured change in self-reported or observer rated depression scores as a continuous or dichotomous measure (e.g. $\geq$ 50% decrease in symptom scores from baseline or remission)

AND/OR

Measured change in use of anti-depressant medication (e.g. proportion of patients taking medication or proportion of patients adhering appropriately to predefined criteria/guidelines), based on self-report or administrative records data.

Table 1. Key characteristics of collaborative care.

A multi-professional approach to patient care
A general practitioner (GP) or family physician and at least one other health professional (e.g. nurse, psychologist, psychiatrist, pharmacist) were involved with patient care, usually acting as a case or care manager to coordinate and/or deliver care for the depressed person
A structured management plan
Evidence based guidelines or treatment protocols. Interventions could include both pharmacological (e.g. antidepressant medication) and non-pharmacological interventions (e.g. patient screening, patient and provider education, counselling, cognitive behaviour therapy)
Scheduled patient follow-ups
An organised approach to patient follow-up that could include one or more scheduled telephone or in-person follow-up appointments to provide specific interventions, facilitate treatment adherence, or monitor symptoms or adverse effects
Enhanced inter-professional communication
Mechanisms to facilitate communication between professionals caring for the depressed person: team meetings, case-conferences, individual consultation/supervision, shared medical records, patient-specific written or verbal feedback between care-givers

Study selection

We identified eligible studies included in the Cochrane review of collaborative care for depression and anxiety [8] and also from eligible studies identified by the updated search of the CENTRAL trials database. Three authors (JH, PB, PC) independently screened non-overlapping subsets of studies against the inclusion criteria for this meta-regression.

Data extraction

Intervention content. Characteristics of collaborative and usual care intervention groups were independently extracted verbatim and coded using a standardised data extraction form and coding manual, specifically tailored to the content of collaborative care interventions (Methods S2).

Patient and process outcomes. The primary patient outcome was reduction in depressive symptoms as measured by observer or patient self-report. Outcomes were extracted for all reported follow-up time points (e.g. six months, twelve months). Most studies reported outcomes at six months follow-up and our analysis was therefore restricted to this time point to maximise both consistency and the number of studies included in the meta-regression. If eligible studies (n = 9) reported outcomes at follow-ups beyond six months we used short term follow-up data closest in time to six months. Where the studies reported two comparisons versus a control group, sample sizes were halved to avoid double counting.

To allow both continuous and dichotomous outcomes to be included in the same meta-regression, we translated dichotomous outcomes into standardised mean differences and standard errors using the *metaeff* Stata command [18].

Collaborative care improves the process of depression care, and use of anti-depressant medications may be a key driver for depressive outcomes. Anti-depressant use as a dichotomous process outcome was extracted; we used risk ratios with log-transformations applied [19].

When studies applied cluster randomisation procedures we accounted for increased Type I error rates by applying the "effective sample sizes" procedure outlined in the Cochrane Handbook [20]. An intraclass correlation coefficient (ICC) of 0.02 [21] was used and sensitivity analyses were performed to explore the impact of adjustments for clustering using an ICC of 0.00 and 0.05 [22]. We also used study sample sizes as a proxy for publication bias [23]. We explored using meta-regression whether there was an inverse relationship between study sample sizes and reported effect sizes. Allocation concealment, an important feature of trials known to reduce risk of bias, was assessed using a binary measure [24].

Analysis

Stata's (Version 12 for Windows) *metan* [25] and *metareg* [26] commands were used to calculate an overall effect size estimate of collaborative care on depressive symptoms and anti-depressant medication use. Consistent with the recommendations of Thompson and Higgins [27], ten covariates were hypothesised to have an effect on these outcomes *a priori* (See Table 2) [11]. In contrast to Bower et al [11] we revised the conceptualisation of enhanced usual care to include an ordinal measure of enhanced usual care in place of primary care provider training (See Methods S2 for the coding and scoring of enhanced usual care).

We used a DerSimonian-Laird [28] random-effects model to calculate the overall effect of collaborative care, accounting for estimated heterogeneity. To quantify the estimated heterogeneity we used the I^2 index, which represents the percentage of estimated between-study variability in the total variability [29]. By convention I^2 values of 25% are considered low, 50% moderate, and 75% high [20]. The main analysis used random-effects meta-regression to estimate a regression coefficient with 95% CIs between study level covariates and outcomes for:

i) Meta-regression model one (multivariable): study level covariates as predictors of depressive symptoms.
ii) Meta-regression model two (multivariable): study level covariates as predictors of anti-depressant use.
iii) Meta-regression model three (univariable; mechanisms of change): anti-depressant use as a predictor of depressive symptoms. This model tested whether use of anti-depressant medication predicted the treatment effect on depressive symptoms.

We explored the potential for confounding or collinearity across the 10 covariates using logistic regression analyses to perform pairwise comparisons. Shared variance between each pair was low ($\leq$0.14), indicating that there is a very small risk of measured confounding or collinearity in our measured variables. To retain statistical power we identified covariates for testing in the multivariable meta-regression models by initially performing a series of separate univariable meta-regression analyses, using a significance criterion of $p \leq 0.10$. The $p \leq 0.10$ threshold was chosen to avoid prematurely discounting potentially important

Table 2. Study level covariates (N = 85 comparisons).

Characteristic	Description	N
Country		
US	Study setting	60
Non-US	Study setting	25
Recruitment method		
Systematic identification	Patients were referred into the study if they were: i) identified from a clinical database as having depression or ii) screened positive for depression on an outcome measure and/or diagnostic clinical interview	69
Referral by clinicians	Patients were referred into the study by their clinician	16
Patient sample		
Anti-depressant medication NOT inclusion criteria	Participants did not have to be on or willing to take anti-depressant medication as part of the study's inclusion criteria	62
Anti-depressant medication part of inclusion criteria	Participants had to be currently taking or willing to take anti-depressant medication as part of the study's inclusion criteria	23
Chronic physical health condition		
Present	Participants with a chronic physical health condition were actively recruited as part of the study's inclusion criteria	19
Absent	Participants with a chronic physical health condition were NOT actively recruited as part of the study's inclusion criteria	66
Case manager professional background		
Mental health professional	Trained in mental health disciplines outside of the context of the trial (i.e. psychologist, psychiatric nurse, social worker)	47
Non-mental health professional	No extensive training in mental health other than that provided by the trial	38
Intervention content		
Medication management	Intervention included a medication management plan to ensure optimal levels of adherence to pharmacotherapy. This does not represent degree of adherence (i.e. anti-depressant use).	38
Psychological or both	Intervention included a recognised psychological treatment model (i.e. behavioural activation, problem solving) either on its own or combined with medication.	47
Number of sessions		
Continuous variable	Based on number of planned sessions in the first six months. If the number of sessions differed based on the treatment modality offered (i.e. participants could choose between medication management or psychological therapy) then a mean score was calculated.	
Supervision frequency		
Ad hoc	No regular patterns of supervision.	29
Scheduled	Supervision occurred on a regular basis (i.e. weekly).	52
Not applicable	Applies to studies whose collaborative care intervention included only the primary care provider but the case manager was a certified mental health practitioner (e.g. psychiatrist, psychologist, psychotherapist).	4
Enhanced usual care		
Ordinal variable (based on summed score, 0 4)	See description provided in Methods S2	
Allocation concealment		
Low risk of bias	Coded according to Cochrane risk of bias tool	39
High risk of bias	Coded according to Cochrane risk of bias tool	4

explanatory variables. Table 2 summarises all ten study level covariates included in both meta-regression models one and two.

Results

Characteristics of included studies

Seventy four trials met our inclusion criteria for the meta-regression (including 85 relevant comparisons, across 21,345 participants); 84 comparisons had data on depressive symptoms (across 21,284 participants), and 59 comparisons had data on anti-depressant use (across, 14, 465 participants). See Figure 1.

Of the 85 comparisons included in the meta-regression 25 (29%) were conducted outside the United States; only 4% were conducted in low to middle income countries (Table S1). Nineteen (22%) comparisons specifically recruited patients with chronic physical disease. As stated in the methods section trials had to meet the four criteria for collaborative care to be included in the review. Key factors that differentiated the type of interventions tested in the meta-regression were case manager background and content of the structured management plan. In 47 (55%) comparisons the case manager was a mental health practitioner, and in 38 (45%) comparisons case managers were drawn from a variety of non-mental health backgrounds. In 39 (46%) comparisons the

Table 3. Characteristics of collaborative care.

Author	Multi-professional approach to patient care		Structured management plan	Number of scheduled follow-ups	Enhanced inter professional communication	
	Medical professional	**Case manager background**			**CM liaison with PCP**	**Supervision frequency**
Adler 2004	Doctor	Non-mental health practitioner	Medication management	6	Shared note system	Scheduled
Araya 2003	Doctor	Mental health practitioner	Both	9	Shared note system	Ad hoc
Bartels 2004	Doctor	Mental health practitioner	Medication management	Not reported	Multiple methods	Not reported
Blanchard 1995	Doctor	Mental health practitioner	Both	12	Verbal	Ad hoc
Bogner 2008	Mixed	Mental health practitioner	Medication management	5	Liaison method	Scheduled
Bogner 2010	Mixed	Non-mental health practitioner	Medication management	5	Liaison method	Scheduled
Bogner 2012	Doctor	Non-mental health practitioner	Medication management	5	Verbal	Ad hoc
Bruce 2004	Doctor	Mental health practitioner	Both	15	Liaison method	Scheduled
Buszewicz 2011	Doctor	Non-mental health practitioner	Both	4	Verbal	Ad hoc
Capoccia 2004	Doctor	non-mental health practitioner	Medication management	10	Shared note system	Scheduled
Chaney 2011	Doctor	Non-mental health practitioner	Medication management	5	Multiple methods	Scheduled
Chew-Graham 2007	Doctor	Mental health practitioner	Both	11	Multiple methods	Scheduled
Ciechanowski 2004	Doctor	Mental health practitioner	Psychological therapy	9	Other	Scheduled
Ciechanowski 2010	Specialist	Mental health practitioner	Psychological therapy	9	Other	Scheduled
Cole 2006	Doctor	Non-mental health practitioner	Both	24	Liaison method	Ad hoc
Datto 2003	Doctor	Mental health practitioner	Medication management	6	Written communication	Scheduled
Davidson 2013	Doctor	Mental health practitioner	Both	11	Verbal	Scheduled
Dietrich 2004	Doctor	Mental health practitioner	Medication management	6	Written communication	Scheduled
Dwight-Johnson 2005	Doctor	Mental health practitioner	Both	7	Multiple methods	Scheduled
Dwight-Johnson 2010	Doctor	Mental health practitioner	Both	12	Liaison method	Scheduled
Dwight-Johnson 2011	Specialist	Mental health practitioner	Psychological therapy	8	Liaison method	Scheduled
Ell 2007	Doctor	Mental health practitioner	Both	12	Liaison method	Ad hoc
Ell 2008	Specialist	Mental health practitioner	Both	21	Multiple methods	Scheduled
Ell 2010	Doctor	Mental health practitioner	Both	18	Liaison method	Scheduled
Finley 2003	Doctor	Non-mental health practitioner	Medication management	8	Multiple methods	Scheduled
Fortney 2007	Doctor	Non-mental health practitioner	Medication management	26	Shared note system	Scheduled
Fritsch 2007	Doctor	Non-mental health practitioner	Medication management	6	Other	Ad hoc
Gensichen 2009	Doctor	Non-mental health practitioner	Both	13	Written communication	Ad hoc

Table 3. Cont.

Author	Multi-professional approach to patient care		Structured management plan	Number of scheduled follow-ups	Enhanced inter professional communication	
	Medical professional	Case manager background			CM liaison with PCP	Supervision frequency
Gjerdingen 2008	Doctor	Mental health practitioner	Medication management	12	Written communication	Ad hoc
Hedrick 2003	Doctor	Mental health practitioner	Both	Not reported	Shared note system	Scheduled
Huffman 2011	Doctor	Mental health practitioner	Medication management	4	Liaison method	Scheduled
Huijbregts 2013	Doctor	Non-mental health practitioner	Both	12	Share note system	Scheduled
Hunkeler 2000	Doctor	Non-mental health practitioner	Both	14	Liaison method	Scheduled
Katon 1995a	Doctor	Mental health practitioner	Both	2	Multiple methods	Not reported
Katon 1995b	Doctor	Mental health practitioner	Both	2	Multiple methods	Not reported
Katon 1996a	Doctor	Mental health practitioner	Both	10	Multiple methods	Scheduled
Katon 1996b	Doctor	Mental health practitioner	Both	10	Multiple methods	Scheduled
Katon 1999	Doctor	Mental health practitioner	Medication management	3	Multiple methods	Not reported
Katon 2001	Doctor	Mental health practitioner	Both	4	Multiple methods	Scheduled
Katon 2004	Doctor	Non-mental health practitioner	Both	7	Multiple methods	Scheduled
Katon 2010	Doctor	Non-mental health practitioner	Both	Not reported	Liaison method	Scheduled
Katzelnick 2000	Doctor	Non-mental health practitioner	Medication management	3	Multiple methods	Ad hoc
Kroenke 2010	Doctor	Non-mental health practitioner	Medication management	4	Other	Scheduled
Landis 2007	Doctor	Mental health practitioner	Medication management	9	Liaison method	Scheduled
Lobello 2010	Doctor	Non-mental health practitioner	Medication management	3	Written communication	Ad hoc
Ludman 2007a	Doctor	Non-mental health practitioner	Medication management	3	Multiple methods	Scheduled
Ludman 2007b	Doctor	Non-mental health practitioner	Both	15	Multiple methods	Scheduled
Ludman 2007c	Doctor	Non-mental health practitioner	Both	25	Multiple methods	Scheduled
Mann 1998	Doctor	Non-mental health practitioner	Medication management	Not reported	Multiple methods	Ad hoc
McCusker 2008	Doctor	Mental health practitioner	Psychological therapy	5	Written communication	Ad hoc
McMahon 2007	Doctor	Mental health practitioner	Medication management	6	Liaison method	Scheduled
Menchetti 2013	Doctor	Non-mental health practitioner	Both	Not reported	Verbal	Scheduled
Morgan 2013	Doctor	Non-mental health practitioner	Both	2	Written communication	Ad hoc
Oslin 2003	Doctor	Mental health practitioner	Medication management	8	Liaison method	Scheduled
Patel 2010	Doctor	Non-mental health practitioner	Both	Not reported	Liaison method	Ad hoc
Piette 2011	Doctor	Mental health practitioner	Psychological therapy	15	Multiple methods	Scheduled

Table 3. Cont.

Author	Multi-professional approach to patient care		Structured management plan	Number of scheduled follow-ups	Enhanced inter professional communication	
	Medical professional	Case manager background			CM liaison with PCP	Supervision frequency
Pyne 2011	Specialist	Non-mental health practitioner	Medication management	Not reported	Shared note system	Scheduled
Richards 2008a	Doctor	Mental health practitioner	Both	10	Multiple methods	Scheduled
Richards 2008b	Doctor	Mental health practitioner	Both	10	Multiple methods	Scheduled
Richards 2012	Specialist	Mental health practitioner	Both	12	Liaison method	Scheduled
Rojas 2007	Doctor	Non-mental health practitioner	Both	8	Not reported	Ad hoc
Rollman 2009	Doctor	Non-mental health practitioner	Both	10	Multiple methods	Scheduled
Ross 2008	Doctor	Mental health practitioner	Medication management	5	Liaison method	Ad hoc
Rost 2002a	Doctor	Non-mental health practitioner	Medication management	6	Written communication	Ad hoc
Rost 2002b	Doctor	Non-mental health practitioner	Medication management	6	Written communication	Ad hoc
Rubenstein 2006	Doctor	Non-mental health practitioner	Medication management		Other	Ad hoc
Simon 2000a	Doctor	Mental health practitioner	Medication management	3	Multiple methods	Scheduled
Simon 2000b	Doctor	Mental health practitioner	Medication management	3	Multiple methods	Scheduled
Simon 2004a	Doctor	Mental health practitioner	Both	3	Multiple methods	Scheduled
Simon 2004b	Doctor	Mental health practitioner	Both	11	Multiple methods	Scheduled
Simon 2011	Doctor	Mental health practitioner	Medication management	4	Shared note system	Scheduled
Smit 2005a	Doctor	Mental health practitioner	Both	4	Written communication	Ad hoc
Smit 2005b	Doctor	Mental health practitioner	Both	4	Written communication	Ad hoc
Smit 2005c	Doctor	Mental health practitioner	Both	8	Written communication	Ad hoc
Strong 2008	Doctor	Non-mental health practitioner	Both	13	Multiple methods	Scheduled
Swindle 2003	Doctor	Mental health practitioner	Medication management	4	Liaison method	Ad hoc
Uebelacker 2011	Doctor	Non-mental health practitioner	Both	8	Written communication	Scheduled
Unutzer 2002	Doctor	Mental health practitioner	Both	15	Shared note system	Scheduled
Vera 2010	Doctor	Mental health practitioner	Medication management	Not reported	Liaison method	Scheduled
Vlasveld 2011	Specialist	Non-mental health practitioner	Both	9	Liaison method	Ad hoc
Wells 2000a	Doctor	Non-mental health practitioner	Medication management	8	Written communication	Ad hoc
Wells 2000b	Doctor	Mental health practitioner	Psychological therapy	Not reported	Written communication	Ad hoc
Wilkinson 2003	Doctor	Non-mental health practitioner	Medication management	5	Not reported	Ad hoc
Williams 2007	Mixed	Non-mental health practitioner	Medication management	7	Liaison method	Scheduled

Table 3. Cont.

Author	Multi-professional approach to patient care		Structured management plan	Number of scheduled follow-ups	Enhanced inter professional communication	
	Medical professional	Case manager background			CM liaison with PCP	Supervision frequency
Yeung 2010	Doctor	Non-mental health practitioner	Medication management	8	Other	Scheduled

CM = case manager; PCP = primary care provider.

intervention included both psychological therapy and antidepressant medication management; 40 (47%) included medication management alone; and 6 (7%) included psychological therapy alone. Table 3 describes characteristics of collaborative care used in the included trials. A reference list of included trials is presented in Results S1.

Meta-analysis of the effect of collaborative care on depressive symptoms and anti-depressant use

Compared with usual care, collaborative care was associated with improvements in depressive symptoms (standardised mean difference, SMD −0.28, 95% CI −0.33 to −0.23; $I^2 = 62.2\%$, 95% CI 52.2% to 70.1%; Figure S1) and increased anti-depressant use (relative risk, RR 1.53, 95% CI 1.40 to1.68; $I^2 = 80.8\%$, 95% CI 75.8% to 84.8%; Figure S2).

Meta-regression model one: predictors of depressive symptoms

The results of the univariable analyses of study-level and patient-aggregate covariates on depressive symptoms are shown in Table 4 and the multivariable analyses are shown in Table 5. Four covariates were identified for inclusion in the multivariable meta-regression model: recruitment by systematic identification using either interviews, outcome measures or electronic medical records (study-level; ß −0.16, 95% CI −0.30 to −0.02), people with a chronic physical condition as an inclusion criterion (study-level; ß −0.17, 95% CI −0.28 to −0.05), psychological interventions, alone or with medication (study-level; ß −0.13, 95% CI −0.23 to −0.03), and scheduled supervision (study-level; ß −0.12, 95% CI −0.23 to −0.02). In the multivariable model only psychological intervention remained as a statistically significant predictor of depressive symptoms (study-level; ß −0.11, 95% CI −0.20 to −0.01). Studies that included psychological interventions (alone or with medication) reported greater improvements in depressive outcomes, compared with those studies that included medication management alone.

The beta coefficient reported for the multivariable predictors of depressive symptoms can be back-transformed from an SMD to a mean difference under certain assumptions for the variance of the effect [30]. We only proceeded to back-transform to the patient health questionnaire-9, for which we observed similar within variability across studies reporting on the same scale, and the beta was equivalent to a decrease of 0.67 (95% CI −1.23 to 0.06). The multivariable model reduced the I^2 statistic from 62.2% (95% CI 52.2% to 70.1%) to 47.8% (95% CI 32.6 to 59.6).

Meta-regression model two: predictors of anti-depressant use

The results of the univariable analyses of study level covariates on antidepressant medication use are shown in Table 6 and multivariable analyses are shown in Table 7. Two study level covariates were identified for inclusion in the multivariable meta-

Table 4. Univariable predictors on depressive symptoms (N = 84).

Variable		Regression Coefficient (95% CI)	SE	P	I^2 (95% CI)
Dichotomous or categorical					
Country	Non-US (vs US)	−0.04 (−0.16 to 0.07)	.06	.47	62.4 (52.5 to 70.3)
Recruitment method	Systematic (vs GP referral)	−0.16 (−0.30 to −0.02)	.07	.03	60.8 (50.3 to 69.1)
Patient sample	Medication inclusion criteria (vs not inclusion criteria)	0.08 (−0.04 to 0.20)	.06	.21	62.3 (52.3 to 70.2)
Chronic physical health condition	Present (vs absent)	−0.17 (−0.28 to −0.05)	.06	.01	58.9 (47.7 to 67.7)
Case manager background	Mental health (vs non-mental health)	0.03 (−0.07 to 0.14)	.05	.53	62.5 (52.6 to 70.3)
Intervention content	Psychological intervention or both (vs medication only)	−0.13 (−0.23 to −0.03)	.05	.01	56.8 (44.9 to 66.1)
Supervision frequency	Scheduled (vs ad hoc)	−0.12 (−0.23 to −0.02)	.05	.02	53.7 (40.7 to 63.9)
	Not applicable (vs ad hoc)	0.10 (−0.13 to 0.33)	.12	.38	
Allocation concealment	High risk (vs low risk)	0.06 (−0.03 to 0.16)	.05	.20	62.0 (51.9 to 70.0)
Continuous					
Enhanced usual care*¶		0.02 (−0.03 to 0.08)	.03	.37	62.0 (51.9 to 70.0)
Number of sessions*¶		−0.01 (−0.02 to 0.00)	.01	.26	50.7 (35.5 to 62.3)

*N of 74 comparisons.
¶model intercepts (constants) not reported.

Table 5. Multivariable predictors of depressive symptoms (N = 84).

Variable	Regression Coefficient (95% CI)	SE	P
Recruitment method (Systematic)	−0.12 (−0.26 to 0.02)	.07	.10
Chronic physical health condition (Present)	−0.10 (−0.22 to 0.02)	.06	.11
Intervention content (Psychological intervention or both)	−0.11 (−0.20 to −0.01)	.05	.03
Supervision frequency (Scheduled)*	−0.08 (−0.19 to 0.02)	.05	.13
Supervision frequency (Not applicable)*	0.06 (−0.15 to 0.28)	.11	.57
Intercept (constant)	−0.05 (−0.20 to 0.10)	.08	.53

I^2 = 47.8% (95% CI 32.6 to 59.6).
*Compared with the reference category, ad hoc supervision.

regression model: studies that recruited participants using systematic identification (RR 1.55, 95% CI 1.22 to 1.97) and studies that included participants with a chronic physical condition (RR 1.45, 95% CI 1.16 to 1.83). In the multivariable meta-regression model studies that recruited participants systematically (RR 1.43, 95% CI 1.12 to 1.81) and included participants with a chronic physical condition (RR 1.32, 95% CI 1.05 to 1.65) remained statistically significant predictors of anti-depressant use. Studies including participants who were systematically identified and those with a chronic physical condition adhered more to their anti-depressant medications. The multivariable model reduced the I^2 statistic from 80.8% (95% CI 75.8% to 84.8%) to 75.2% (95% CI 68.1% to 80.7%).

Sensitivity analyses using intraclass correlation coefficients of 0.00 and 0.05 for cluster trials did not impact greatly on the multivariable meta-regression findings (see Results S2 and Results S3). The subgroup analysis exploring the relationship between sample size and effect size for both depressive symptoms and medication use was statistically non-significant, thus decreasing the likelihood that our findings are susceptible to publication bias (Results S4).

Meta-regression model three: the effect of change in anti-depressant use on depressive symptoms

Increased anti-depressant use was not associated with improvement in depressive symptoms (ß −0.13, 95% CI −0.27 to 0.004, p = 0.06).

Discussion

Overall, collaborative care successfully improves both patient outcomes and the process of care for depression. Studies that included psychological interventions, (alone or with medication management), as part of collaborative care were associated with greater improvements in depressive symptoms compared with studies that only included medication management alone. Use of antidepressants was increased in studies that included participants with a chronic physical health condition and in studies that recruited participants through a process of systematic identification.

Strengths and limitations

Our analyses were based on a priori decisions about covariates likely to moderate the treatment effect of collaborative care [11] and included the largest and most comprehensive dataset about

Table 6. Univariable predictors of antidepressant use (N = 59).

Variable		Relative risk (95% CI)	SE	P	I^2 (95% CI)
Dichotomous or categorical					
Country	Non-US (vs US)	0.89 (0.71 to 1.13)	.11	.34	80.1 (74.8 to 84.3)
Recruitment method	Systematic (vs GP referral)	1.55 (1.22 to 1.97)	.19	<.001	77.3 (71.0 to 82.2)
Patient sample	Medication inclusion criteria (vs not inclusion criteria)	0.85 (0.68 to 1.07)	.10	.16	80.6 (75.5 to 84.6)
Chronic physical health condition	Present (vs absent|)	1.45 (1.16 to 1.83)	.17	.001	78.2 (72.2 to 82.9)
Case manager background	Mental health (vs non-mental health)	1.06 (0.85 to 1.31)	.12	.61	80.9 (75.9 to 84.9)
Intervention content	Psychological intervention or both (vs medication only)	0.92 (0.74 to 1.14)	.10	.44	81.1 (76.2 to 85.0)
Supervision frequency	Scheduled (vs ad hoc)	1.03 (0.82 to 1.29)	.12	.83	81.3 (76.4 to 85.2)
	Not applicable (vs ad hoc)	0.94 (0.44 to 2.02)	.37	.87	
Allocation concealment	High risk (vs low risk)	0.89 (0.72 to 1.09)	.09	.25	80.9 (75.9 to 84.9)
Continuous					
Enhanced usual care		0.93 (0.85 to 1.03)	.05	.17	81.0 (76.0 to 84.9)
Number of sessions*¶		0.99 (0.97 to 1.01)	.01	.54	78.2 (71.9 to 83.1)

*N of 53 comparisons.
¶model intercepts (constants) not reported.

Table 7. Multivariable predictors of antidepressant use (N = 59).

Variable	Relative risk (95% CI)	SE	P
Recruitment method (systematic)	1.42 (1.12 to 1.81)	.17	.004
Chronic physical health condition (Present)*	1.32 (1.05 to 1.65)	.15	.02
Intercept (constant)	1.08 (0.88 to 1.32)	.11	.46

I^2 = 75.2% (95% CI 68.1% to 80.7%).
*Compared with the reference category, physical health condition absent.

collaborative care. By searching extensively, we were able to include almost twice as many trials as previous reviews, and this substantially enhanced our ability to quantify and explore heterogeneity with a greater level of statistical power, thus reducing the chance of spurious findings [31]. In addition, the large number of studies gives us more confidence in the asymptotic meta-analysis methods employed [32], even if the study effects are not normally distributed [33]. The high levels of estimated heterogeneity are a positive finding since it appears heterogeneity levels are being consistently underestimated in meta-analyses [34]. Although there is a link between meta-analysis size and heterogeneity levels and we would expect to detect high levels given the size of our review [34], as we do, the large between-study variability implies that there might be other study or patient-level variables that could explain some of it (e.g. depression severity, ethnicity of patients, fidelity to intervention, quality of case manager training, and level of engagement in psychological treatment).

Additionally, meta-regression can be weakened by other statistical considerations and poor reporting. For example, we were not able to include demographic variables in the regression models due to a lack of variability, and we were unable to model a dose response relationship between treatment effects and case management sessions because most trials did not report data about the frequency, intensity, and duration of psychological treatments. We contacted authors for this information but this process did not overcome this limitation pointing to the need for more comprehensive reporting about the delivery of treatments in psychological therapy trials. More severely depressed patients are more responsive to psychological [35] and pharmacological interventions [36] but we were unable to replicate these analyses in trials of collaborative care because depression severity was inconsistently reported; contacting authors did not overcome this issue. Failure to include these covariates may have biased our results [37]. This limitation also highlights the need for more consistent and comprehensive reporting about the content of complex mental health interventions and efforts to strengthen reporting and specification of complex behaviour change are a step forward to overcoming this limitation [38].

In the absence of individual patient data we had to rely on analyses of mean study effects which are prone to bias ('ecological fallacy': deducing for an individual from a group mean), which are difficult to interpret since the relationships within- and between-studies might differ, making evidence from such analyses inconclusive [27]. In addition, we could not use a single structural equation model to properly account for mediating and moderating effects and the relationships between antidepressant use and depressive symptoms.

Most trials included in this review only reported short-term follow-up limiting opportunities to conduct sensitivity analyses of moderators of long term effectiveness of collaborative care. The absence of long term follow-up data among the group of trials included in this review resembles the findings of Deshauer et al., who screened more than 2000 records for classic placebo-controlled RCTs of selective serotonin reuptake inhibitors and identified only six studies with follow-up of 6 months or greater [39]. There is a clear need to build longer term follow-up into trials of treatment of depression given that depression is episodic and the ultimate goal of treatment is to bring about sustained recovery. Additionally, most trials did not report if the trial population included patients with comorbid chronic physical health conditions, further reducing the number of comparisons entered into the regression models. Furthermore, it is reasonable to assume that all studies that included older adults will have included patients with unreported comorbidity, potentially rendering comparisons of collaborative care in chronic physical health conditions redundant. However, our analysis suggests that presence of a chronic physical health condition as a study inclusion criteria remained a key moderator of medication adherence irrespective of the presence of unreported comorbidities, suggesting that this issue has substantive significance, and does not represent confounding.

We analysed ten theoretically plausible covariates that might determine the effectiveness of collaborative care on both depressive symptoms and medication use using an initial p value of 0.10. Assuming statistical independence then approximately one in ten of our tests was susceptible to type I error but we did not adjust for multiple testing. However, we felt justified in this approach. Although adopting a more conservative approach to hypothesis testing using multiplicity adjustments would have decreased our chances of making a Type I error, we would have also increased our chances of Type II errors (i.e. false negatives), and thus rejected important predictors of the effectiveness of collaborative care outcomes [40].

Comparisons with the previous meta-regression analysis

A novel finding of our meta-regression is that including psychological therapy, either alone or with antidepressant medication, conferred additional benefit, at least for depressive symptoms. Compared with previous analyses [11] we included a greater number of trials (+50) in our analysis which means that our analysis is the first to be powered to detect this finding. In addition, we showed that studies that systematically identified patients were important moderators of anti-depressant medication use. This finding may also be due to increased statistical power generated by our meta-regression. Additionally, we also showed that the presence of a chronic physical condition moderated use of anti-depressant medications – trials that included patients with chronic physical conditions reported increased use of anti-depressant medication. This patient characteristic was not explored in the previous meta-regression.

Contrary to the findings of a previous meta-regression [11], case-manager background did not predict reduction in depressive symptoms. Despite improvements there are still shortages of psychologists and psychotherapists, especially in low and middle-income countries [41], but case management of depression in the context of collaborative care might not need be delivered by a mental health professional. Indeed there is emerging evidence, mainly from the United States, that nurse-led collaborative care is more effective than usual care for treating depression in people with chronic physical disease [42], suggesting that non-mental health trained primary care nurses are as well placed as mental health professionals to work as case managers for certain types of patients. However, where case managers are drawn from non-mental health professions there may need to be more emphasis on ensuring that there are satisfactory arrangements in place for regular specialist supervision.

Clinical supervision of psychological therapists can positively affect the process of treatment, leading to greater confidence, self-awareness, and competence among therapists [43], and, in the context of brief psychological treatment, possibly improved patient outcomes [44]. Our initial univariable analysis adds weight to previous findings [11] that compared with ad hoc supervision the availability of scheduled case manager supervision from a mental health specialist predicted improved depressive symptom outcomes. This finding has important implications for patient benefit given that large scale epidemiological studies have shown that depression is under-treated because of inadequate anti-depressant medication management by health care providers, along with poor clinical supervision and patient follow-up [45]. Inadequate anti-depressant treatment of depression is more pronounced in people with chronic physical conditions [46]. Recurrence of symptoms is also common, but patients who continue treatment with anti-depressants reduce the risk of recurrence by 70% compared with those who discontinue treatment [47], although it is not clear whether reduction in relapse represents true long term efficacy or avoidance of relapse precipitated by antidepressant withdrawal [48]. Additionally, few patients respond to an initial 20 mg dose of citalopram and only about 40% of patients achieve remission after receiving the full therapeutic dosage of an anti-depressant medication [49]. Furthermore, up to 20% of patients remain depressed after completing an initial phase of treatment [50]. Regular supervision within collaborative care could thus help to overcome therapeutic impasse by supporting case managers to identify and manage patients who do not initially respond to or discontinue treatment by facilitating changes to anti-depressant dosage, augmentation of medication with another therapy, or recommending switching to another treatment.

Implications for policy and practice

Our findings show that structured management plans that included psychological interventions either as a standalone therapy or in combination with antidepressant medication predicted reductions in depressive symptoms more so than collaborative care that only offered patients anti-depressant medication. While the additional effects associated with psychological treatment were small this result does highlight the importance of patient choice in the delivery of health care for depression. Across a diverse range of psychiatric conditions and health care settings patients have reported a 3-fold preference for psychological treatment over pharmacological treatment, underscoring the need to link treatment strategies to patient preference [51].

We showed that certain types of patients appear to be better at taking anti-depressant medications than others. In the absence of collaborative care depression is under-treated with anti-depressant medication in older adults with chronic physical conditions [46]. However, our findings show that this patient group showed improved levels of anti-depressant use compared with those without chronic physical conditions. It may be that patients with depression and chronic physical conditions are primed to respond well to structured management programmes that include anti-depressant medication because they are well versed in using medications to self-manage their chronic illness. However the burden of treatment for patients with complex, chronic physical and mental comorbidities may reduce their capacity to collaborate in their care [52].

Novel to this review was our finding that compared with recruitment by clinicians, trials that systematically identified patients were associated with increased use of anti-depressant medication. This finding goes beyond methodological considerations about how to effectively recruit patients into mental health trials. Patients referred to mental health services by clinicians tend to be patients with most to gain as they may be more severely depressed. However, the fact that we found that systems based approaches to patient identification predicted increased use of anti-depressant medication highlights the fact that population approaches to disease management can identify different types of patients who may have additional capacity to benefit, further underlining the importance of structured approaches to depression care.

Future work and conclusion

Given the premise that collaborative care is an organisational framework within which different combinations of psychological and pharmacological interventions can be used a key unanswered question relates to how interventions can be tailored, adjusted, or changed to meet the needs of patients. Most collaborative care trials have only measured adherence to anti-depressants but not frequency of changes to medication dosage or augmentation of medication with another therapy. Given that use of anti-depressant medication might be a proxy for why collaborative care is effective it is critical that future trials include process measures that can evaluate adjustment and augmentation of medication similar to those used in the Teamcare trial [53]. Additionally, meta-analysis using individual rather than study-level data would increase opportunities to detect differential treatment effects across individuals in randomised trials, and allows for more complex modelling of the association of treatment effects and patient characteristics [54].

In conclusion, these results update and expand on a previous analysis of factors that differentiate collaborative care trials that improve patient outcomes and/or the process of care from those that do not. Psychological therapy is an active ingredient in collaborative care with or without anti-depressant medication, emphasising the importance of building flexible collaborative care models that include different combinations of pharmacological and non-pharmacological therapies that meet patients' treatment preferences. Furthermore, patients systematically identified and those with chronic physical conditions are likely to adhere more to pharmacological treatments. Using systems based approaches to identify patients with depression highlights the importance of borrowing elements from chronic disease management models to improve the process of depression care.

Supporting Information

Figure S1 Forest plot of effect of collaborative care on depressive symptoms. *Meta-analysis of individual trial and* *pooled effects. Random effects model used. 95% CI = 95% confidence intervals.*

Figure S2 Forest plot of effect of collaborative care on antidepressant use. *Meta-analysis of individual trial and pooled effects. Random effects model used. 95% CI = 95% confidence intervals.*

Table S1 Characteristics of included studies.

Methods S1 Central Search Strategy.

Methods S2 Meta-regression coding manual.

Checklist S1 PRISMA Checklist.

Results S1 Reference list of included studies.

Results S2 Sensitivity analysis: Cluster Intraclass correlation coefficient of 0.00.

Results S3 Sensitivity analysis: Cluster Intraclass correlation coefficient of 0.05.

Results S4 Sensitivity analysis: Relationship between sample size and effect size.

Acknowledgments

PC is the guarantor of this work and, as such, had full access to all the data in the study and takes responsibility for the integrity of the data and the accuracy of the data analysis.

Author Contributions

Conceived and designed the experiments: PC JH EK PB. Analyzed the data: JH EK PC PB JA. Wrote the paper: PC JH EK PB. Edited the manuscript: WW LG SG DR CD KL JA.

References

1. Ferrari AJ, Charlson FJ, Norman RE, Patten SB, Freedman G, et al. (2013) Burden of Depressive Disorders by Country, Sex, Age, and Year: Findings from the Global Burden of Disease Study 2010. PLoS Med 10: e1001547.
2. Moussavi S, Chatterji S, Verdes E, Tandon A, Patel V, et al. (2007) Depression, chronic diseases, and decrements in health: results from the World Health Surveys. Lancet 370: 851–858.
3. Wagner EH, Austin BT, Michael Von K (1996) Organizing Care for Patients with Chronic Illness. The Milbank Quarterly 74: 511–544.
4. Bodenheimer T, Wagner EH, Grumbach K (2002) Improving primary care for patients with chronic illness. JAMA 288: 1775–1779.
5. Furukawa TA, Yoshimura R, Harai H, Imaizumi T, Takeuchi H, et al. (2009) How many well vs. unwell days can you expect over 10 years, once you become depressed? Acta Psychiatrica Scandinavica 119: 290–297.
6. Tsai AC, Morton SC, Mangione CM, Keeler EB (2005) A meta-analysis of interventions to improve care for chronic illnesses. American Journal of Managed Care 11: 478–488.
7. Gunn J, Diggens J, Hegarty K, Blashki G (2006) A systematic review of complex system interventions designed to increase recovery from depression in primary care. BMC Health Serv Res 6: 88.
8. Archer J, Bower P, Gilbody S, Lovell K, Richards D, et al. (2012) Collaborative care for depression and anxiety problems. Cochrane Database Syst Rev 10: CD006525.
9. Gilbody S, Bower P, Whitty P (2006) Costs and consequences of enhanced primary care for depression: systematic review of randomised economic evaluations. Br J Psychiatry 189: 297–308.
10. Katon W, Unutzer J (2006) Collaborative care models for depression: time to move from evidence to practice. Arch Intern Med 166: 2304–2306.
11. Bower P, Gilbody S, Richards D, Fletcher J, Sutton A (2006) Collaborative care for depression in primary care. Making sense of a complex intervention: systematic review and meta-regression. Br J Psychiatry 189: 484–493.
12. Liberati A, Altman DG, Tetzlaff J, Mulrow C, Gøtzsche PC, et al. (2009) The PRISMA Statement for Reporting Systematic Reviews and Meta-Analyses of Studies That Evaluate Health Care Interventions: Explanation and Elaboration. Annals of Internal Medicine 151: W-65.
13. Royle P, Waugh N (2005) A simplified search strategy for identifying randomised controlled trials for systematic reviews of health care interventions: a comparison with more exhaustive strategies. BMC Medical Research Methodology 5: 23.
14. Korff MV, Goldberg D (2001) Improving outcomes in depression. BMJ 323: 948–949.
15. Weingarten SR, Henning JM, Badamgarav E, Knight K, Hasselblad V, et al. (2002) Interventions used in disease management programmes for patients with chronic illnesswhich ones work? Meta-analysis of published reports. BMJ 325: 925.
16. Gilbody S, Whitty P, Grimshaw J, Thomas R (2003) Educational and organizational interventions to improve the management of depression in primary care: a systematic review. JAMA 289: 3145–3151.
17. Boerma WG, Verhaak PF (1999) The general practitioner as the first contacted health professional by patients with psychosocial problems: a European study. Psychol Med 29: 689–696.
18. Kontopantelis E, Reeves D (2009) METAEFF: Stata module to perform effect sizes calculations for meta-analyses. Statistical Software Components.
19. Lipsey MW, Wilson D (2001) Practical Meta-Analysis. Thousand Oaks: Sage Publictions Inc.
20. Higgins JPT, Green S (2011) Cochrane Handbook for Systematic Reviews of Interventions Version 5.1.0: Cochrane Collaboration.
21. Adams G, Gulliford MC, Ukoumunne OC, Eldridge S, Chinn S, et al. (2004) Patterns of intra-cluster correlation from primary care research to inform study design and analysis. Journal of clinical epidemiology 57: 785–793.
22. Donner A, Klar N (2002) Issues in the meta-analysis of cluster randomized trials. Statistics in medicine 21: 2971–2980.
23. Pereira TV, Horwitz RI, Ioannidis JA (2012) Empirical evaluation of very large treatment effects of medical interventions. JAMA 308: 1676–1684.
24. Hewitt C, Hahn S, Torgerson DJ, Watson J, Bland JM (2005) Adequacy and reporting of allocation concealment: review of recent trials published in four general medical journals. BMJ 330: 1057–1058.
25. Harris R, Bradburn M, Deeks J, Harbord R, Altman D, et al. (2008) metan: fixed- and random-effects meta-analysis. Stata Journal 8: 3–28.
26. Harbord RM, Higgins JPT (2008) Meta-regression in Stata. Stata Journal 8: 493–519.
27. Thompson SG, Higgins JP (2002) How should meta-regression analyses be undertaken and interpreted? Stat Med 21: 1559–1573.
28. DerSimonian R, Laird N (1986) Meta-analysis in clinical trials. Controlled clinical trials 7: 177–188.
29. Higgins JP, Thompson SG (2002) Quantifying heterogeneity in a meta-analysis. Stat Med 21: 1539–1558.
30. Kontopantelis E, Reeves D (2009) MetaEasy: A Meta-Analysis Add-In for Microsoft Excel. Journal of Statistical Software 30.
31. Peduzzi P, Concato J, Kemper E, Holford TR, Feinstein AR (1996) A simulation study of the number of events per variable in logistic regression analysis. J Clin Epidemiol 49: 1373–1379.
32. Brockwell SE, Gordon IR (2001) A comparison of statistical methods for meta-analysis. Statistics in medicine 20: 825–840.
33. Kontopantelis E, Reeves D (2012) Performance of statistical methods for meta-analysis when true study effects are non-normally distributed: A simulation study. Statistical methods in medical research 21: 409–426.
34. Kontopantelis E, Springate DA, Reeves D (2013) A Re-Analysis of the Cochrane Library Data: The Dangers of Unobserved Heterogeneity in Meta-Analyses. PLoS One 8: e69930.
35. Driessen E, Cuijpers P, Hollon SD, Dekker JJ (2010) Does pretreatment severity moderate the efficacy of psychological treatment of adult outpatient depression? A meta-analysis. J Consult Clin Psychol 78: 668–680.
36. Kirsch I, Deacon BJ, Huedo-Medina TB, Scoboria A, Moore TJ, et al. (2008) Initial severity and antidepressant benefits: a meta-analysis of data submitted to the Food and Drug Administration. PLoS Med 5: e45.
37. Negassa A, Hanley JA (2007) The effect of omitted covariates on confidence interval and study power in binary outcome analysis: a simulation study. Contemp Clin Trials 28: 242–248.
38. Michie S, Richardson M, Johnston M, Abraham C, Francis J, et al. (2013) The Behavior Change Technique Taxonomy (v1) of 93 Hierarchically Clustered Techniques: Building an International Consensus for the Reporting of Behavior Change Interventions. Annals of Behavioral Medicine 46: 81–95.
39. Deshauer D, Moher D, Fergusson D, Moher E, Sampson M, et al. (2008) Selective serotonin reuptake inhibitors for unipolar depression: a systematic review of classic long-term randomized controlled trials. Canadian Medical Association Journal 178: 1293–1301.

40. Rothman KJ (1990) No adjustments are needed for multiple comparisons. Epidemiology 1: 43–46.
41. Saraceno B, van Ommeren M, Batniji R, Cohen A, Gureje O, et al. (2007) Barriers to improvement of mental health services in low-income and middle-income countries. The Lancet 370: 1164–1174.
42. Ekers D, Murphy R, Archer J, Ebenezer C, Kemp D, et al. (2013) Nurse-delivered collaborative care for depression and long-term physical conditions: A systematic review and meta-analysis. J Affect Disord 149: 14–22.
43. Milne D, James I (2000) A systematic review of effective cognitive-behavioural supervision. British Journal of Clinical Psychology 39: 111–127.
44. Bambling M, King R, Raue P, Schweitzer R, Lambert W (2006) Clinical supervision: Its influence on client-rated working alliance and client symptom reduction in the brief treatment of major depression. Psychotherapy Research 16: 317–331.
45. Salisbury C, Johnson L, Purdy S, Valderas JM, Montgomery AA (2011) Epidemiology and impact of multimorbidity in primary care: a retrospective cohort study. British Journal of General Practice 61: e12–e21.
46. Kendrick T, Dowrick C, McBride A, Howe A, Clarke P, et al. (2009) Management of depression in UK general practice in relation to scores on depression severity questionnaires: analysis of medical record data. BMJ 338: b750.
47. Dickens C, Katon W, Blakemore A, Khara A, McGowan L, et al. (2012) Does depression predict the use of urgent and unscheduled care by people with long term conditions? A systematic review with meta-analysis. Journal of Psychosomatic Research 73: 334–342.
48. El-Mallakh R, Briscoe B (2012) Studies of Long-Term Use of Antidepressants. CNS Drugs 26: 97–109.
49. Mathur R, Hull SA, Badrick E, Robson J (2011) Cardiovascular multimorbidity: the effect of ethnicity on prevalence and risk factor management. British Journal of General Practice 61: e262–e270.
50. Bower P, Macdonald W, Harkness E, Gask L, Kendrick T, et al. (2011) Multimorbidity, service organization and clinical decision making in primary care: a qualitative study. Family Practice 28: 579–587.
51. RK M, SW W, AD P, JA W, MW O (2013) Patient preference for psychological vs pharmacologic treatment of psychiatric disorders: a meta-analytic review. Journal of Clinical Psychiatry 74: 595–602.
52. May C, Montori VM, Mair FS (2009) We need minimally disruptive medicine. BMJ 339: b2803.
53. Katon WJ, Lin EH, Von Korff M, Ciechanowski P, Ludman EJ, et al. (2010) Collaborative care for patients with depression and chronic illnesses. N Engl J Med 363: 2611–2620.
54. Riley RD, Lambert PC, Abo-Zaid G (2010) Meta-analysis of individual participant data: rationale, conduct, and reporting. BMJ 340: c221.

13

Higher Quality of Life and Lower Depression for People on ART in Uganda as Compared to a Community Control Group

Faith Martin[1]*, Steve Russell[1], Janet Seeley[2,3]

1 School of International Development (DEV), University of East Anglia, Norwich, United Kingdom, **2** London School of Hygiene and Tropical Medicine, London, United Kingdom, **3** Uganda Research Unit on AIDS, Medical Research Council/Uganda Virus Research Institute, Entebbe, Uganda

Abstract

Provision of antiretroviral treatment (ART) to people living with HIV (PLWH) has increased globally. Research measuring whether ART restores subjective well-being to "normal" levels is lacking, particularly in resource limited settings. The study objectives are to compare quality of life and depression symptoms for PLWH on ART to a general community population and to explore factors to explain these differences, including socio-economic status and the impact of urban or rural residence. PLWH on ART (n = 263) were recruited from ART delivery sites and participants not on ART (n = 160) were recruited from communities in Wakiso District, Uganda. Participants were interviewed using the translated World Health Organisation Quality of Life brief measure, the Hopkins Symptom Checklist depression section, and questions about socio-economic status, residence as urban or rural and, for PLWH on ART, self-reported adherence and use of HIV counselling. Compared to the community sample and controlling for location of residence, PLWH on ART had significantly higher quality of life (QOL) for physical, psychological and environment domains, but not the social domain. These differences were not due to socio-economic status alone. Depression scores were significantly lower for PLWH on ART. Both comparisons controlled for the effect of location of residence. People on ART self-reported high adherence and the majority had used HIV counselling services. Our findings show better QOL amongst PLWH on ART compared to a general community sample, which cannot be explained solely by differences in socio-economic status nor location of residence. The general community sample results point towards the challenges of life in this setting. Access to health services may underpin this difference and further research should explore this finding, in addition to identification of psychological mechanisms that relate to better QOL. ART provision infrastructure has clear benefits. Further work should consider sustainability and replication for other health conditions.

Editor: Jessica E. Haberer, Massachusetts General Hospital, United States of America

Funding: The research was funded by the UK Government Economic and Social Research Council (ESRC) (project number: RES-063-23-2663), Medical Research Council and Department for International Development. The funders had no role in study design, data collection and analysis, decision to publish, or preparation of the manuscript.

Competing Interests: The authors have declared that no competing interests exist.

* Email: psmfm@bath.ac.uk

Introduction

The impact of antiretroviral therapy (ART) on the health of people living with HIV (PLWH) is well documented [1–4]. Over the last decade, the measurement of the effects of ART on quality of life (QOL) has been increasingly a focus of research, predominantly in industrialised countries [5–7]. As the roll-out of ART has increased in resource-limited settings, researchers have also begun to explore the impact of ART on QOL and more general well-being in those settings. A literature review of these studies show that PLWH on ART have significantly better physical health, emotional well-being, mental health and daily function compared to PLWH who are not on ART [1]. Similarly, ART is associated with lower depression compared to PLWH not on ART; as people's health and hope are restored, they can work again and engage socially [8]. However it remains unclear the extent to which PLWH on ART achieve similar well-being as people in the general community who are not on ART.

A better understanding of the well-being for PLWH on ART, compared to the general population, is important first as this provides an indicator of needs and intervention success. Identification of either low QOL or high depression may point to ongoing unmet needs. Second, achievement of good QOL over longer term may provide a motivator for ongoing adherence to ART [9,10]. Finally, depression specifically is highly relevant owing to the global burden of the condition [11]. High depression may indicate a treatment need of high relevance to PLWH as depression is a barrier to adequate ART adherence [12].

QOL and depression are affected by a number of factors, including gender, age, religious beliefs and socio-economic status (SES) [13]. SES is more strongly associated to QOL in resource-limited settings [14], such as Uganda. SES may impact QOL through access to healthcare and fulfilment of basic needs [15]. The American Psychological Association draws researchers' attention to the importance of SES in relation to HIV/AIDS, advising considering SES particularly in research around well-being [16]. Differences in quality of life related to health may be mediated by SES: the impact of HIV on QOL may be explained by differences in SES associated with health status, such as inability to work owing to poor health.

While treatment can make HIV a manageable chronic condition [17] and may allow people to "resume relatively normal lives" [1,9], there is limited information on the QOL and depression of PLWH on ART compared to a general community sample. Subjective QOL is not easily predicted by health status, as people may psychologically adapt to changes in health [18]. Additionally, in some resource-limited settings where substantial donor funding has been allocated to HIV services compared to other health services, it is possible that PLWH on ART have access to better counselling support and treatment than the general population [19,20], as well as new sources of social support at clinics, such as meeting new people and involvement with HIV related community groups [21]. These resources may generate positive QOL effects compared to others in the general population.

ART could mean that PLWH continue to experience QOL below that of a general community sample, as they are still living with a serious condition and may experience long-term reduced health or side-effects [22], social exclusion or depression owing to losses experienced, and reduced life-expectancy [23]. Alternatively, ART could mean that PLWH experience QOL and depression at the same level as the general community sample, as their health may be returned to a more "normal" level with minimal side effects [24], health may mean a return of ability to work [25], signs of illness may be less visible meaning reduced concerns around stigma, and counselling and psychological adjustment may help maintain mood [9,26]. Finally, ART could mean that PLWH experience higher QOL and less depression than the general community, as they may have access to new social support and health care services as a result of being HIV positive. Counselling or social support may provide new perspectives on life and skills that enhance well-being and psychological adjustment [9,27]. This may be particularly relevant in a resource limited setting, where access to services and care may be limited for the general population. Both differing levels of resources and the effect of psychological adjustment and coping render it difficult to predict QOL in PLWH on ART.

Reviewing the evidence of the impact of ART on PLWH globally, a limited number of studies have compared QOL or depression between PLWH on ART and a general sample. Typically studies report higher depression in those with HIV than without [28,29], although ART is linked to reduced depression in PLWH [24]. Lower QOL is reported in those with HIV compared to a general population sample, for example comparing PLWH on ART to a general sample in Vietnam [30] and in Malawi [31]. These studies include either people on ART for a short duration or made no selection based on ART duration. The reviewed research leaves questions of the impact of duration of treatment longer than 12 months unanswered. Notable exceptions to the pattern of worse outcomes in PLWH are recent findings from Uganda and South Africa, which showed greater subjective QOL and functional ability in older (aged over 50 years) PLWH on ART compared to those without HIV, explained in part by better access to healthcare for PLWH [20,21,32]. It is of interest whether these findings only apply to older adults.

The principal aim of this paper is to compare well-being for PLWH on ART to a general community sample in the resource-limited setting of Wakiso, Uganda. Specifically, subjective QOL and an indicator of depression are compared between PLWH who have been on ART for at least one year and a general community sample. In addition, the potential mediating role of SES is addressed.

Methods

Study site

Data were collected between January 2011 and March 2012 in Wakiso District, central Uganda. Three types of ART delivery sites in the District were selected to recruit participants: the HIV clinic at the government hospital in Entebbe; three government health centres outside Entebbe that have referral links to Entebbe; and the Entebbe branch of a well-established non-governmental organisation, The AIDS Support Organisation (TASO).

Wakiso District, which encircles the capital city Kampala, was selected as the site for ease of access to the study population (the research project and team were based at the Medical Research Council/Uganda Virus Research Institute [MRC/UVRI], Entebbe) and because of the presence of established government and non-government treatment providers. This region includes both more urban and more rural communities; however, this distinction is not a simple one as there is substantial peri-urban development and people may travel between communities.

Sample

For the PLWH on ART sample, participants must have been on ART for more than one year to be eligible. A list of eligible patients was compiled for each facility, which was then stratified by age and gender. The sample was selected randomly from the ART delivery sites using systematic random sampling intervals. The participants from the general population were randomly recruited from nearby villages, first stratified by gender, using resident lists from communities which had been part of an earlier unrelated MRC/UVRI study. It must be noted that HIV status was not determined in the control sample. The data collected herein are part of a wider study "Life on antiretroviral therapy: People's adaptive coping and adjustment to living with HIV as a chronic condition in Wakiso District, Uganda", funded by the UK Economic and Social Research council (grant number RES-062-23-2663). Sampling for the control group was completed using an existing list of residents in several communities held by the Medical Research Council from previous studies. Sampling was not stratified by age nor by urban vs rural variations.

Data collection measures

Measures assessed quality of life, mood and socio-economic status. In addition, participants provided information about location of residence as urban or rural, their age, gender, household size, years of education, religion, marital status, use of medication and HIV counselling and self-reported adherence over the last three days and if they had missed pills more than three times in the last month [33].

The fifteen item depression section of the Hopkins Symptom Check List (DHSCL) [34] was used. Scores range from 15 to 60, with higher scores indicating more symptoms of depression. This measure is commonly used as a screening tool for depression and has been validated for use in a range of cultures [35–37]. It is validated for use in Uganda in the Luganda language and has good predictive validity to detect depression and good internal consistency [38]. The measure has a cut-off score to indicate likely presence of depression. The Hopkins checklist has been researched to identify a cut-off point that indicates the likely presence of depression. This cut-off point has been found to be related to context, culture and measurement version. For example a mean score greater than 1.75 is used in Norway [39] and 1.03 for pregnant women with HIV in Tanzania [40]. Studies using the Ugandan version of the measure (as used in this study) have validated and used a cut-off of above 30 (or an individual's mean score of 2) to indicate probable depression [41,42]. This same method is used here to allow comparisons to other studies in Uganda.

To assess quality of life, the World Health Organisation (WHO) Quality of Life measure the WHOQOL-BREF was used [43]. Twenty-six items assess four domains of quality of life: 1) physical health, 2) psychological, 3) social relationships and 4) environment. Higher scores indicate better quality of life. Domain scores range from 4–20. This measure was selected as it provides an estimate of quality of life extending beyond health-related quality of life alone and has been shown to be valid cross-culturally [43]. The measure was translated into Luganda using the WHO guidelines and achieved adequate validity and internal consistency, comparable to other translated versions [44].

Participants were also asked to complete items forming a socio-economic status (SES) score. SES scores were created from variables of owning one's home, having electricity, having piped water, having a good toilet (flush), having a house with a good roof (iron/tile) and having a paid job (skilled manual labour, formal business, professional or service job). The SES scores were created through inverse frequency weighting, where rarest items are given greater weighting in the score (weights for each variable are derived by dividing total sample size by number of participants who have the item, these are then summed to create the overall score). Higher scores indicate greater assets and socio-economic status.

Ethical considerations

Ethical approval for the study was obtained from the Uganda Virus Research Institute and the University of East Anglia, UK. Overall approval was granted by the Uganda National Council for Science and Technology. Informed consent was gained from participants in written format, or witnessed oral consent was used, endorsed by thumb print. These consent procedures were ethically approved.

Analysis

Statistical data were analysed using PASW Statistics SPSS version 18. Differences between the characteristics of the HIV and control group were compared, using t-tests or the appropriate non-parametric equivalent (Mann-Whitney U). ANCOVA was used to compare depression and QOL scores between the groups. ANCOVA was chosen to covary for any variables where there were significant differences between the groups' characteristics. ANCOVA was only conducted after checking for homogeneity of regression for the covariate at each level of the independent variable. Homogenity of regression was assessed by calculating the interaction terms for the independent variable and covariate. Effect sizes for differences in relation to HIV group were calculated using a standard method to include consideration of the variance of the covariate [45].

Correlation analysis was performed using Pearson's r, as data were found to be normally distributed, and was used to explore the relationship between variables. Group sizes were unequal comparing the HIV group and control group; therefore, corrections for unequal variances are reported where necessary (reflected in the reported degrees of freedom). Effect sizes are included (Cohen's *d*) where appropriate.

Mediation analysis was used to test the significance of the indirect effects of the independent variable or "IV" (HIV group or control group) on the dependent variables or "DV" (WHOQOL domains) through a potential mediator or M (socio-economic status). Mediation analysis addresses the degree to which differences between the groups' QOL may be due to the impact of SES. The mediated or indirect effect is the product of effect of IV on M (a) and the effect of M on the DV (b), partialling out the effects of the IV on the DV [46]. The direct effect (c') is the relationship between IV and DV, taking account of the mediated effect. The total effect (c) is the total relationship between IV and DV. Mediation analysis used bootstrapping to estimate the indirect (or mediated effect) size, which were considered significant when the 95% confidence interval did not include zero [47,48]. The SPSS Macro was used to calculate the model components [49]. There is no agreed upon way of calculating how much of the variables effect is due to mediation [50]. The method used here is to calculate the proportion of the total effect that is mediated (creating a percentage by dividing indirect effect by total effect, subtracting this from one and multiplying by 100).

Results

Demographic differences between HIV and control group

Table 1 shows the comparison between demographic data for the PLWH on ART group or "HIV group" ($n = 263$) and control group ($n = 160$). Prior to exploring any differences in outcomes of depression and quality of life scores between the groups, it was essential to ensure that the groups were comparable in terms of other variables that may have an impact on these outcomes. Comparisons of marital status ($\chi^2(2) = 5.24$ $p = 0.07$), gender ($\chi^2(1) = 3.16$ $p = 0.076$), religion ($\chi^2(1) = 0.21$ $p = 0.65$), education level ($\chi^2(2) = 1.23$ $p = 0.54$) and age (t(239.5, equal variances not assumed) = 0.016 $p = 0.99$) revealed no significant differences between HIV and control group. As such, there is no requirement to control for these variables when comparing QOL or depression scores for the two groups.

Total household size was significantly different ($t(283) = 2.309$, $p = 0.022$, mean difference 0.72, 95% CI 0.10–1.33). When household size was correlated with WHOQOL scores and depression scores, only correlation with the WHOQOL psychological domain (domain 2) was significant ($r = -0.1$, $p = 0.042$). This was a weak correlation. There were significant differences in urban compared to rural residences of the two groups, although this division is a simplification as there is peri-urban development. Those in the HIV group were more likely to be living in urban regions than those in the control ($\chi^2(1) = 43.357$, $p < 0.0001$). As such, comparisons between HIV group and depression and WHOQOL outcomes included location of residence as a covariate.

Socio-economic status (SES) was significantly different between the two groups ($t(421) = 2.589$, $p = 0.01$). SES was significantly higher for people with HIV, although this was a small difference (effect size $d = 0.26$). SES correlated significantly with depression ($r = -0.11$, $p = 0.031$). The correlations between SES and physical health (WHOQOL domain 1, $r = 0.10$, $p = 0.035$), WHOQOL psychological (domain 2, $r = 0.14$, $p = 0.003$) and environment (WHOQOL domain 4, $r = 0.20$, $p < 0.001$) were significant, although only demonstrating a weak relationship. Mediation analysis was conducted to take into account the impact of SES on group differences for the WHOQOL domains and depression symptoms. Although social relationships (WHOQOL domain 3) did not correlate significantly with SES ($r = 0.09$, $p = 0.052$), mediation analysis was conducted for completion.

Table 1. Demographic details of the HIV and Control groups.

Variable	HIV (n = 263)	CONTROL (n = 160)	p value
Mean Age in years (s.d.)	39.8 (9.76)	39.8 (15.22)	0.99
Mean number of people living in household (s.d.)	4.6 (2.68)	5.3 (3.33)	0.022
Socio-economic status (s.d.)	6.4 (4.32)	5.3 (3.96)	0.01
	Frequency (%)	Frequency (%)	
Urban	113	19	<0.0001
Rural	150	141	
Number female	177 (67.3)	94 (58.8)	0.076
Education level			
None	32 (12.2)	17 (10.6)	0.54
Primary	144 (54.8)	93 (58.1)	
Junior	3 (1.1)	4 (2.5)	
Senior school	62 (27.3)	40 (25.0)	
Further education	12 (4.6)	6 (3.8)	
Religion			
Christian	226 (85.9)	140 (87.5)	0.65
Muslim	37 (14.1)	20 (12.5)	
Marital status			
Single	60 (22.8)	27 (16.9)	0.07
Married	155 (58.9)	112 (70.0)	
Other	48 (18.3)	21 (13.1)	

ART and HIV counselling use in HIV group

All 263 participants in the HIV group were taking ART at the time of the study, having started ART more than one year prior to the start of the study. Of the HIV group, 250/263 (95.1%) had received HIV counselling. Self-reported adherence revealed 19 participants (7.2%) reported missed pills in the last 3 days and 12 (4.6%) reported having missed their pills more than three times in the last month.

Comparing depression between HIV and control group

Mean scores on the DHSCL were calculated by group. The HIV group's mean score was 22.0 (s.d. 5.50), compared to 24.9 (s.d. 6.44) for the control group. The mean difference is −2.92 (95% CI −4.17–−1.67), with higher scores in the control group, indicating more symptoms of depression. There was a significant difference between the two groups for depression scores after controlling for the effect of location of residence ($F(1,393) = 4.315$, $p = 0.038$). The effect of the covariate was also significant ($F(1,393) = 4.076$, $p = 0.044$). Taking account of the covariate variance, the effect size for HIV group was 0.50 (95% CI 0.29–0.71).

Chi-square test revealed that depression and group were associated, as χ^2 (df-1) = 10.82, p = 0.001, phi = 0.161 (small effect size). The results in Table 2 illustrate how proportionately more people in the control group are potentially depressed.

Comparing Quality of Life between HIV and control group

Table 3 provides mean scores on WHOQOL domains by HIV and control group. ANCOVA revealed that scores were significantly higher in the HIV group physical health (WHOQOL domain 1), after controlling for the effect of location of residence ($F(1,419) = 5.123, p = 0.024$). The effect size, taking into account the covariate, was medium (d = 0.43, 95%CI 0.23–0.63). The covariate was not significantly related to physical health QOL ($F(1,419) = 3.486, p = 0.062$).

For domain 2 (psychological) ANCOVA revealed significantly higher scores for the HIV group after controlling for the effect of location of residence ($F(1,419) = 6.591, p = 0.011$). The effect size, taking into account the covariate, was large (d = 0.80, 95%CI 0.60–1.00). The covariate was not significantly related to psychological QOL ($F(1,419) = 1.765, p = 0.185$).

For domain 3, social relationships, ANCOVA revealed no significant differences between the groups after controlling for the effect of location of residence ($F(1,419) = 0.73, p = 0.786$). The covariate was not significantly related to social relationship QOL ($F(1,419) = 2.874, p = 0.091$).

For domain 4, environment, ANCOVA revealed significantly higher scores for the HIV group after controlling for the effect of location of residence ($F(1,419) = 14.518, p < 0.001$). The effect size, taking into account the covariate, was medium (d = 0.75, 95%CI 0.55–0.95). The covariate was not significantly related to environment QOL ($F(1,419) = 2.550, p = 0.111$).

Mediation analysis: HIV group and WHOQOL in relation to SES

Mediation analysis was completed to explore the degree to which SES is affecting the relationship between case and quality of life or depression symptoms. In all cases, the effect of HIV group (independent variable) on the mediator SES was 1.0869. Table 4 provides the summary analysis.

For all comparisons, the relationship between HIV group (case or control) and the WHOQOL domain or depression remained significant when the effect of SES was accounted for: there is no full mediation of HIV group and QOL or depression by SES.

Table 2. Indicated depression by HIV or control group.

Depression indicated	HIV group (%)	Control group (%)
Yes	24 (9.6)	31 (21.1)
No	226 (90.4)	116 (78.9)

There was only partial mediation by SES for WHOQOL 2 (psychological) and 4 (environment) domains. However, the effect of SES on the HIV group to QOL relationship was very small. The proportion of the total effect that was mediated was calculated (Table 4). This illustrates the minimal proportion of the relationship between HIV group and QOL that was found to be mediated by SES, with between 3.6 and 5.9% of the relationship between IV and DV mediated by SES.

Discussion

Compared to a general population sample, greater QOL was seen for PLWH on ART for physical, psychological and environment domains after controlling for the effect of location of residence. Social relationship (WHOQOL domain 3) scores were not significantly different in relation to group. Although socio-economic status was higher in the PLWH on ART, this accounted for at most 6% of variance in QOL scores. Mean depression scores (after controlling for the effect of location of residence) and number of people reaching a threshold for possible depression diagnosis were lower for PLWH on ART. PLWH on ART were found to achieve better well-being than the general community sample.

At first glance these results seem counter-intuitive: that people with a chronic, incurable illness should have better QOL and lower symptoms of depression than the general sample. One possibility is that these results may tell us about the lives of the general sample in Uganda. Many people live in harsh economic and social conditions, and experience living costs that outstrip income [51], and gender inequalities can make women's lives and relationships particularly difficult [26]. Access to affordable essential services remains a problem for many and PLWH on ART appear to have better access to these services.

The HIV sample reported generally high levels of adherence. Self-reported adherence was used, and this may be an inaccurate estimate [52]. Most of the HIV sample had received HIV counselling (although the quality of this is unknown). Other studies show high adherence levels on ART, where available, in sub-Saharan African settings [53,54]. The QOL and depression results presented here are therefore for a sample of people who appear to be adhering to ART and using services. A different pattern of results may be observed comparing PLWH on ART with lower adherence or with lower access to counselling services. Adherence to ART and the impact of ART on QOL and depression may change as the length of time a person is taking ART increases [55]. Longitudinal studies should explore how QOL and depression may alter over time and taking into account levels of adherence.

This study is one of the first studies in sub-Saharan Africa to provide a direct comparison between an HIV and non-HIV group, showing the rates of depression for the general population are higher. QOL scores, if viewed as a percentage of scale maximum, ranged across the domains from 71% to 83% for PLWH on ART and 62% to 74.5% for the general sample. These ranges are similar to findings that QOL among non-western populations is generally around 60–80% of scale maximum [56]. Although there were significant differences in depression scores overall, the two groups' mean depression scores were not clinically different (the means for both groups were below the clinical cut-off). However, we found significantly more people scoring above the cut-off for likely depression in the general sample as compared to the PLWH on ART group. Typically studies find higher depression in PLWH compared to the general population; however, the findings here may reflect the positive impact of ART and counselling. Twenty-one percent of participants in the control sample reached DHSCL scores indicating potential depression, compared to only 9.6% of the HIV sample. Previous research found similar rates of depression symptoms with a national prevalence in Uganda of 29.3% [42] and 8.1% in an HIV sample [41]. As the rate of attendance at HIV counselling was very high in our sample, it was not possible to explore any effect of counselling on reported mood.

PLWH were receiving counselling, care and treatment from specialised HIV services provided by the state and non-governmental organisations, notably TASO. HIV service infrastructure has received a great deal of investment since 2004/5, substantively enhanced by donor funding. These services may impact QOL domains, including offering access to health care (environment domain) and benefits of health care (physical). In contrast the sample from the general population are unlikely to have been accessing specialised treatment and counselling services.

Table 3. WHOQOL Scores by HIV and Control group.

WHOQOL Domain	HIV group mean (s.d.)	Control group mean (s.d.)	Mean difference	95% CI of mean difference	Effect size (d)
1 Physical health	14.4 (2.15)	13.3 (3.17)	1.09*	0.54–1.65	0.43
2 Psychological	16.6 (1.80)	14.9 (2.52)	1.69*	1.24–2.13	0.80
3 Social relationships	14.6 (2.75)	14.0 (3.16)	0.65 (n.s.)	0.08–1.23	-
4 Environment	14.2 (2.04)	12.4 (2.74)	1.74**	1.24–2.23	0.75

** indicates significantly different at $p<0.01$,

* indicates significance at $p<0.05$, based on ANCOVA results. Reported effect sizes take into account the variance relating to the covariate (location of residence).

Table 4. Summary of Mediation analysis of socio-economic status and the relationship between HIV case and WHOQOL domains (Unstandardised co-efficients are shown).

Dependent variable	Direct effect of HIV group on DV (*c'*)	Indirect effect (*ab*)	95% CI of indirect effect	Total effect (*c*)	Proportion %
Depression	2.7895**	0.1301	−0.3882–0.008	2.9196**	4.45609
WHOQOL 1 (Physical health)	1.0404**	0.0534	−0.0030–0.1698	1.094**	4.89945
WHOQOL 2 (Psychological)	1.6267**	0.0587*	0.0078–0.1607	1.685**	3.45994
WHOQOL 3 (Social relationships)	0.5903*	0.0619	−0.0016–0.1963	0.6522*	9.49095
WHOQOL 4 (Environment)	1.6338**	0.1018*	0.0241–0.2316	1.736**	5.88710

* significant at $p<0.05$.
**significant at $p<0.01$ Proportion calculated as $(1-(c'/c))*100$.

Inequalities of service provision for PLWH compared to other conditions or the general population have been found elsewhere [57], and a study in South Africa recently found greater QOL in older adults with HIV compared to those without HIV, explained by better access to healthcare for PLWH [20]. ART facilities provide something akin to "islands of excellence in seas of under provision" [58]. Individuals in both the case and control groups live in difficult circumstances and this study did not collect detailed data regarding service access. However, through contact with ART clinics, PLWH had access to a service which gave them the opportunity to talk about their problems in counselling sessions or with their in-group of PLWH. This may relate to the higher reported QOL and should be investigated in further research.

Research exploring psychological adjustment and the concept of "post-traumatic growth" suggests that following health shocks and/or treatment, people may experience a renewed sense of well-being [59]. Gratitude for a new chance at life, a refreshed sense of priorities and a shift in standards against which QOL is judged can all lead to increased subjective QOL following illness [60]. Studies with PLWH in various settings, including Uganda, have found descriptions of this renewed sense of meaning and gratitude [61,62]. It may be that these adjustment processes underpin observed differences, together with different access to resources.

It must be noted that not all PLWH on ART experience good QOL. Identification of people with high reported QOL could be used as peer counsellors to support those who are faring less well on ART or could be used to help motivate those who are refusing/struggling with adherence to ART. The lower QOL and lower mood in the community sample also suggests a need for provision of psychosocial intervention more widely. Greater understanding of the factors contributing to outcomes in the general community is required to help target any such intervention and explore wider policy development regarding improvement of well-being.

Limitations

This study has several limitations. Although not statistically significant, there were more women and single people in the PLWH on ART group. Further research could explore the relative relevance of these variables to well-being outcomes.

ANCOVA was conducted to take into account the covariate of location of residence. The urban-rural dichotomy does not take into account the many differences between the sites, where development initiatives have led to the provision of services in the rural environments and infrastructure that may be more similar to a peri-urban environment. Additionally, although location of residence may be in a more urban area for example, work may take place in a more rural environment or vice versa. As such, a more detailed examination of the impact of participants' environment would be of benefit.

Although SES was measured with a scale specifically designed for this population, SES is difficult to measure. The measure here included assets and employment items. Alternatives such as a longer assets index or measure of expenditure versus income may have revealed different results.

Self-reported adherence was used to estimate adherence. Adherence is difficult to measure accurately and alternative, objective or more detailed measures of adherence should be included in future research. In addition, data relating to counselling only concerned attendance at counselling. Further research should consider the quality and content of this intervention to properly understand its effect on QOL and depression.

It is probable that some of the general population sample are HIV positive and untreated, because HIV prevalence is estimated at 7.3% [63] and many people are un-tested. It was not possible to account for this in the data analysis. No data were collected around objective health measures or types of treatment, therefore it is not possible to know the extent to which differences in health QOL were due to better health in the ART group. It is well known that although people with poor health typically have lower QOL than those without health problems [43], the relationship between health status and QOL is complex, particularly in relation to chronic conditions [64]. Further research should explore the relative roles of objective health indicators and psychological adjustment in relation to QOL judgements. The generalizability of findings is unclear, although our results add to an emerging evidence base in sub-Saharan African nations were HIV treatment is accessible that shows better well-being amongst PLWH (on ART) compared to a general sample [20,21,32].

Conclusions

PLWH on ART were experiencing higher QOL and lower depression scores than the general community sample. The precise mechanisms driving these results need to be investigated. It may be that PLWH on ART experience better health than the control group, particularly as this sample reported good adherence. PLWH on ART may have better access to healthcare resources than the general community and may receive not only ART but also treatment for other illness, for example, access to antibacterial medications which treat common infections. As such, access to ART may also provide better access to healthcare overall. Further research could directly explore and measure these mechanisms to quantify their impact on QOL and depression. The needs of the general community sample and factors associated with their lower QOL also require further research and potential intervention.

As HIV care is rolled out to lower level health centres in Uganda and elsewhere and gradually integrated into the general health system, it is useful to reflect on the particular benefits that PLHW in our study may have derived from the infrastructure that has been put in place because of HIV. People with other chronic conditions, such as hypertension, might also benefit from such regular social and medical support, but in a financially resourced constrained world the provision of such services may decline, with consequences for ART adherence as well as the QOL of PLHV.

Acknowledgments

We are grateful to all the study participants for spending time with us and sharing their experiences, and to the staff at The AIDS Support Organisation (TASO), and the government hospital and health centres, for facilitating this research. We thank the Medical Research Council/ Uganda Virus Research Institute Research Unit on AIDS in Entebbe for support.

Author Contributions

Analyzed the data: FM SR JS. Wrote the paper: FM SR JS.

References

1. Beard J, Feeley F, Rosen S (2009) Economic and quality of life outcomes of antiretroviral therapy for HIV/AIDS in developing countries: A systematic literature review. AIDS Care 21: 1343–1356.
2. Hogg RS, Heath KV, Yip B, Craib KJ, O'Shaughnessy MV, et al. (1998) Improved survival among hiv-infected individuals following initiation of antiretroviral therapy. JAMA 279: 450–454.
3. Brinkhof MWG, Pujades-Rodriguez M, Egger M (2009) Mortality of Patients Lost to Follow-Up in Antiretroviral Treatment Programmes in Resource-Limited Settings: Systematic Review and Meta-Analysis. PLoS ONE 4: e5790.
4. Monforte AdA, Testa L, Adorni F, Chiesa E, Bini T, et al. (1998) Clinical outcome and predictive factors of failure of highly active antiretroviral therapy in antiretroviral-experienced patients in advanced stages of HIV-1 infection. AIDS 12: 1631–1637.
5. Mannheimer SB, Matts J, Telzak E, Chesney M, Child C, et al. (2005) Quality of life in HIV-infected individuals receiving antiretroviral therapy is related to adherence. AIDS Care 17: 10–22.
6. Liu C, Ostrow D, Detels R, Hu Z, Johnson L, et al. (2006) Impacts of HIV infection and HAART use on quality of life. Quality of Life Research 15: 941–949.
7. Preau M, Leport C, Salmon-Ceron D, Carrieri P, Portier H, et al. (2004) Health-related quality of life and patient-provider relationships in HIV-infected patients during the first three years after starting PI-containing antiretroviral treatment. AIDS Care 16: 649–661.
8. Wagner GJ, Ghosh-Dastidar B, Garnett J, Kityo C, Mugyenyi P (2012) Impact of HIV antiretrovirals therapy on depression and mental health among clients with HIV in Uganda. Psychosomatic Medicine 74: 883–890.
9. Russell S, Seeley J (2010) The transition to living with HIV as a chronic condition in rural Uganda: Working to create order and control when on antiretroviral therapy. Social Science and Medicine 70: 375–382.
10. Mbonye M, Seeley J, Ssembajja F, Birungi J, Jaffar S (2013) Adherence to antiretroviral therapy in jinja, Uganda: a six-year follow-up study. PLoS ONE 8: e78243.
11. Ferrari AJ, Charlson FJ, Norman RE, Patten SB, Freedman G, et al. (2013) Burden of Depressive Disorders by Country, Sex, Age, and Year: Findings from the Global Burden of Disease Study 2010. PLoS Med 10: e1001547.
12. Starace F, Massa A, Amico KR, Fisher JD (2006) Adherence to antiretroviral therapy: An empirical test of the information-motivation-behavioral skills model. Health Psychology 25: 153–162.
13. Camfield L, Skevington SM (2008) On Subjective Well-being and Quality of Life. Journal of Health Psychology 13: 764–775.
14. Diener E, Sandvik E, Seidlitz L, Diener M (1993) The relationship between income and subjective well-being: Relative or absolute? Social Indicators Research 28: 195–223.
15. Peltzer K, Phaswana-Mafuya N (2008) Health-related quality of life in a sample of HIV-infected South Africans. African Journal of AIDS Research 7: 209–218.
16. APA (n.d.) HIV/AIDS & Socioeconomic Status. American Psychological Association, accessed online November 2013. Available: http://www.apa.org/pi/ses/resources/publications/factsheet-hiv-aids.pdf.
17. McGrath JW, Winchester MS, Kaawa-Mafigiri D, Walakira E, Namutiibwa F, et al. (2014) Challenging the Paradigm: Anthropological Perspectives on HIV as a Chronic Disease. Medical Anthropology: null-null.
18. Ubel PA, Loewenstein G, Jepson C (2003) Whose quality of life? A commentary exploring discrepancies between health state evaluations of patients and the general public. Quality of life Research 12: 599–607.
19. Kunihira NR, Nuwaha F, Mayanja R, Peterson S (2010) Barriers to use of antiretroviral drugs in Rakai district of Uganda. African Health Sciences 10: 120–129.
20. Nyirenda M, Chatterji S, Falkingham J, Mutevedzi P, Hosegood V, et al. (2012) An investigation of factors associated with the health and well-being of HIV-infected or HIV-affected older people in rural South Africa. BMC Public Health 12: 259.
21. Negin J, Nyirenda M, Seeley J, Mutevedzi P (2013) Inequality in Health Status Among Older Adults in Africa: The Surprising Impact of Anti-Retroviral Treatment. Journal of Cross-Cultural Gerontology 28: 491–493.
22. Bucciardini R, Wu AW, Floridia M, Fragola V, Ricciardulli D, et al. (2000) Quality of life outcomes of combination zidovudine-didanosine-nevirapine and zidovudine-didanosine for antiretroviral-naive advanced HIV-infected patients. AIDS 14: 2567–2574.
23. Remien RH, Mellins CA (2007) Long-term psychosocial challenges for people living with HIV: let's not forget the individual in our global response to the pandemic. AIDS October 21: S55–S63.
24. Jelsma J, Maclean E, Hughes J, Tinise X, Darder M (2005) An investigation into the health related quality of life of individuals living with HIV who are receiving HAART. AIDS Care 17: 579–588.
25. Blalock AC, McDaniel J, Farber EW (2002) Effect of employment on quality of life and psychological functioning in patients with HIV/AIDS. Psychosomatics 43: 400–404.
26. Seeley J (2014) HIV and East Africa. Thirty Years in the Shadow of an Epidemic. Abingdon, UK: Routledge.
27. Bekele T, Rourke SB, Tucker R, Greene S, Sobota M, et al. (2012) Direct and indirect effects of perceived social support on health-related quality of life in persons living with HIV/AIDS. AIDS Care 25: 337–346.
28. Collins PY, Holman AR, Freeman MC, Patel V (2006) What is the relevance of mental health to HIV/AIDS care and treatment programs in developing countries? A systematic review. AIDS August 20: 1571–1582.
29. Gibbie T, Hay M, Hutchison CW, Mijch A (2007) Depression, social support and adherence to highly active antiretroviral therapy in people living with HIV/AIDS. Sexual Health 4: 227–232.
30. Tran BX, Ohinmaa A, Nguyen LT, Nguyen TA, Nguyen TH (2011) Determinants of health-related quality of life in adults living with HIV in Vietnam. AIDS Care 23: 1236–1245.
31. Fan AP-C, Kuo H-CC, Kao DY-T, Morisky DE, Chen Y-MA (2011) Quality of life and needs assessment on people living with HIV and AIDS in Malawi. AIDS Care 23: 287–302.
32. Scholten F, Mugisha J, Seeley J, Kinyanda E, Nakubukwa S, et al. (2011) Health and functional status among older people with HIV/AIDS in Uganda. BMC Public Health 11: 886.
33. Oyugi JH, Byakika-Tusiime J, Charlebois E, Kityo C, Mugerwa R, et al. (2004) Multiple validated measures of adherence indicate high levels of adherence to generic HIV antiretroviral therapy in a resource limited setting. JAIDS Journal of Acquired Immune Deficiency Syndromes 36: 1100–1102.
34. Derogatis LR, Lipman RS, Rickels K, Uhlenhuth EH, Covi L (1974) The Hopkins Symptom Checklist (HSCL): a self-report symptom inventory. Behav Sci 19: 1–15.
35. Lee B, Kaaya SF, Mbwambo JK, Smith-Fawzi MC, Leshabari MT (2008) Detecting depressive disorder with the Hopkins Symptom Checklist-25 in Tanzania. Int J Soc Psychiatry 54: 7–20.
36. Cepeda-Benito A, Gleaves DH (2000) Cross-ethnic equivalence of the Hopkins Symptom Checklist-21 in European American, African American, and Latino College Students. Cultural Diversity and Ethnic Minority Psychology 6: 297–308.
37. Fawzi MC, Pham T, Lin L, Nguyen TV, Ngo D, et al. (1997) The validity of posttraumatic stress disorder among Vietnamese refugees. Journal of Traumatic Stress 10: 101–108.
38. Bolton P, Wilk CM, Ndogoni L (2004) Assessment of depression prevalence in rural Uganda using symptom and function criteria. Social Psychiatry & Psychiatric Epidemiology 39: 442–447.
39. Teodorescu D-S, Siqveland J, Heir T, Hauff E, Wentzel-Larsen T, et al. (2012) Posttraumatic growth, depressive symptoms, posttraumatic stress symptoms, post-migration stressors and quality of life in multi-traumatized psychiatric outpatients with a refugee background in Norway. Health and Quality of Life Outcomes 10: 84.
40. Kaaya SF, Fawzi MCS, Mbwambo JK, Lee B, Msamanga GI, et al. (2002) Validity of the Hopkins Symptom Checklist-25 amongst HIV-positive pregnant women in Tanzania. Acta Psychiatrica Scandinavica 106: 9–19.
41. Kinyanda E, Hoskins S, Nakku J, Nawaz S, Patel V (2011) Prevalence and risk factors of major depressive disorder in HIV/AIDS as seen in semi-urban Entebbe district, Uganda. BMC Psychiatry 11: 205.
42. Kinyanda E, Woodburn P, Tugumisirize J, Kagugube J, Ndyanabangi S, et al. (2011) Poverty, life events and the risk for depression in Uganda. Soc Psychiatry Psychiatr Epidemiol 46: 35–44.

43. Skevington SM, Lotfy M, O'Connell KA, Group W (2004) The World Health Organization's WHOQOL-BREF quality of life assessment: psychometric properties and results of the international field trial. A report from the WHOQOL group. Quality of Life Research 13: 299–310.
44. Martin F, Russell S, Seeley J (2013) The WHOQOL BREF questionnaire in Luganda: Validation with sample including people living with HIV in Uganda. DEV Reports and Policy Paper Series. The School of International Development, University of East Anglia, UK.
45. Lipsey M, Wilson DB (2001) Practical Meta-analysis. London: Sage.
46. MacKinnon DP (2008) Introduction to Statistical Medication Analysis. Hove, East Sussex: Taylor Francis.
47. Rucker DD, Preacher KJ, Tormala ZL, Petty RE (2011) Mediation analysis in social psychology: Current practices and new recommendations. Social and Personality Psychology Compass 5: 359–371.
48. Preacher KJ, Hayes AF (2004) SPSS and SAS procedures for estimating indirect effects in simple mediation models. Behavior Research Methods 36: 717–731.
49. Preacher KJ, Hayes AF (2008) Asymptotic and resampling strategies for assessing and comparing indirect effects in multiple mediator models. Behavior Research Methods 40: 879–891.
50. Hayes AF, Preacher KJ, Myers TA (2011) Mediation and the estimation of indirect effects in political communication research. Sourcebook for political communication research: Methods, measures, and analytical techniques: 434–465.
51. Ministry of Finance (2010) Uganda National Report. In: Ministry of Finance PaED, editor. Kampala: Republic of Uganda. Accessed online 14/09/13. Available: http://www.un.org/wcm/webdav/site/ldc/shared/Uganda.pdf.
52. Shi L, Liu J, Fonseca V, Walker P, Kalsekar A, et al. (2010) Correlation between adherence rates measured by MEMS and self-reported questionnaires: a meta-analysis. Health Qual Life Outcomes 8: 99.
53. Ware NC, Idoko J, Kaaya S, Biraro IA, Wyatt MA, et al. (2009) Explaining adherence success in sub-Saharan Africa: an ethnographic study. PLoS Medicine/Public Library of Science 6: e11.
54. Mills EJ, Nachega JB, Buchan I, et al. (2006) Adherence to antiretroviral therapy in sub-saharan africa and north america: A meta-analysis. JAMA 296: 679–690.
55. Byakika-Tusiime J, Crane J, Oyugi J, Ragland K, Kawuma A, et al. (2009) Longitudinal Antiretroviral Adherence in HIV+ Ugandan Parents and Their Children Initiating HAART in the MTCT-Plus Family Treatment Model: Role of Depression in Declining Adherence Over Time. AIDS and Behavior 13: 82–91.
56. Cummins R (1996) The domains of life satisfaction: an attempt to order chaos. Social Indicators Research 38: 303–328.
57. Men C, Meessen B, van Pelt M, Van Damme W, Lucas H (2012) "I wish I had AIDS": a qualitative study on access to health care services for HIV/AIDS and diabetic patients sin Cambodia. Health, Culture and Society 2.
58. Ooms G, Van Damme W, Baker BK, Zeitz P, Schrecker T (2008) The 'diagonal'approach to Global Fund financing: a cure for the broader malaise of health systems. Global Health 4.
59. Hefferon K, Grealy M, Mutrie N (2009) Post-traumatic growth and life threatening physical illness: A systematic review of the qualitative literature. British journal of health psychology 14: 343–378.
60. Schwartz CE, Sprangers MA (2009) Reflections on genes and sustainable change: toward a trait and state conceptualization of response shift. Journal of clinical epidemiology 62: 1118–1123.
61. Russell S, Seeley J, Ezati E, Wamai N, Were W, et al. (2007) Coming back from the dead: living with HIV as a chronic condition in rural Africa. Health Policy and Planning: 1–4.
62. Mutabazi-Mwesigire D, Seeley J, Martin F, Katamba A (2014) Perceptions of quality of life among Ugandan patients living with HIV: a qualitative study. BMC Public Health 14: 343.
63. Ministry of Health (2011) Uganda AIDS Indicator Survey. Kampala, Uganda: Ministry of Health
64. Schwartz CE, Sprangers MA (2000) Adaptation to changing health: Response shift in quality-of-life research: American Psychological Association.

Longitudinal Associations between Adolescent Psychotic Experiences and Depressive Symptoms

Sarah A. Sullivan[1]*, Nicola Wiles[1], Daphne Kounali[1], Glyn Lewis[2], Jon Heron[1], Mary Cannon[3], Liam Mahedy[1], Peter B. Jones[4], Jan Stochl[4], Stan Zammit[1,5]

1 Centre for Academic Mental Health, School of Social and Community Medicine, University of Bristol, Bristol, United Kingdom, **2** Division of Psychiatry, University College London, London, United Kingdom, **3** Department of Psychiatry, Royal College of Surgeons in Ireland, Dublin, Ireland, **4** Department of Psychiatry, Cambridge Neuroscience, University of Cambridge, Cambridge, United Kingdom, **5** Institute of Psychological Medicine and Clinical Neurosciences, University of Cardiff, Cardiff, United Kingdom

Abstract

Background: Psychotic experiences are prevalent in community samples and are highly correlated with depressive symptoms. This study aimed to investigate the longitudinal associations between psychotic experiences and depressive symptoms between adolescence and young adulthood.

Method: Prospective cohort study with a 6 year follow-up in a community sample of 7632 adolescents and young adults. Depressive symptoms were assessed with the Short Moods and Feelings Questionnaire and psychotic experiences with a semi-structured clinical interview at 12 and 18 years. Longitudinal and cross-sectional associations were investigated with regression and structural equation models.

Results: Depressive symptoms and psychotic experiences were associated at each time-point (12 years $r = 0.486$ [95% CI 0.457, 0.515]; 18 years $r = 0.286$ [95% CI 0.233, 0.339]) and there were longitudinal within-phenotype associations (depressive symptoms $r = 0.252$ [95% CI 0.205, 0.299]; psychotic experiences $r = 0.662$ [95% CI 0.595, 0.729]). There was an across-phenotype association between psychotic experiences at 12 and depressive symptoms at 18 $r = 0.139$ [95% CI 0.086, 0.192; $p < 0.001$], but no association between depressive symptoms at 12 and psychotic experiences at 18 $r = -0.022$ [95% CI −0.032, 0.077; $p = 0.891$].

Conclusions: Longitudinal across-phenotype associations were substantially weaker than cross-sectional associations or within-phenotype longitudinal associations. Whilst psychotic experiences at 12 years were associated with a small increase in depression at 18 years, depression at 12 years was not associated with psychotic experiences at 18 years once across-phenotype cross-sectional and within-phenotype longitudinal associations were accounted for. This suggests that the biological mechanisms underlying depression at this age do not increase subsequent risk of psychotic experiences once they resolve.

Editor: Marieke Wichers, Maastricht University, Netherlands

Funding: The UK Medical Research Council (Grant ref:74882), the Wellcome Trust (Grant ref:076467) and the University of Bristol provide core support for ALSPAC. This study was funded by MRC grant G0701503. The funders had no role in study design, data collection and analysis, decision to publish, or preparation of the manuscript.

Competing Interests: The authors have declared that no competing interests exist.

* Email: sarah.sullivan@bristol.ac.uk

Introduction

Psychotic experiences (PEs) are reported by approximately 5–7% of individuals in community samples [1,2]. They are of relevance to schizophrenia given that these are key symptoms of the disorder, but their predictive value is low. However, given their associations with impaired functioning, and frequent co-morbidity with other psychopathologies, particularly depression [3–12], they are of public health importance. The relationship between PEs and depression over time is likely to be complex, but understanding this may help gauge the extent to which presence of PEs leads to depression and vice versa, or whether they are different manifestations of a common pathology.

The strong correlation between PEs and depression[6,10] means that examining the continuities and discontinuities of these phenotypes from early adolescence through early adulthood using standard analytical procedures is problematic. For example, confounding by co-morbid psychopathology could occur whereby an association between depression at time 1 and PEs at time 2 could arise because many people with depression at time 1 already have PEs at time 1. Furthermore, measures of depression and PEs are subject to measurement error, and with repeated assessments similar errors occurring at each time point could result in associations between constructs over time due to correlation of residual errors (i.e. variation in the measurement of PEs and depression due to factors other than variation in presence of psychopathology). This could occur, for example, as a result of personality characteristics that cause a respondent to always over-report symptoms.

Whilst there is evidence from longitudinal studies to support the hypothesis that PEs are associated with later depression [9,10,13–15] and that depression is associated with later PEs [16,17] these previous studies have not examined whether depression increases the risk of PEs (and vice versa) independently of the within psychopathology association of PEs (or depression) over time.

In an elegant study [18] the independent effects of depression and PEs over time were examined using a path analysis of PEs and depression measured at 4 time-points over 2 years in 138 adolescents being treated for major depression. Although there were strong cross-sectional correlations at each time-point, depression and PEs were not associated longitudinally. However, this study may have had limited statistical power to find evidence of longitudinal associations given the sample size, whilst measurement error from correlated residuals may have resulted in over-estimation of cross-sectional associations.

Structural equation modelling (SEM) minimizes the problem of residual errors by modelling associations between latent traits rather than observed variables, and also allows examination of associations whilst allowing for the correlation between phenotypes. To our knowledge there has been only one other study [19] to investigate the association between mood and psychotic symptoms using structural equation modelling. This study investigated the longitudinal association between depressed mood and paranoia in 301 patients with psychosis over 12 months and found that depressed mood was associated with an increased longitudinal risk of paranoia but there was no evidence that paranoia was prospectively associated with depressed mood.

We hypothesised that PEs and depression would not be associated over time, once the effect of persistent PEs or depression had been accounted for. Our aims were: i) to use SEM to estimate the extent to which depression and PEs are associated over time whilst accounting for cross-sectional (across-phenotype) and longitudinal (within-phenotype) effects, and minimising residual error, and ii) to compare our results using an SEM approach with those when using standard regression models.

Materials and Methods

Avon Longitudinal Study of Parents and Children (ALSPAC)

The study sample consists of ALSPAC (http://www.bristol.ac.uk/alspac/) participants. All pregnant women resident in the former Avon Health Authority in South West England with an estimated delivery date of between 1st April 1991 and 31st December 1992 were invited to participate. The children of 15,247 pregnancies were recruited. Of this sample of 15,458 foetuses, 14,701 were live births and alive at 1 year [20,21].

The sample is representative of those born at that time in the former county of Avon during this period [22].

Ethics

Ethical approval for the study was obtained from the ALSPAC Ethics and Law Committee and the Southmead, Frenchay, UBHT and Weston Research Ethics Committees. Written consent was obtained from participants to allow use of anonymized linked data for research by bona fide scientists.

Dataset

We used a sub sample (n = 7632) of participants with data on at least one measure of; depressive symptoms (DS) or PEs at 12 or 18 years. The dataset represents approximately 52% of the original cohort. See Appendix S1 for a comparison of variables in the whole ALSPAC cohort and those included in the study dataset.

Missing Data

Missing data patterns were examined. Multiple imputation in the Stata statistical package [23] was used to impute missing data using multiple imputation by fully conditional specification using chained equations [24,25] (see Table S2). All analyses were carried out on the imputed dataset (n = 7632).

Outcome and Exposure Measures

PEs at 12 and 18 years. PEs were assessed using a semi-structured interview (PLIKSi) that has been described elsewhere [26,27]. At 12 years participants were asked about PEs over the previous 6 months and at 18 years participants were asked about PEs since the age of 12. Questions were asked about unusual experiences and 12 core psychotic experiences (Appendix S1). The assessment of each core symptom began with a structured stem question enquiring whether the experience had occurred. 'Maybe' or 'yes' responses were followed by cross-questioning to establish whether experiences were psychotic. If the interviewer did not consider that the experience was psychotic after cross-questioning a rating of not present was made. Each experience was therefore rated by the interview as either; not present, suspected or definitely present.

The average Kappa values for inter-rater reliability were 0.72 and 0.83 for the 12 year and 18 year interviews respectively. Test-retest agreement at 18 years was 0.74.

Depressive symptoms (DSs) at 12 and 18 years. Self-reported DSs were assessed using the Short Moods and Feeling Questionnaire (SMFQ) [28] which asked about symptoms over the previous 2 weeks. The standard version consists of 13 questions but the version used in this analysis consists of only 12. Question 4 "teenager felt restless" was not used because previous work has found that this question was poorly understood [29]. Each question had 3 possible responses; 0 never, 1 sometimes, 2 always. The possible score range for each participant was therefore 0 to 24. A higher score indicated more depressive symptoms. At each time point responses to the twelve SMFQ items were divided into three groups (A, B and C) resulting in three continuous sum-scores. Group A was formed of items 1, 5, 8 and 11; B from items 2, 6, 9, and 12; and C from items 3, 7, 10 and 13). Reasons for this approach have been described previously[30].

Potential Confounders

We adjusted for gender and two proxy measures of social class (maternal education and maternal marital status at birth). Marital status was dichotomised into never married and married presently or previously. Maternal education was dichotomised into lower (CSE, GCSE, vocational) and higher (A level, degree or above).

Statistical Analysis

i) Standard regression models. Logistic regression models were used to investigate the cross-sectional association between PEs and DSs at each time-point, and the longitudinal association between DSs at 12 years and PEs at 18 years, adjusted for PEs at 12 years, DSs at 18 years, and confounders. Linear regression was used to investigate the association between PEs at 12 years and DSs at 18, adjusted for DSs at 12 years, PEs at 18 and other confounders. PEs were coded as 1 for PE suspected or definitely present detected during the clinical interview or a positive response to a stem question and 0 for no PE detected during the clinical interview or a no response to a stem question. If a stem question was positively responded to but not detected during the clinical interview it was still coded as 1.

ii) Structural equation model. SEM comprises of a measurement model employing confirmatory factor analysis, and a structural element [31]. The measurement model consists of four factors (latent variables) represented in Figure 1 as ovals. Model estimation problems resulted from the scarcity of many of the PEs, therefore three indicators were generated for PEs at each time-point; total hallucinations, total delusions including thought disorder, and total unusual experiences. Unusual experiences were included because of evidence that they are associated with increased risk of PEs at 18 [27]. Hallucinations and delusions indicators had four response categories (no, yes to ≥1 stem question, ≥1 interview-rated as suspected, ≥1 interviewer-rated as definite). Stem question responses were included to increase the number of outcomes. We considered that even if positive responses to stem questions were not interviewer-rated they would still add useful information to the PEs factors. There is evidence[32] that psychotic experiences described by participants but not clinically rated are associated with clinical psychosis. We also have evidence (details from corresponding author on request) that responding positively to a stem question but not being interviewer-rated at age 12 is associated with an interview rated PE at 18. Also any variance in the stem questions variable not shared with other indicators would be extraneous to the factor. Unusual experiences had three response categories (no, interview-rated as suspected, interview-rated as definitely present). The three scales created from the SMFQ (see DSs section above) were used as continuous indicators for latent traits at each time-point.

In order to enable identification of the measurement model the PEs and DSs factors at 12 and 18 were allowed to co-vary, but the indicators and errors were not. To enable scaling of the factors, the variance of each was set to 1[31]. The indicators for the PEs factors were categorical and therefore did not have error terms. The error terms (E1-6) shown in Figure 1 represent omitted causes and score unreliability not contained within the DS factors, whilst the error terms E7 and E8 represent variance in the outcomes (PE18 and DS18) not explained by the model. Cross-sectional, across-phenotype associations, longitudinal, within phenotype associations, and longitudinal, across-phenotype associations were investigated in the structural model (Figure 1). Potential confounders were adjusted for in the cross-sectional, across-phenotype path of the model at age 12.

A maximum likelihood estimator (with robust standard errors) was used because it is robust to non-normally distributed continuous variables.

Since the period of assessment for each outcome at 18 years was different (see Methods) the SEM model was repeated but only including those with PEs at 18 that had occurred within the previous year (n = 88 excluded It would have been preferable to limit PEs to those which had occurred within the previous 6 months in order to make the outcome periods identical, however these data were not available.

Model Fit

Model fit was assessed using RMSEA and CFI/TLI statistics obtained by re-fitting the model using data from complete cases only (n = 2891) because the range of model fit diagnostics available in Mplus for imputed data is limited.

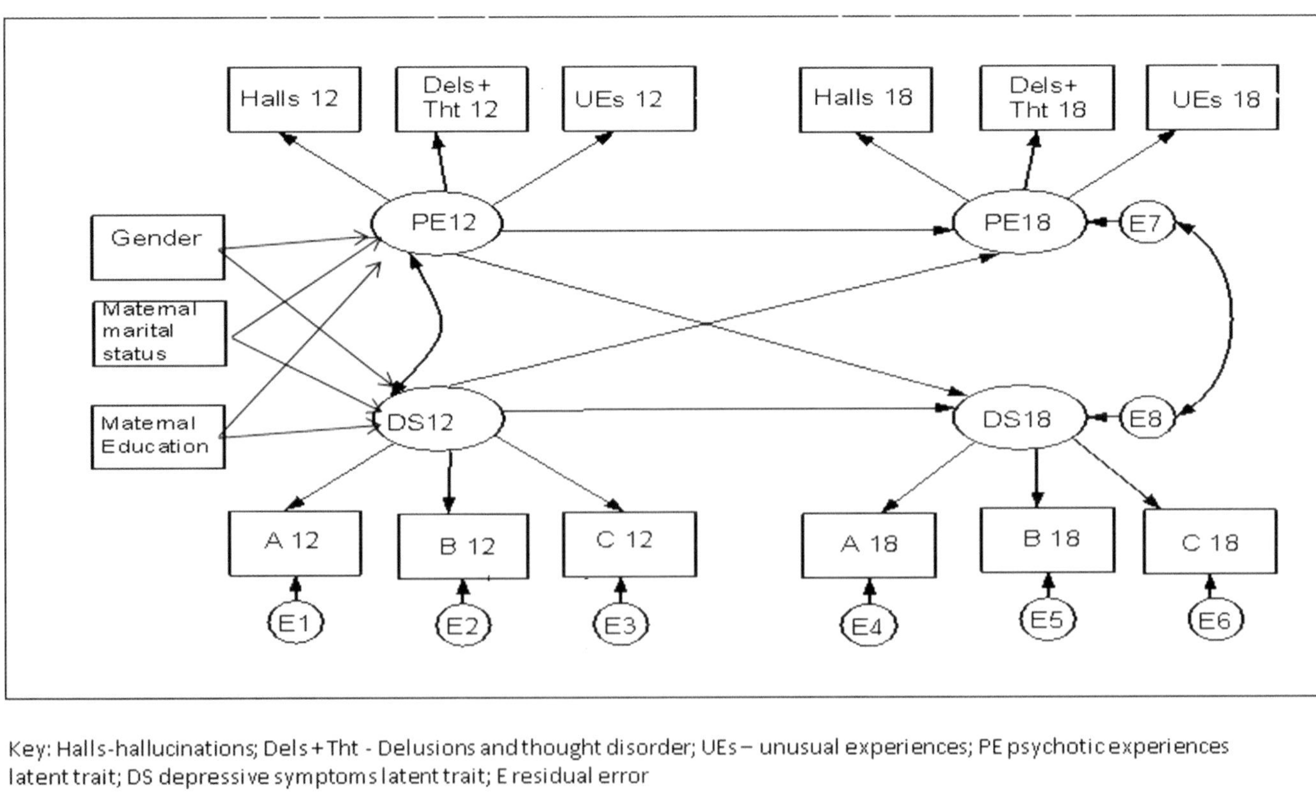

Figure 1. Structural Model.

Post-Hoc Analyses

We tested associations between factors with either DS18 or PE18 as the primary outcome, in order to test the conditioning effect of the other primary outcome factor. The results of this analysis are shown in Figure S1.

Results

Descriptive Data

Compared to those excluded because of missing data, study participants were less likely to be male (51.3% versus 47.9%) or have a mother who was unmarried (19.1% versus 14.3%) or with lower education (64.6% versus 57.3%) at their birth (Table S1).

Mean DS score increased between 12 (mean SMFQ score = 3.44) and 18 years (mean = 5.76) by approximately 0.6 of a standard deviation. The proportion of those experiencing suspected or definite PEs was smaller at 18 years (hallucinations 9.1%, delusions 3.3% and unusual experiences 15.6%) than at 12 years (12.2%, 7.4% and 15.8% respectively) (Table 1).

Relationship between PEs and depression

Using linear and logistic regression on observed data, there was strong evidence that PEs and DSs were associated cross-sectionally, both at 12 and 18 years. DSs at age 12 were associated with PEs at age 18, even after adjusting for baseline PEs, DSs at age 18, and potential confounders. Similarly, PEs at age 12 were associated with DSs at age 18, even after adjusting for baseline DSs, PEs at age 18, and potential confounders (see Table 2 and Figure S2).

In the confirmatory factor analysis, the standardised loadings of each indicator on each factor were high (see Table S3). The correlation between PEs and DS factors at 12 years was 0.46 (95% CI 0.43, 0.49) and between PEs and DS factors at 18 years was 0.38 (95% CI 0.34, 0.42). In general, loadings for the DS indicators on the DS factors were higher than for the PE indicators on the PE factors.

In the SEM analysis using latent constructs of PEs and DSs, cross-sectional associations at each time-point and longitudinal within-phenotype associations were strong (see Table 3). However, whilst there was strong evidence that PEs at 12 were associated with DSs at 18 years ($p \leq 0.0001$) there was no evidence that DSs at 12 were associated with PEs at 18 ($p = 0.891$). The RMSEA statistic for this model was 0.038 (95% CI 0.034, 0.043), the CFI statistic was 0.961, and the TLI statistic was 0.949, which all suggested adequate model fit [33]. Repeating this model but including those with PEs at 18 only if their experiences were present during the previous year (see Methods) produced results that were materially unchanged to those above (available on request).

Discussion

Main Findings

Our hypothesis that there would be no across-phenotype association between psychotic experiences and depression over time once the effects of persistent psychotic experiences and depression had been accounted for was supported for one pathway but not the other.

With standard regression modelling we found strong evidence that PEs at age 12 were associated with depressive symptoms at age 18 even after adjusting for concurrent depressive symptoms at age 12 and persistence of PEs at age 18. We also observed a similarly strong relationship between depressive symptoms at age 12 and PEs at age 18.

However, when using an SEM approach we found little evidence that those who had high depressive symptom scores at 12 were more likely to experience PEs at 18 if their depressive symptoms had resolved by this age, whereas those with PEs at 12 were slightly more likely to experience depressive symptoms at 18 even if their PEs had resolved by 18 years. The most likely explanation for the association we observed between depressive symptoms at 12 and PEs at 18 when using standard regression modelling, inconsistent with our findings when using SEM, is measurement error resulting from the combination of: i) the association between depressive symptoms at 12 and depressive symptoms at 18, and ii) the strong cross-sectional association between PEs and depressive symptoms at both 12 and 18 years.

These findings lead to three main conclusions. Firstly, the method of statistical analysis used is important when dealing with repeated measures of strongly correlated data. As we have observed here it is possible to come to different conclusions about whether depressive symptoms at age 12 increase risk of PEs at age 18 independently of the effects of persisting depression when using standard regression techniques compared to using an SEM approach. Regression models with observed data cannot adequately deal with the problem of correlation between outcomes and exposures. Secondly, early adolescent depression is not associated with increased risk of developing PEs once the co-existence of depression and PEs is accounted for. It is perhaps not unexpected that depression is associated with PEs; for example

Table 1. Depressive symptom and psychotic experience data (n = 7632).

	12 years	18 years
SMFQ scores (range 0–24) mean (SD)	3.44 (3.7)	5.76 (4.9)
Total hallucinations		
Suspected n (%)	458 (6.0%)	298 (3.9%)
Definite n (%)	473 (6.2%)	397 (5.2%)
Total delusions and thought disorder		
Suspected n (%)	427 (5.6%)	183 (2.4%)
Definite n (%)	137 (1.8%)	69 (0.9%)
Unusual Experiences		
Suspected n (%)	679 (8.9%)	473 (6.2%)
Definite n (%)	527 (6.9%)	717 (9.4%)

Table 2. Cross-sectional & longitudinal associations between PEs and depression n = 7632.

Exposure	Outcome	N (% with outcome)	OR[a]	CI	P
DS12	PE12	1075 (14.0%)	1.04	1.03, 1.06	0.0001
DS18	PE18	723 (9.4%)	1.02	1.01, 1.04	≤0.0001
DS12	PE18	723 (9.4%)	1.04[b]	1.03, 1.05	≤0.0001
			Beta[a]	CI	P
PE12	DS12		2.91	1.68, 4.13	≤0.0001
PE18	DS18		2.48	1.26, 3.69	≤0.0001
PE12	DS18		1.61[c]	0.83, 2.39	≤0.0001

[a]adjusted for gender, maternal marital status and maternal education.
[b]additionally adjusted for PE12 and DS18.
[c]additionally adjusted for Dep12 and PE18.
Key: PE12 psychotic experiences at 12 years; PE18 psychotic experiences at 18 years; DS12 depressive symptoms at 12 years; DS18 depressive symptoms at 18 years.

increased feelings of self-consciousness that occur in depression could manifest as paranoid ideation or delusions at their extreme. Our findings suggest that disrupted biological (and non-biological) mechanisms underlying depression do not exert long-term effects on risk of PEs once they resolve. Thirdly, there is evidence that early adolescent PEs do infer a slightly increased risk of later depression. One possible explanation for this is that PEs may cause long-term problems with loss of trust in others, impaired self-confidence, and social isolation, and if these persist even if PEs do not, they could increase the risk of subsequent depression.

Comparison with Previous Research

One previous study of adolescents [17] and one study of adults [34] found evidence of longitudinal associations between depressive symptoms and later PEs. When using standard regression models we also found evidence of this association. However, such models are potentially problematic when dealing with such complex relationships.

Whilst we observed evidence of an association between PEs at baseline and depression at follow-up, three other studies did not [6,18,19]. However, these studies had substantially smaller sample sizes (n = 1037, n = 138 and n = 301) than in our study which may have reduced the statistical power to detect any association, particularly as the association we observed was a relatively small effect. Two of these studies [6,18] used self-report assessments of PEs rather than semi-structured interviews, random measurement error may have resulted in estimates closer to the null. The follow-up period in the two longitudinal studies [18,19] was substantially shorter (24 and 12 months) than the follow-up period in our study. It is possible that the latency period between psychotic experiences and depression is lengthy which may explain why we were able to detect this association with our follow-up period of 6 years.

In order to explain the continuities and discontinuities of psychopathology over time homotypic and heterotypic theories of continuity have been proposed [35,36]. Homotypic continuity suggests that depression and PEs represent a single disease process which persists over time, whereas heterotypic continuity proposes that depression and PEs either represent the same underlying disease process which may be manifested differently across development, or that one psychopathology is a risk factor for the other. Our findings are more consistent with the latter concept given that: i) we observe strong within-phenotype associations over time even after adjusting for the other psychopathology, and ii) we observe some evidence that PEs are associated with an increased risk of depression over time independently of any cross-sectional associations between these two phenotypes.

Not all PEs arise within the context of depression, and there are likely to be important differences in the pathogenic mechanisms underlying these two phenotypes in community samples. Depression scores increase during adolescence whilst frequency of PEs decreases, consistent with this belief. It is possible that PEs arising outside the context of depressive symptoms index aetiological mechanisms underlying schizophrenia more strongly than PEs arising within the context of depression. We are not able to test this hypothesis here, though if it were possible to identify individuals for whom PEs were more likely to reflect mechanisms of interest

Table 3. Associations between psychotic experiences and depressive symptom latent traits over time – β coefficients and 95% confidence intervals and p values (n = 7632).

Exposure	Outcome	Standardised β coefficient	95% CI	Wald p value
PE12	PE18	0.662	0.595, 0.729	≤0.0001
DS12	PE18	0.004	−0.050, 0.059	0.891
DS12	DS18	0.252	0.205, 0.299	≤0.0001
PE12	DS18	0.139	0.089, 0.192	≤0.0001
DS12	PE12	0.486	0.457, 0.515	≤0.0001
DS18	PE18	0.286	0.233, 0.339	≤0.0001

Key: PE12 latent trait of psychotic experiences at 12 years; PE18 latent trait of psychotic experiences at 18 years; DS12 latent trait of depressive symptoms at 12 years. DS18 latent trait of depressive symptoms at 18 years.

for disorders such as schizophrenia, this would have important implications for research in this field.

Strengths and Limitations

Our study has three major strengths. First, the use of a semi-structured interview to assess PEs and the advantage of detailed repeated measures data on both PEs and depressive symptoms. Second, the large population sample has enabled more precise estimation of associations between depression and PEs than previous studies to date. Third, the use of SEM has allowed us to examine both within and across-phenotype relationships of PEs and depressive symptoms over time whilst minimising problems arising from correlated data.

There are also a number of limitations. First, selection bias resulting from sample attrition associated with factors associated with the outcome, the exposure, or both is a concern. However attrition from the ALSPAC cohort is similar to that from other similar sized cohorts[37] and sensitivity analyses conducted using a complete cases dataset (i.e. with data on all exposures, outcomes and confounders) and a dataset including imputed data produced the same findings, suggesting that our findings are unlikely to be due to attrition bias. Second, the combination of hallucinations, delusions and unusual experiences to produce three indicators to generate a factor for PEs at each time-point assumes equal validity for each of the experiences combined into one indicator. This assumption was necessary to ensure model fit, but if validities are unequal a degree of measurement error may account for some of the variance of each of the PEs factors. Third, we only had access to data on PEs and depressive symptoms at 12 and 18 years and therefore are only able to generalise our findings to associations between these psychopathologies in early adolescence and early adulthood Fourth, our data allowed us to detect across-phenotype associations at each time-point but not whether one phenotype occurred first and caused the other shortly afterwards. For instance PEs may have occurred and due to the resulting social isolation cause depression within a few days or weeks.

In the context of these limitations it is important for future studies with data on both PEs and depressive symptoms, measured repeatedly over time, to further investigate their complex relationship during adolescent development. Our findings demonstrate the importance of using appropriate statistical methods to deal with problems arising from strong co-morbidity of phenotypes if the aim is to understand more about the long-term relationships between these phenotypes, and their influence on progression to clinical disorder over time.

Supporting Information

Figure S1 Post hoc analyses.

Figure S2 Structural equation model and coefficients.

Table S1 Comparison of variables in the ALSPAC cohort and the study dataset.

Table S2 Pattern of missing data.

Table S3 Factor loadings.

Appendix S1 Unusual experiences and psychotic experiences questions.

Acknowledgments

We are extremely grateful to all the families who took part in this study, the midwives for their help in recruiting them, and the whole ALSPAC team, which includes interviewers, computer and laboratory technicians, clerical workers, research scientists, volunteers, managers, receptionists and nurses.

Author Contributions

Conceived and designed the experiments: SAS NW DK GL JH MC LM PBJ JS SZ. Performed the experiments: SAS NW DK GL JH MC LM PBJ JS SZ. Analyzed the data: SAS LM JH. Contributed reagents/materials/analysis tools: JH LM. Contributed to the writing of the manuscript: SAS NW DK GL JH MC LM PBJ JS SZ.

References

1. van Os J, Linscott RJ, Myin-Germeys I, Delespaul P, Krabbendam L (2009) A systematic review and meta-analysis of the psychosis continuum: evidence for a psychosis proneness-persistence-impairment model of psychotic disorder. PsycholMed 39: 179–195.
2. Linscott RJ, van OJ (2010) Systematic reviews of categorical versus continuum models in psychosis: evidence for discontinuous subpopulations underlying a psychometric continuum. Implications for DSM-V, DSM-VI, and DSM-VII 1. AnnuRevClinPsychol 6: 391–419.
3. Altman H, Collins M, Mundy P (1997) Subclinical hallucinations and delusions in nonpsychotic adolescents. Journal of Child Psychology and Psychiatry 38: 413–420.
4. Olfson M, Lewis-Fernandez R, Weissman MM, Feder A, Gameroff MJ, et al. (2002) Psychotic symptoms in an urban general medicine practice. American Journal of Psychiatry 159: 1412–1419.
5. van Os J, Hanssen M, Vijl RV, Ravelli A (2000) Strauss (1969) revisited: a psychosis continuum in the general population? Schizophrenia Research 45: 11–20.
6. Debbane M, Van der Linden M, Gex-Fabry M, Eliez S (2009) Cognitive and emotional associations to positive schizotypy during adolescence. Child Psychology and Psychiatry 50: 326–334.
7. Barrantes-Vidal N, Fananas L, Rosa A, Caparros B, Dolors Riba M, et al. (2003) Neurocognitive, behavioural and neurodevelopmental correlates of schizotypy clusters in adolescents from the general population. Schizophrenia Research 61: 293–302.
8. Yung AR, Nelson B, Baker K, Buckby JA, Baksheev G, et al. (2009) Psychotic-like experiences in a community sample of adolescents: implications for the continuum model of psychosis and prediction of schizophrenia 2. AustNZJPsychiatry 43: 118–128.
9. Polanczyk G, Moffitt TE, Arseneault L, Cannon M, Ambler A, et al. (2010) Etiological and Clinical Features of Childhood Psychotic Symptoms: Results From a Birth Cohort. Archives of General Psychiatry 67: 328–338.
10. van Rossum I, Dominguez M, Lieb R, Wittchen H, Van Os J (2011) Affective dysregulation and reality distortion: A 10-year prospective study of their association and clinical relevance. Schizophr Bull 37: 561.
11. Kelleher I, Keeley H, Corcoran P, Lynch F, Fitzpatrick C, et al. (2012) Clinicopathological significance of psychotic experiences in non-psychotic young people: evidence from four population-based studies. British Journal of Psychiatry 201: 26–32.
12. Kelleher I, Lynch F, Harley M, Molloy C, Roddy S, et al. (2012) Psychotic Symptoms in Adolescence Index Risk for Suicidal Behavior Findings From 2 Population-Based Case-Control Clinical Interview Studies. Archives of General Psychiatry 69: 1277–1283.
13. Dhossche D, Ferdinand R, van der Ende J, Hofstra MB, Verhulst F (2002) Diagnostic outcome of self-reported hallucinations in a community sample of adolescents. Psychol Med 32: 619–627.
14. Scott J, Martin G, Welham J, Bor W, Najman J, et al. (2009) Psychopathology During Childhood and Adolescence Predicts Delusional-Like Experiences in Adults: A 21-Year Birth Cohort Study. American Journal of Psychiatry 166: 567–574.
15. Cannon M, Caspi A, Moffitt TE, Harrington H, Taylor A, et al. (2002) Evidence for early-childhood, pan-developmental impairment specific to schizophreniform disorder: results from a longitudinal birth cohort. Archives of General Psychiatry 59: 449–456.
16. Wiles N, Zammitt S, Bebbington P, Singleton N, Meltzer H, et al. (2006) Self reported psychotic symptoms in the general population: results from the logitudinal study of the British National Psychiatric Morbidity Survey. British Journal of Psychiatry 188: 519–526.

17. Weiser M, Lubin G, Caspi A, Rabinowitz J, Shmushkevitz M, et al. (2008) Dysthymia in male adolescents is associated with increased risk of later hospitalization for psychotic disorders: a historical-prospective cohort study. Early Intervention in Psychiatry 2: 67–72.
18. Wigman JTW, Lin A, Vollebergh WAM, van Os J, Raaijmakers QAW, et al. (2011) Subclinical psychosis and depression: Co-occurring phenomena that do not predict each other over time. Schizophrenia Research 130: 277–281.
19. Fowler D, Hodgekins J, Garety P, Freeman D, Kuipers E, et al. (2011) Negative cognition, depressed mood and paranoia: A longitudinal pathway analysis using structural equation modelling. Schizophr Bull 38: 1063–1073.
20. Boyd A, Golding J, Macleod J, Lawlor DA, Fraser A, et al. (2012) Cohort profile: The 'Children of the 90s' - the index offspring of the Avon Longitudinal Study of Parents and Children. Int J Epidemiol April 16: 1–17.
21. Fraser A, Macdonald-Wallis C, Tilling K, Boyd A, Golding J, et al. (2013) Cohort Profile: The Avon Longitudinal Study of Parents and Children: ALSPAC mothers cohort. International Journal of Epidemiology 42: 97–110.
22. Golding J, Pembrey M, Jones R (2001) ALSPAC-the Avon Longitudinal Study of Parents and Children. I Study methodology. Paediatric & Perinatal Epidemiology 15: 74–87.
23. StataCorp LPR (2009) Stata Statistical Software. College Station TX.
24. van Buuren S, Boshuizen HC, Knook DL (1999) Multiple imputation of missing blood pressure covariates in survival analysis. Statistics in Medicine 18: 681–694.
25. Little RJA RD (2002) Statistical analysis with missing data. New York: Wiley.
26. Horwood J, Salvi G, Thomas K, Duffy L, Gunnell D, et al. (2008) IQ and non-clinical psychotic symptoms in 12-year-olds: results from the ALSPAC birth cohort. British Journal of Psychiatry 193: 185–191.
27. Zammit S, Kounali D, Cannon M, David A, Gunnel D, et al. (2013) Prevalence and prediction of psychotic experiences, prodromal syndromes and psychotic disorder at age 18 in a longitudinal, population-based cohort study. Am J Psychiatry in press.
28. Angold A, Costello EJ, Messer SC, Pickles A, Winder F, et al. (1995) The development of a short questionnaire for use in epidemiological studies of depression in children and adolescents. International Journal of Methods in Psychiatric Research 5: 1–12.
29. Sharp C, Goodyer IM, Croudace TJ (2006) The Short Mood and Feelings Questionnaire (SMFQ): A unidimensional item response theory and categorical data factor analysis of self-report ratings from a community sample of 7-through 11-year-old children. Journal of Abnormal Child Psychology 34: 379–391.
30. Joinson C, Heron J, Lewis G, Croudace T, Araya R (2011) Timing of menarche and depressive symptoms in adolescent girls from a UK cohort. British Journal of Psychiatry 198: 17–23.
31. Klein R B (2011) Principles and Practice of Structural Equation Modeling. New York, London: The Guilford Press.
32. van Nierop M, Van Os J, Gunther N, Myin-Germeys I, De Graaf R, et al. (2012) Phenotypically continuous with clinical psychosis, discontinuous in need for care: evidence for an extended psychosis phenotype. Schizophr Bull 38: 231–238.
33. Hu LT, Bentler PM (1999) Cutoff Criteria for Fit Indexes in Covariance Structure Analysis: Conventional Criteria Versus New Alternatives. Structural Equation Modeling-a Multidisciplinary Journal 6: 1–55.
34. Wiles NJ, Zammit S, Bebbington P, Singleton N, Meltzer H, et al. (2006) Self-reported psychotic symptoms in the general population - Results from the longitudinal study of the British National Psychiatric Morbidity Survey. British Journal of Psychiatry 188: 519–526.
35. Rutter M, Kim-Cohen J, Maughan B (2006) Continuities and discontinuities in psychopathology between childhood and adult life. J Child Psychol Psychiatry 47: 276–295.
36. Maughan B, Collishaw S, Stringaris A (2013) Depression in childhood and adolescence. J Can Acad Child Adolesc Psychiatry 22: 35–40.
37. Zammit S, Odd D, Horwood J, Thompson A, Thomas K, et al. (2009) Investigating whether adverse prenatal and perinatal events are associated with non-clinical psychotic symptoms at age 12 years in the ALSPAC birth cohort. Psychological Medicine 39: 1457–1467.

Association of Brain-Derived Neurotrophic Factor Gene Val66Met Polymorphism with Primary Dysmenorrhea

Lin-Chien Lee[1,2,3]¶, Cheng-Hao Tu[1,3,4]¶, Li-Fen Chen[1,3], Horng-Der Shen[5], Hsiang-Tai Chao[6,7], Ming-Wei Lin[5,8]*, Jen-Chuen Hsieh[1,3]*

1 Institute of Brain Science, National Yang-Ming University, Taipei, Taiwan, **2** Department of Physical Medicine and Rehabilitation, Cheng Hsin General Hospital, Taipei, Taiwan, **3** Integrated Brain Research Unit, Division of Clinical Research, Department of Medical Research, Taipei Veterans General Hospital, Taipei, Taiwan, **4** Department of Education and Research, Taipei City Hospital, Taipei, Taiwan, **5** Division of Basic Research, Department of Medical Research, Taipei Veterans General Hospital, Taipei, Taiwan, **6** Department of Obstetrics and Gynecology, Taipei Veterans General Hospital, Taipei, Taiwan, **7** Department of Obstetrics and Gynecology, Faculty of Medicine, School of Medicine, National Yang-Ming University, Taipei, Taiwan, **8** Institute of Public Health, National Yang-Ming University, Taipei, Taiwan

Abstract

Primary dysmenorrhea (PDM), the most prevalent menstrual cycle-related problem in women of reproductive age, is associated with negative moods. Whether the menstrual pain and negative moods have a genetic basis remains unknown. Brain-derived neurotrophic factor (BDNF) plays a key role in the production of central sensitization and contributes to chronic pain conditions. BDNF has also been implicated in stress-related mood disorders. We screened and genotyped the *BDNF* Val66Met polymorphism (rs6265) in 99 Taiwanese (Asian) PDMs (20–30 years old) and 101 age-matched healthy female controls. We found that there was a significantly higher frequency of the Met allele of the *BDNF* Val66Met polymorphism in the PDM group. Furthermore, *BDNF* Met/Met homozygosity had a significantly stronger association with PDM compared with Val carrier status. Subsequent behavioral/hormonal assessments of sub-groups (PDMs = 78, controls = 81; eligible for longitudinal multimodal neuroimaging battery studies) revealed that the *BDNF* Met/Met homozygous PDMs exhibited a higher menstrual pain score (sensory dimension) and a more anxious mood than the Val carrier PDMs during the menstrual phase. Although preliminary, our study suggests that the *BDNF* Val66Met polymorphism is associated with PDM in Taiwanese (Asian) people, and *BDNF* Met/Met homozygosity may be associated with an increased risk of PDM. Our data also suggest the *BDNF* Val66Met polymorphism as a possible regulator of menstrual pain and pain-related emotions in PDM. Absence of thermal hypersensitivity may connote an ethnic attribution. The presentation of our findings calls for further genetic and neuroscientific investigations of PDM.

Editor: Reiner A. Veitia, Institut Jacques Monod, France

Funding: This research was supported by the Taipei Veterans General Hospital (V100D-001, V100D-001-1, V100D-001-2, V100E3-002, V101E3-002, and V102E3-002), Cheng-Hsin General Hospital (101-33), National Science Council (NSC 100-2314-B-010-006-MY3, NSC 100-2629-B-010-001, NSC 101-2629-B-010-001, NSC 101-2911-I-009-101, and NSC 102-2629-B-010-001), Yen Tjing Ling Medical Foundation (CI-100-5), and The Aim for the Top University Plan of the Ministry of Education for National Yang-Ming University. The funders had no role in study design, data collection and analysis, decision to publish, or preparation of the manuscript.

Competing Interests: The authors have declared that no competing interests exist.

* Email: jchsieh@ym.edu.tw (JCH); mwlin@ym.edu.tw (MWL)

¶ These authors contributed equally to this work.

Introduction

Primary dysmenorrhea (PDM), defined as pain associated with menstruation in the absence of organic disease, affects 90% of adolescent girls and more than 50% of menstruating women worldwide [1–4]. The related suffering is described as severe and distressing by 10–20% of the subjects with this condition [2–4]. Despite the unclear pathogenesis of PDM, myometrial hypercontractility and vasoconstriction are the two most widely accepted mechanisms [5,6]. In addition, prostaglandins, chemokines, cytokines, growth factors, oxytocin, leukotrienes, and vasopressin, either within the uterus itself or in menstrual fluid or peripheral blood, are potential contributors to altered uterine physiology [7–10]. Furthermore, PDM can be associated with hampered daily function [11], decreased self-rated overall health [12], and negative moods (e.g., depressive and anxious symptoms) [13,14]. However, to our knowledge there is no report in the literature discussing possible genetic causes of PDM in terms of the pain experience and associated emotions.

Brain-derived neurotrophic factor (BDNF), a member of neurotrophin family, supports neuronal growth, differentiation and survival in the peripheral and central nerve systems, and induces long-lasting changes in synaptic plasticity [15,16]. BDNF is considered a pain modulator because of its involvement in activity-dependent synaptic plasticity within the pain circuitry. With a pro-nociceptive role, BDNF generates the hyperalgesic responses in inflammatory models of pain [17]. BDNF also plays a key role in the production of central sensitization and contributes to chronic pain conditions [17,18]. Moreover, BDNF is potentially involved in stress-related mood disorders [19], e.g., major depression. Stress [19] or chronic pain [20] decreases the expression of BDNF in brain structures that control mood and contributes to depression.

Natural fluctuations of circulating sex hormones across the menstrual cycle are supposed to be associated with mood and cognition alterations in women. BDNF serves as a mediator of sex hormone effects in the hippocampus, and interaction between estrogen and hippocampal BDNF may underlie the menstrual cycle-related problems [21,22]. Estrogen regulates *BDNF* gene expression in the brain of animal models, directly by interaction between estrogen receptor and *BDNF* [23]; and indirectly by GABAergic interneurons modulation [24]. During the estrus phase with low estrogen level, *BDNF* Met/Met homozygous mice exhibited increased anxiety-related behaviors because of decreased BDNF availability and affected BDNF signaling [22]. *BDNF* genotype may therefore alter risk for the development, and could play a role in the diagnosis and treatment of menstrual cycle-related problems, specifically PDM.

The *BDNF* Val66Met polymorphism (rs6265) leads to the substitution of methionine (Met) for valine (Val) at codon 66 of the proBDNF protein. The Met allele leads to a reduced activity-dependent secretion of BDNF from neurons and impaired BDNF signaling [25]. The *BDNF* Val66Met polymorphism (rs6265) might be implicated in both chronic pain conditions and mood disorders. It has been reported that the Met allele carriers, compared to the Val homozygotes, displayed augmented cortical processing of experimental pain in chronic low back pain patients, whilst reduced pain processing without the co-existence of chronic pain [26]. The authors proposed a possible epigenetic modulation that enhances *BDNF* Val66Met polymorphism sensitivity in these chronic pain patients to experimentally induced mildly painful stimuli. Animal models with *BDNF* Met allele exhibited increased anxiety-related behaviors under stress, and this phenomenon implicates an effect of the gene (*BDNF* genotype) × environment (stress) interaction on the mood [25,27]. Although the findings were controversial, previous human studies of *BDNF* Val66Met polymorphism had reported that only *BDNF* Met/Met homozygosity was associated with heightened anxiety [28,29] and an increased risk of depression [30].

In this study, we firstly set out to explore whether the *BDNF* Val66Met polymorphism (rs6265) could be associated with a higher risk of PDM among Taiwanese (Asian) people. Secondly, we reasoned that *BDNF* Met/Met homozygous PDMs might exhibit heightened menstrual pain perception and more negative emotions as compared to Val carrier PDMs. The relationships between *BDNF* Val66Met polymorphism genotypes and the pain- and emotion-related clinical manifestations of PDM, and the psychophysical assessments (pain sensitivity to experimentally induced thermal skin pain) were examined.

Methods

Participants

The inclusion criteria for the PDM group were the followings: (1) 20–30 year-old Taiwanese (Asian) females; (2) a regular menstrual cycle of approximately 27–32 days; (3) a history of PDM longer than 6 months; (4) cramping pain during the menstrual period in the last 6 months rated higher than 4 on a visual analog scale (0 = not at all, 10 = the worst pain imaginable); and (5) right-handedness, as confirmed by the Edinburgh Handedness Inventory. The inclusion criteria for the healthy control females were similar to the PDM group, except that the controls did not experience menstrual pain. The exclusion criteria for all the participants were a history of head injury, pathological pituitary gland disease, organic pelvic disease, psychiatric disorder, immediate plans for pregnancy or a positive pregnancy test, a history of childbirth, and having a metal/pacemaker implant. The participants had not used oral contraceptives within 6 months prior to the study. No analgesics had been taken within 24 hours before the study. All the subjects in the PDM group underwent pelvic ultrasonography to exclude secondary dysmenorrhea caused by organic pelvic diseases, such as endometriosis or adenomyosis. All the participants were clinically examined and diagnosed in the Gynecology clinic by a gynecologist (HTC).

Altogether, 306 PDMs and 199 controls were originally screened between August 31, 2011 and September 30, 2013 as intended for multimodal imaging genetics studies (magnetic resonance imaging and magnetoencephalography). During the screening stage, 207 PDMs and 98 controls were excluded due to one or a combination of the following factors: an irregular menstrual cycle, a prolonged or shortened menstrual cycle, inconsistent pain intensity, pelvic abnormalities by ultrasonography, or being unwilling to complete the entire series of genetic, hormonal, behavioral, and multimodal neuroimaging studies. Eventually, a total of 99 PDMs and 101 healthy controls (matched for age and educational level) were enrolled. All these subjects also participated in multimodal imaging genetics experiments (the data will be reported elsewhere). All the experiments were completed within three menstrual cycles due to difficulties in scheduling the brain scanning within one menstrual cycle. The overall study was conducted in accordance with the Declaration of Helsinki and was approved by the Institutional Review Board of Taipei Veterans General Hospital. The participants provided written informed consent.

Genotyping

Blood samples for genotyping were obtained during the initial examination. Whole blood collected in 10 mL EDTA tubes was stored in 4°C fridge, and DNA extraction was subsequently performed using the Puregene kit following the manufacturer's guidelines (Gentra Systems, Minneapolis, MN). Commercial TaqMan single-nucleotide polymorphism assays (Applied Biosystems, Foster City, CA) were used for genotyping. The polymerase chain reaction amplification was conducted in total volume of 1 L using the following amplification protocol: 50°C for 2 min, 95°C for 10 min, and 40 cycles of 94°C for 15 sec and 62°C for 1 min. Fluorescence measurements were performed using the ABI HT7900 (Applied Biosystems, Foster City, CA), and allele calling was performed with the SDS 2.2 software package (Applied Biosystems). Genotypes were independently assigned to the subjects by two technicians blinded to the subjects' information.

Serum Hormone Measurements

The sera extracted from the blood samples drawn during the menstrual phase (within 1–3 days after the start of menstrual flow) and periovulatory phase (12–16 days after the start of menstrual flow) were stored for batch analysis using commercialized assays (UniCel DxC 800 Synchron Clinical Systems, Beckman Coulter, Inc., Brea, CA). The total serum concentrations were assayed using a chemiluminescence immunoassay technique for the estradiol and progesterone, and a radioimmunoassay technique for the testosterone.

Behavioral AssessmentsMenstrual pain experience. The PDMs completed the McGill Pain Questionnaire during the initial examination and again during the menstrual phase to assess the recalled overall and current experiences of menstrual pain, respectively.

Personality traits and quality of life. All the participants in the two groups completed the Basic Personality Inventory [31] and the SF-36 (quality of life) [32] during the initial examination to assess personality traits and quality of life, respectively.

Assessment of anxiety, depressive mood and pain catastrophizing. To evaluate the psychological status across the menstrual cycle, all the participants in the two groups completed self-reported psychological measurements during the menstrual phase and periovulatory phase. Ovulation was confirmed using a urinary luteinizing hormone test [33–35]. The psychological battery included the Spielberger State-Trait Anxiety Inventory [36], the Beck Anxiety Inventory [37], the Beck Depression Inventory [38], and the Pain Catastrophizing Scale [39]. The order of the assessments was balanced across the subjects for the menstrual phase and periovulatory phase. Multimodal neuroimaging studies were conducted during these two phases; the results will be reported elsewhere.

Quantitative sensory testing for central sensitization. To examine central sensitization throughout the menstrual cycle, as previously reported in studies on white populations [40–44], we performed a thermal quantitative sensory testing (thermal sensation and pain thresholds) according to the established protocol of an ascending limit approach for heat pain and a descending limit approach for cold pain [45]. Heat and cold stimuli (TSA 2001-II, MEDOC, Israel) were administered to the bilateral periumbilical areas (T11-dermatome, referral area of menstrual pain) and forearm extensor areas (C7-dermatome, remote control area) during the menstrual phase and periovulatory phase. The baseline temperature was set at 32°C, and all the thresholds were obtained with a ramped stimulation method (1°C/sec). The perception thresholds for cold and warm were determined first, followed by the pain thresholds for cold and heat. The mean thresholds were calculated by averaging three consecutive measurements. The limits of the temperature range were set between 0 and 50°C.

Statistical Analysis

SPSS Statistics 20.0 (SPSS Inc., Chicago, IL) was used for all the analyses. The data are presented as the means ± standard deviation. The results were considered significant at $P<0.05$ (two-tailed). We did not apply multiple corrections for all these inventories since they access different sensory, affective, cognitive, and physiological dimensions of pain, and the discrete physical and mental impacts of social life. In the first stage of the analysis, the Hardy-Weinberg equilibrium of the *BDNF* genotype distribution and the relationship between genotype and PDM were examined using the chi-square test. We then conducted the second stage of the analysis by investigating the associations between the *BDNF* Val66Met polymorphism and behavioral/hormonal manifestations. The Val/Val and Val/Met subjects were treated as a single genotype category (*BDNF* Val carriers) and compared with the *BDNF* Met/Met homozygotes in the subsequent analyses. This strategy was corroborated by our findings that there were no essential differences in any of the behavioral/hormonal assessments between the *BDNF* Val/Val and *BDNF* Val/Met subjects in the PDM and control groups (all $P>0.05$). Between-group (PDM vs. control) and between-genotype (Met/Met homozygotes vs. Val carriers) differences in demographic characteristics and McGill Pain Questionnaire scores were examined using a two-sample t-test or the Mann-Whitney U test. A two-way analysis of variance (ANOVA) of the Basic Personality Inventory and SF-36 data was conducted for the main effects of group (PDM vs. control) and *BDNF* genotype (Met/Met homozygotes vs. Val carriers), as well as the interaction between them. For the assessments of behavior, quantitative sensory testing and serum hormone levels during the two phases, a general linear model with a repeated measures design was first applied to examine the possible effects of group (PDM vs. control), genotype (Met/Met homozygotes vs. Val carriers), menstrual cycle (menstrual phase vs. periovulatory phase) and the interactions between these factors. To further determine whether different *BDNF* genotypes were associated with different psychological attributes of state anxiety, trait anxiety, Beck Anxiety Inventory, Beck Depression Inventory, and Pain Catastrophizing Scale scores across the menstrual cycle for the respective PDM and control group, repeated-measures ANOVAs were conducted on each psychological measurement to compare the PDM and control groups.

Results

Demographic Characteristics (Table 1)

There were no significant differences between the PDM and control groups in age, age at menarche, years of menstruating or average days of one menstrual cycle ($P>0.05$). The PDM group had been experiencing moderate cyclic menstrual pain (recalled overall McGill Pain Questionnaire-pain rating index: 33.3±12.96) for 2 (1.8±0.82) days per month for approximately 10 (9.2±2.70) years.

Of all the PDMs and controls who received genetic testing, 21 PDMs were excluded from the genetic-behavioral-hormonal-multimodal neuroimaging studies for the following reasons: appendicitis after recruitment (n = 1), fifth ventricle in the brain (n = 2), arteriovenous malformation in the brain (n = 1), MRI claustrophobia (n = 2), irregular menstrual cycle after recheck (n = 1), and withdrawal with incomplete behavioral/hormonal data (n = 14). Twenty controls were excluded from the genetic-behavioral-hormonal-multimodal neuroimaging studies for the following reasons: intracranial arachnoid cyst (n = 1), irregular menstrual cycle after recheck (n = 1), development of systemic lupus erythematosus after recruitment with anti-lupus medications (n = 1), undisclosed prior head injury (n = 1), and withdrawal with incomplete data (n = 16). The participants with the aforementioned problems and incidental MRI brain findings were excluded from further genetic-behavioral-hormonal and multimodal neuroimaging analyses. The demographic data of the remaining participants (PDM = 78, control = 81) retained similar features of the original samples ($P>0.05$).

Genotypes and Allele Distributions (Table 2)

Participants in the two groups were all successfully genotyped. The genotype distributions of the *BDNF* Val66Met (rs6265) for both groups were in Hardy-Weinberg equilibrium ($P>0.05$; Table 2). A sample size of 200 (99 PDMs, 101 controls) achieved 64% statistical power to detect an effect size of 0.184 using a 2-degree-of-freedom chi-square test with a significance level of 0.05. The PDM group differed significantly from the control group in *BDNF* genotypes ($P = 0.034$) and alleles ($P = 0.013$) distributions. There was a significant excess of the Met allele in the PDM group compared with the control group (Table 2). The PDM prevalence difference in all *BDNF* Met/Met homozygotes (63.8%) vs. all Val carriers (43.7%) attained high significance ($P = 0.012$). Treating the *BDNF* Val allele carriers as the baseline, the odds ratio for *BDNF* Met/Met homozygosity was 2.27 (95% confidence interval = 1.21–4.27) ((PDM-Met/Met × control-Val-carriers)/(PDM-Val-carriers × control-Met/Met)). It implied that those carrying the *BDNF* Met/Met genotype had an increased risk of PDM. The *BDNF* Val66Met polymorphism had no association with the age of onset (Val carriers, 14.2±1.76 years of age; Met homozygotes, 13.9±1.56) or duration of menstrual pain per cycle (Val carriers, 1.8±0.86 days; Met/Met homozygotes, 1.8±0.75) in the PDM group.

For the behavioral/hormonal assessments (PDM = 78, control = 81; eligible for multimodal neuroimaging studies), the subgroups retained the original group features in terms of the

Table 1. Demographic data of the original genotyping groups and the behavioral/hormonal sub-groups.

	PDM		Control	
	Genotyping	**Behavioral/hormonal**	**Genotyping**	**Behavioral/hormonal**
Subject number	99	78	101	81
Age	23.3 (2.33)	23.4 (2.41)	23.8 (2.35)	23.9 (2.38)
Age at menarche	12.0 (1.27)	12.0 (1.25)	12.2 (1.05)	12.3 (1.08)
Years of menstruating	11.3 (2.57)	11.4 (2.66)	11.5 (2.46)	11.6 (2.56)
Days of one menstrual cycle	29.5 (1.12)	29.4 (1.18)	29.6 (1.20)	29.6 (1.23)
Years of dysmenorrhea history	9.2 (2.70)	9.3 (2.79)		
Days of menstrual pain per cycle	1.8 (0.82)	1.9 (0.83)		
MPQ: recalled pain rating index	33.3 (12.96)	34.5 (13.17)		
MPQ: recalled pain intensity	3.1 (1.21)	3.1 (1.17)		

Abbreviations: MPQ, McGill Pain Questionnaire; PDM, primary dysmenorrhea. The data are presented as the means (SD).

genotype and allele distributions (Table S1). No differences in demographic data were noted between the *BDNF* Met/Met homozygotes and the Val carriers in the sub-groups (all $P>0.05$).

Differences in Behavioral Assessments

Menstrual pain experience (Table 3). During the menstrual phase, differences in pain rating index ($P=0.131$) and present pain intensity ($P=0.925$) of McGill Pain Questionnaire were not demonstrated between the *BDNF* Met/Met homozygous PDMs and the Val carrier PDMs. However, the *BDNF* Met/Met homozygous PDMs scored significantly higher on the sensory subscale of McGill Pain Questionnaire compared with the Val carriers ($P=0.017$).

Personality traits and quality of life (Table 4). There was a significant main effect of group (but no significant main effect of *BDNF* genotype or interaction between group and *BDNF* genotype) on the anxiety ($F=10.975$, $R^2=0.068$, $P=0.001$), depression ($F=8.875$, $R^2=0.056$, $P=0.003$), and hypochondriasis ($F=27.314$, $R^2=0.154$, $P<0.001$) dimensions of Basic Personality Inventory. Significant group effect was noted also on physical ($F=31.554$, $R^2=0.173$, $P<0.001$) and mental ($F=40.455$, $R^2=0.211$, $P<0.001$) components of SF-36. Regardless of genotype, the PDMs (compared with the controls) scored significantly higher on the anxiety, depression, and hypochondriasis dimensions of Basic Personality Inventory and significantly lower on the physical and mental components of SF-36.

Anxiety, depressive mood and pain catastrophizing (Table 5). For the analyses of the entire cohort, there was a significant main effect of group on the state anxiety ($F=27.089$, $R^2=0.152$, $P<0.001$), trait anxiety ($F=17.593$, $R^2=0.106$, $P<0.001$), Beck Anxiety Inventory ($F=59.864$, $R^2=0.284$, $P<0.001$), Beck Depression Inventory ($F=17.810$, $R^2=0.106$, $P<0.001$), and Pain Catastrophizing Scale ($F=72.171$, $R^2=0.334$, $P<0.001$) scores, with a significant interaction between menstrual cycle and group on the state anxiety ($F=24.269$, $R^2=0.138$, $P<0.001$), Beck Anxiety Inventory ($F=70.943$, $R^2=0.320$, $P<0.001$), Beck Depression Inventory ($F=32.477$, $R^2=0.177$, $P<0.001$), and Pain Catastrophizing Scale ($F=4.412$, $R^2=0.030$, $P=0.037$) scores. There was also a significant main effect of menstrual cycle on the state anxiety ($F=16.459$, $R^2=0.098$, $P<0.001$), Beck Anxiety Inventory ($F=60.690$, $R^2=0.287$, $P<0.001$), Beck Depression Inventory ($F=28.713$, $R^2=0.160$, $P<0.001$), and Pain Catastrophizing Scale ($F=4.514$, $R^2=0.030$, $P=0.035$) scores and a significant main effect of *BDNF* genotype on the state anxiety ($F=6.207$, $R^2=0.039$, $P=0.014$) and Beck Anxiety Inventory ($F=4.974$, $R^2=0.032$, $P=0.027$) scores. Significant interactions between menstrual cycle and *BDNF* genotype ($F=7.595$, $R^2=0.048$, $P=0.007$), as well as among menstrual cycle, group and *BDNF* genotype ($F=4.509$, $R^2=0.029$, $P=0.035$), on the Beck Anxiety Inventory score were noted.

In the individual group analyses, the PDM group exhibited a significant main effect of menstrual cycle on state anxiety ($F=33.144$, $R^2=0.309$, $P<0.001$), Beck Anxiety Inventory ($F=85.498$, $R^2=0.536$, $P<0.001$), Beck Depression Inventory ($F=45.579$, $R^2=0.381$, $P<0.001$), and Pain Catastrophizing Scale ($F=7.556$, $R^2=0.095$, $P=0.008$) scores, as well as a significant interaction between menstrual cycle and *BDNF* genotype on the Beck Anxiety Inventory score ($F=7.743$, $R^2=0.095$, $P=0.007$) (Table 5). In view of R^2 statistics, the significant interaction between menstrual cycle and *BDNF* genotype should mainly be attributed to the main effect of menstrual cycle in the PDM group. By contrast, the control group exhibited neither significant main effects nor interactions (Table S2). Compared with the controls, the PDMs reported significantly higher state anxiety, trait anxiety, Beck Anxiety Inventory, Beck Depression Inventory, and Pain Catastrophizing Scale scores during either the menstrual phase or periovulatory phase. The PDMs had significantly higher state anxiety, Beck Anxiety Inventory, Beck Depression Inventory, and Pain Catastrophizing Scale scores, but not trait anxiety score, during the menstrual phase than the periovulatory phase. The controls demonstrated no significant between-phase differences in any of the psychological measurements. The Met/Met homozygous PDMs, compared with the Val carrier PDMs, manifested higher Beck Anxiety Inventory scores during the menstrual phase, but not during the periovulatory phase. In the controls, an absence of between-genotype differences was noted in all the psychological measurements.

Quantitative sensory testing results (Table S3). Because there was no right-left difference in any of the measured thresholds in each subject (all $P>0.05$), we averaged the bilateral values for the corresponding dermatome areas for the group comparisons. No main effect of menstrual cycle, group, *BDNF* genotype or interactions between them was noted for any of the measured thresholds. In brief, we detected no regional or generalized central sensitization of superficial (skin) pain in the Taiwanese (Asian) participants.

Table 2. *BDNF* rs6265 genotype distributions and allele frequency.

	Genotype (n, %)				Allele frequency		
	G/G (Val/Val)	G/A (Val/Met)	A/A (Met/Met)	*P*	Val	Met	*P*
PDM (n = 99)	24, 24.2%	38, 38.4%	37, 37.4%	0.034	43.4%	56.6%	0.013
Control (n = 101)	33, 32.7%	47, 46.5%	21, 20.8%		55.9%	44.1%	

Abbreviations: *BDNF*, brain-derived neurotrophic factor; PDM, primary dysmenorrhea; A, adenine; G, guanine; Val, Valine; Met, Methionine.

Serum Hormone Levels (Table S4)

There was a significant main effect of menstrual cycle, but no main effect of group or *BDNF* genotype, on the serum estradiol ($F = 85.604$, $R^2 = 0.393$, $P < 0.001$), progesterone ($F = 8.937$, $R^2 = 0.063$, $P = 0.003$), and testosterone ($F = 31.150$, $R^2 = 0.190$, $P < 0.001$) levels. The serum gonadal hormone levels were significantly higher during the periovulatory phase than during the menstrual phase, regardless of group or *BDNF* genotype.

Discussion

The Association of *BDNF* Val66Met Polymorphism with PDM

To our knowledge, this is the first study to report a significant association between the *BDNF* Val66Met polymorphism and PDM. The genotype distributions and allele frequencies of the *BDNF* Val66Met polymorphism exhibit substantial ethnic differences, which may consequently affect the results of genetic association studies. The Met allele frequency in Asian populations (40–50%) is significantly higher than that of white populations (25–32%) [15,46]. The *BDNF* genotype distribution and allele frequency of the overall sample (Met allele frequency: 50.25%) in our study concur with previous reports on Asian populations [47,48]. The finding that Taiwanese PDMs exhibit a significantly higher *BDNF* Met/Met prevalence and *BDNF* Met allele frequency implies that young *BDNF* Met/Met homozygous Taiwanese females may have an increased risk of PDM (Table 2).

The Role of *BDNF* Val66Met Polymorphism as a Regulator of Menstrual Pain

In animal studies, BDNF functions either as a pro-nociceptive or an anti-nociceptive role in the brainstem pain modulatory system (midbrain periaqueductal gray and rostral ventromedial medulla). On one hand, BDNF mRNA and protein levels are upregulated in the dorsal root ganglion, spinal cord and brainstem pain modulatory system under peripheral noxious stimulation. BDNF herein exerts pro-nociceptive effects and contributes to descending pain facilitation and chronic pain hypersensitivity [49,50]. On the other hand, BDNF can manifest protective anti-nociceptive effects under repeated painful conditions as a result of multiple mechanisms, including a direct neurotransmitter-like effect or processes of neural plasticity in the anti-nociceptive systems, induction of serotonin-related analgesia, and a modulatory effect at the supraspinal level [51]. BDNF can therefore be consociated with both an enhancement of nociceptive impact, and a dampened response to protect the brain from pain overstimulation [51]. Thus, the overall effect of BDNF on pain perception and experience depends on the net interaction output of these apparently contrasting activities at different neural structures in which BDNF is produced, secreted, and left to act [17,50,51]. The *BDNF* Val66Met polymorphism can lead to impaired BDNF signaling in the brainstem pain modulatory system and it may be associated with altered menstrual pain modulation in PDMs. The aforementioned dual effects of BDNF on pain may explain in part the diversity of the results of behavioral and psychological assessments, as demonstrated that *BDNF* genotype expressed an effect on the sensory dimension scores but not on the other dimension scores and the total scores (pain rating index) of McGill Pain Questionnaire reported during the menstrual phase.

PDM is not only associated with irritable bowel syndrome and fibromyalgia but is also viewed as a harbinger of these conditions [52,53]. Central sensitization-induced viscero-visceral [44] and viscero-somatic hyperalgesia [40] outside the uterine referral area during early life can be a mechanism contributing to these chronic

Table 3. *BDNF* rs6265 genotype effect on McGill Pain Questionnaire scores of PDMs during the menstrual phase.

	Met/Met	Val carrier	*P*
Subject number	29	49	
Pain rating index	32.3 (13.47)	26.7 (12.02)	0.131
Sensory	18.5 (6.21)	14.7 (6.13)	0.017
Affective	4.2 (3.57)	3.4 (2.29)	0.554
Evaluative	2.4 (2.02)	2.1 (2.01)	0.613
Miscellaneous	7.2 (3.72)	6.5 (3.81)	0.418
Present pain intensity	2.7 (1.02)	2.6 (1.01)	0.925

Abbreviations: *BDNF*, brain-derived neurotrophic factor; PDM, primary dysmenorrhea; Val, valine; Met, methionine. The data are presented as the means (SD).

pain conditions later in life. In PDMs with comorbid irritable bowel syndrome, treating menstrual pain helps to relieve the pain associated with irritable bowel syndrome [54]. A role for BDNF protein in chronic pain conditions such as irritable bowel syndrome [55] and fibromyalgia [56–58] has been suggested. It has been postulated that BDNF protein strengthens the synaptic plasticity within the pain modulatory circuitry and contributes to descending pain facilitation and the subsequent visceral pain and hypersensitivity [50]. It has been reported that irritable bowel syndrome was associated with the up-regulation of BDNF in the intestinal mucosa and that colonic BDNF expression correlated with the severity of abdominal pain [55]. Fibromyalgia has been reported to be associated with the up-regulation of BDNF in the cerebrospinal fluid [56], and the extent of this up-regulation was correlated with the duration of chronic pain. However, it remains to be explored whether *BDNF* Val66Met polymorphism substantially modulates the process of central sensitization and whether a specific genotype(s) renders PDMs more vulnerable to the development of irritable bowel syndrome and fibromyalgia later in life.

Personality Traits and Quality of Life of PDMs

Compared with the controls, the PDMs manifested significantly higher levels of depressive mood, anxiety, and hypochondriasis as their personality traits (Table 4). These findings are in line with previous studies [59,60]. However, these levels did not reach the degree of clinical severity, such as an anxiety disorder, that is mandatory for psychiatric intervention. The PDMs reported a significantly lower quality of life, encompassing both physical and mental components, compared with the controls (Table 4). The absence of main effects of genotype or the interaction between group and genotype in both the Basic Personality Inventory and SF-36 assessments connotes that the *BDNF* Val66Met polymorphism does not directly influence personality traits and quality of life. Rather, menstrual pain per se is the dominant factor influencing these two life facets. Such dysmenorrhea-associated dysfunction, in its severe and protracted form, may through chronification eventually impact women's long-term health as profoundly as chronic diseases [12].

The Possible Role of *BDNF* Val66Met Polymorphism as a Regulator of Emotions in PDM

The PDMs exhibited more prominent negative moods (anxiety and depression) and pain catastrophizing compared with the controls (Table 5 and Table S2). Women with high pain catastrophizing scores may have altered cognitive-affective processing of menstrual pain-laden emotional orientations, which may precipitate depression, anxiety and altered pain experience [61]. Although the interaction between the *BDNF* genotype and menstrual cycle for Beck Anxiety Inventory scores in the PDM group was not substantial, we found an effect of the gene (*BDNF* genotype) × environment (menstrual pain) interaction on the Beck Anxiety Inventory scores when considering menstrual pain as an environmental stressor. Additionally, the *BDNF* Met/Met homozygous PDMs displayed higher anxiety during the menstrual phase compared with the Val carrier PDMs (Table 5). It is noteworthy that the *BDNF* Val66Met polymorphism produced no significant effects on mood across the menstrual cycle in the control group. These findings collectively connote that the *BDNF* Val66Met polymorphism is modestly associated with the supraspinal modulation of menstrual pain-laden emotional processing. Although *BDNF* Val66Met polymorphism alone may not effectuate depressive and anxious moods, it may represent a predisposing factor, and chronic stress like cyclic menstrual pain is necessary for the detection [62]. Our arguments are in agreement with a meta-analysis that concluded that *BDNF* Met/Met homozygous Asians are predisposed to a sub-significantly higher risk of anxiety disorders [28].

The possible mechanisms underlying the modulatory function of the *BDNF* Val66Met polymorphism on mood may be manifold. According to the neurotrophic model for stress-related mood disorders [19], Met/Met homozygotes may exhibit a deficient expression of BDNF in the mood control areas of the brain during stress (e.g., chronic pain [20]), which may predispose vulnerable subjects to mood disorders [63]. This hypothesis is corroborated by animal studies in which Met/Met homozygotes exhibited defective activity-dependent BDNF secretion from neurons and manifested anxiety-related behaviors in stressful settings [25]. Furthermore, declines in estrogen (as a positive regulator that enhances BDNF expression) during the menstrual phase may lead to a decreased expression of BDNF in the brain, which in turn could hamper the BDNF signaling in the mood-controlling networks of susceptible subjects [21,22]. This study did not reveal a group or genotype main effect (or the interaction between them) on gonadal hormones (Table S4). Thus, the role of estrogen as a regulator of PDM-related emotions remains elusive.

Absence of Central Sensitization to Experimental Skin Pain

Having a sample size many times greater than those reported in the literature [40–43], we found no group (PDM vs. control), menstrual cycle (menstrual phase vs. periovulatory phase), or genotype (*BDNF* Met/Met homozygotes vs. Val carriers) effects on pain sensitivity to experimental skin thermal stimuli (Table S3).

Table 4. ANOVA results of Basic Personality Inventory and SF-36 assessments, stratified by group and *BDNF* genotype.

	PDM		Control		Main effect		Interaction
	Met/Met	**Val carrier**	**Met/Met**	**Val carrier**	**Group (*P*)**	**Genotype (*P*)**	**Group*Genotype (*P*)**
Subject number	29	49	17	64			
Basic Personality Inventory							
Depression	3.2 (2.72)	3.7 (3.44)	2.4 (2.47)	1.7 (1.87)	0.003	0.887	0.240
Anxiety	6.1 (3.25)	4.9 (3.42)	3.4 (3.10)	3.9 (2.70)	0.001	0.480	0.135
Social introversion	3.5 (2.49)	3.4 (2.86)	4.1 (2.28)	3.7 (2.57)	0.357	0.688	0.776
Self depreciation	2.1 (2.14)	2.5 (2.70)	2.1 (1.64)	2.6 (2.40)	0.929	0.283	0.835
Interpersonal problems	4.8 (2.43)	4.2 (2.22)	4.5 (3.06)	3.5 (2.71)	0.269	0.082	0.709
Impulse expression	4.6 (3.29)	4.4 (3.03)	4.2 (3.55)	4.5 (2.97)	0.878	0.945	0.681
Deviation	2.4 (1.93)	2.5 (2.34)	2.3 (1.49)	2.1 (1.95)	0.393	0.830	0.653
Hypochondriasis	4.6 (3.25)	4.7 (2.84)	2.4 (1.41)	2.2 (1.92)	<0.001	0.986	0.757
Persecutory ideas	2.7 (2.11)	2.8 (2.03)	2.8 (1.74)	2.0 (2.15)	0.393	0.342	0.205
Thinking disorder	1.8 (1.94)	1.9 (1.63)	1.6 (1.62)	1.5 (1.80)	0.363	0.926	0.837
SF-36							
Physical component	46.3 (10.10)	45.2 (10.12)	52.6 (5.64)	54.7 (4.08)	<0.001	0.727	0.243
Mental component	46.2 (7.51)	46.5 (7.19)	53.1 (4.95)	53.7 (4.69)	<0.001	0.668	0.915

Abbreviations: ANOVA, analysis of variance; *BDNF*, brain-derived neurotrophic factor; SF-36, 36-Item Short-Form Health Survey; PDM, primary dysmenorrhea; Val, valine; Met, methionine. The data are presented as the means (SD).

Table 5. Results of repeated-measures ANOVA of psychological measurements: effects of menstrual cycle and *BDNF* genotype in the PDM group.

	Met/Met	Val carrier	Main effect		Interaction
			Phase (*P*)	Genotype (*P*)	Phase*Genotype (*P*)
Subject number	29	49			
State anxiety					
MENS	45.5 (9.68)	41.1 (8.61)	<0.001	0.052	0.495
POV	38.9 (7.84)	36.0 (5.60)			
Trait anxiety					
MENS	45.6 (10.10)	44.0 (8.21)	0.056	0.386	0.886
POV	44.3 (9.37)	42.4 (8.55)			
Beck anxiety					
MENS	14.9 (6.95)	10.9 (6.82)	<0.001	0.138	0.007
POV	6.3 (5.96)	6.3 (5.78)			
Beck depression					
MENS	13.8 (10.52)	11.3 (9.73)	<0.001	0.429	0.295
POV	6.1 (7.27)	5.7 (6.94)			
Pain catastrophizing					
MENS	22.6 (11.05)	19.6 (12.58)	0.008	0.383	0.512
POV	18.8 (9.27)	17.3 (12.35)			

Abbreviations: ANOVA, analysis of variance;
BDNF, brain-derived neurotrophic factor;
PDM, primary dysmenorrhea; MENS, menstrual phase;
POV, periovulatory phase;
Val, valine; Met, methionine.
The data are presented as the means (SD).

Our findings are at odds with published studies (based on very small samples of 10–22 PDMs and 10–31 controls; most studies had 10 of each) that dysmenorrheic white women, compared with non-dysmenorrheic ones, exhibit heightened pain sensitivity or central sensitization (either regional or generalized) to experimental somatic [40–43] and visceral stimuli [44]. Notwithstanding, other studies on dysmenorrheic white women have also yielded conflicting results [43,64]. Our results indicate that additional factors contributing to the diversity of the clinical manifestations of PDM may include different genetic constitutions (in the context of ethnicity) and the diverse nature and quality of experimental pain caused by different stimuli [65]. Future studies employing imaging genetics [66] in combination with more comprehensively designed psychophysical experiments (including deep somatic pain and visceral pain assessments) on a larger sample may be helpful to elucidate the supraspinal (brain) mechanisms that underlie the presence or absence of central sensitization in the context of ethnic differences. It should be born in mind that such mechanisms of presence or absence of central sensitization may occur at different level of the neuraxis of the central nervous system.

Limitations and Further Considerations

Our study indicates an association of the *BDNF* Val66Met polymorphism with PDM, and our data suggest, yet not strongly affirm, a possible role of *BDNF* Val66Met polymorphism as a regulator of menstrual pain and pain-related emotions in PDM. The discordance between genetic association and clinical manifestations in our study has been corroborated by a previous study on Taiwanese that reported the genetic association of the *BDNF* Val66Met polymorphism with a higher risk of geriatric depression, but not with the disease severity (depression and cognitive deficit) [30]. Some possible explanations are suggested below. Firstly, we speculate that the overall manifestations of pain experience of PDM may be determined in part by the net output of contrasting pro- and anti-nociceptive effect of BDNF in the pain circuitry, that may result in the discordance between the genetic risk predisposition and pain-emotional expressions. This can be better appreciated in the context that PDM, dissimilar with major affective disorders and neurological diseases, usually does not manifest intense mood liability and functional disability except the severe form that leads to absenteeism from school and work. Secondly, the *BDNF* Val66Met polymorphism, as an individual gene, may not play a dominant role in the overall expressions of menstrual pain and pain-related emotions, in which polygenic interactions and regulations (e.g., genes related to the serotonergic and dopaminergic systems) are most likely involved [67–69]. Thirdly, the behavioral assessments we used may not perfectly reflect the pain- and emotion-related experiential facets of PDM. Fourthly, functional variants within the coding or regulatory regions of the *BDNF*, other than the *BDNF* Val66Met polymorphism, might also contribute to the clinical manifestations of PDM. The *BDNF* G-712A polymorphism, a genetic variant located in the putative promoter region [70], has been reported to be associated with major depression in Chinese [71]. Lastly, the *BDNF* Val66Met polymorphism may not be directly involved in the pathogenesis of PDM, and the association between the *BDNF* Val66Met polymorphism and PDM may be through linkage disequilibrium with other genetic variants of the *BDNF* or nearby genes.

The sample sizes in the current report are relatively small due to the rigorous inclusion/exclusion criteria and the demanding processes of associated longitudinal multimodal neuroimaging studies for each participant. We consider the novel findings reported in this study as preliminary. However, our observations do echo the recent mandate for a thorough revisit of PDM [4,52], and invite further studies of larger sample size for the genetic and neuroscientific underpinnings of the clinical (pain and related emotions) and psychophysical (pain sensitivity) manifestations of PDM females.

Conclusions

Our data suggest that the *BDNF* Val66Met polymorphism is associated with PDM in Taiwanese (Asian) people. *BDNF* Met/Met homozygous young Taiwanese females may have an increased risk of PDM. The putative role of *BDNF* Val66Met polymorphism as a supraspinal regulator of menstrual pain and pain-laden emotions remains to be further verified. Absence of thermal hypersensitivity may connote an ethnic attribution. Ethnicity of different genetic constitutions should be taken into consideration in future PDM research.

Supporting Information

Table S1 *BDNF* rs6265 genotype distributions and allele frequency in the behavioral/hormonal sub-groups.

Table S2 Results of repeated-measures ANOVA of psychological measurements: effects of menstrual cycle and *BDNF* genotype in the control group.

Table S3 Results of repeated-measures ANOVA of quantitative sensory testing: effects of group, *BDNF* genotype and menstrual cycle.

Table S4 Results of repeated-measures ANOVA of gonadal hormone levels: effects of group, *BDNF* genotype and menstrual cycle.

Acknowledgments

We extend particular appreciation to Ian-Ting Chu, Intan Low, Wei-Chi Li, Feng-Xuan Jian, and Shin-Hua Lin for their technical and experimental help.

Author Contributions

Conceived and designed the experiments: LCL CHT LFC JCH. Performed the experiments: LCL CHT. Analyzed the data: LCL CHT MWL JCH. Contributed reagents/materials/analysis tools: HDS MWL. Wrote the paper: LCL CHT MWL JCH. Clinical Assessment: HTC. Final approval: JCH.

References

1. French L (2005) Dysmenorrhea. Am Fam Physician 71: 285–291.
2. Davis AR, Westhoff CL (2001) Primary dysmenorrhea in adolescent girls and treatment with oral contraceptives. J Pediatr Adolesc Gynecol 14: 3–8.
3. Fedorowicz Z, Nasser M, Jagannath VA, Beaman JH, Ejaz K, et al. (2012) Beta2-adrenoceptor agonists for dysmenorrhoea. Cochrane Database Syst Rev 5: Cd008585.
4. Berkley KJ (2013) Primary dysmenorrhea: an urgent mandate. Pain: Clinical Updates XXI NO3: 1–8.
5. Guo SW, Mao X, Ma Q, Liu X (2013) Dysmenorrhea and its severity are associated with increased uterine contractility and overexpression of oxytocin receptor (OTR) in women with symptomatic adenomyosis. Fertil Steril 99: 231–240.
6. Akerlund M (1994) Vascularization of human endometrium. Uterine blood flow in healthy condition and in primary dysmenorrhoea. Ann N Y Acad Sci 734: 47–56.
7. Ma H, Hong M, Duan J, Liu P, Fan X, et al. (2013) Altered cytokine gene expression in peripheral blood monocytes across the menstrual cycle in primary dysmenorrhea: a case-control study. PLoS One 8: e55200.
8. Abu JI, Konje JC (2000) Leukotrienes in gynaecology: the hypothetical value of anti-leukotriene therapy in dysmenorrhoea and endometriosis. Hum Reprod Update 6: 200–205.
9. Akerlund M (2006) Targeting the oxytocin receptor to relax the myometrium. Expert Opin Ther Targets 10: 423–427.
10. Tzafettas J (2006) Painful menstruation. Pediatr Endocrinol Rev 3 Suppl 1: 160–163.
11. Sundell G, Milsom I, Andersch B (1990) Factors influencing the prevalence and severity of dysmenorrhoea in young women. Br J Obstet Gynaecol 97: 588–594.
12. Barnard K, Frayne SM, Skinner KM, Sullivan LM (2003) Health status among women with menstrual symptoms. J Womens Health (Larchmt) 12: 911–919.
13. Alonso C, Coe CL (2001) Disruptions of social relationships accentuate the association between emotional distress and menstrual pain in young women. Health Psychol 20: 411–416.
14. Dorn LD, Negriff S, Huang B, Pabst S, Hillman J, et al. (2009) Menstrual symptoms in adolescent girls: association with smoking, depressive symptoms, and anxiety. J Adolesc Health 44: 237–243.
15. Verhagen M, van der Meij A, van Deurzen PA, Janzing JG, Arias-Vasquez A, et al. (2010) Meta-analysis of the BDNF Val66Met polymorphism in major depressive disorder: effects of gender and ethnicity. Mol Psychiatry 15: 260–271.
16. Lommatzsch M, Zingler D, Schuhbaeck K, Schloetcke K, Zingler C, et al. (2005) The impact of age, weight and gender on BDNF levels in human platelets and plasma. Neurobiol Aging 26: 115–123.
17. Merighi A, Salio C, Ghirri A, Lossi L, Ferrini F, et al. (2008) BDNF as a pain modulator. Prog Neurobiol 85: 297–317.
18. Latremoliere A, Woolf CJ (2009) Central sensitization: a generator of pain hypersensitivity by central neural plasticity. J Pain 10: 895–926.
19. Duman RS, Monteggia LM (2006) A neurotrophic model for stress-related mood disorders. Biol Psychiatry 59: 1116–1127.
20. Duric V, McCarson KE (2006) Persistent pain produces stress-like alterations in hippocampal neurogenesis and gene expression. J Pain 7: 544–555.
21. Spencer JL, Waters EM, Milner TA, Lee FS, McEwen BS (2010) BDNF variant Val66Met interacts with estrous cycle in the control of hippocampal function. Proc Natl Acad Sci U S A 107: 4395–4400.
22. Bath KG, Chuang J, Spencer-Segal JL, Amso D, Altemus M, et al. (2012) Variant brain-derived neurotrophic factor (Valine66Methionine) polymorphism contributes to developmental and estrous stage-specific expression of anxiety-like behavior in female mice. Biol Psychiatry 72: 499–504.
23. Solum DT, Handa RJ (2002) Estrogen regulates the development of brain-derived neurotrophic factor mRNA and protein in the rat hippocampus. J Neurosci 22: 2650–2659.
24. Blurton-Jones M, Kuan PN, Tuszynski MH (2004) Anatomical evidence for transsynaptic influences of estrogen on brain-derived neurotrophic factor expression. J Comp Neurol 468: 347–360.
25. Chen ZY, Jing D, Bath KG, Ieraci A, Khan T, et al. (2006) Genetic variant BDNF (Val66Met) polymorphism alters anxiety-related behavior. Science 314: 140–143.
26. Vossen H, Kenis G, Rutten B, van Os J, Hermens H, et al. (2010) The genetic influence on the cortical processing of experimental pain and the moderating effect of pain status. PLoS One 5: e13641.
27. Yu H, Wang DD, Wang Y, Liu T, Lee FS, et al. (2012) Variant brain-derived neurotrophic factor Val66Met polymorphism alters vulnerability to stress and response to antidepressants. J Neurosci 32: 4092–4101.
28. Frustaci A, Pozzi G, Gianfagna F, Manzoli L, Boccia S (2008) Meta-analysis of the brain-derived neurotrophic factor gene (BDNF) Val66Met polymorphism in anxiety disorders and anxiety-related personality traits. Neuropsychobiology 58: 163–170.
29. Montag C, Basten U, Stelzel C, Fiebach CJ, Reuter M (2010) The BDNF Val66Met polymorphism and anxiety: support for animal knock-in studies from a genetic association study in humans. Psychiatry Res 179: 86–90.
30. Hwang JP, Tsai SJ, Hong CJ, Yang CH, Lirng JF, et al. (2006) The Val66Met polymorphism of the brain-derived neurotrophic-factor gene is associated with geriatric depression. Neurobiol Aging 27: 1834–1837.
31. Holden RR, Fekken GC, Reddon JR, Helmes E, Jackson DN (1988) Clinical reliabilities and validities of the Basic Personality Inventory. J Consult Clin Psychol 56: 766–768.
32. Ware J, Snow K, Kosinski M, Gandek B (1993) SF-36 Health Survey Manual and Interpretation Guide. Boston, MA: The Health Institute, New England Medical Center.
33. Hwang RJ, Chen LF, Yeh TC, Tu PC, Tu CH, et al. (2008) The resting frontal alpha asymmetry across the menstrual cycle: a magnetoencephalographic study. Horm Behav 54: 28–33.

34. Hwang RJ, Wu CH, Chen LF, Yeh TC, Hsieh JC (2009) Female menstrual phases modulate human prefrontal asymmetry: a magnetoencephalographic study. Horm Behav 55: 203–209.
35. Tu CH, Niddam DM, Yeh TC, Lirng JF, Cheng CM, et al. (2013) Menstrual pain is associated with rapid structural alterations in the brain. Pain 154: 1718–1724.
36. Spielberger C, Gorsuch R, Lushene R, Vagg P, Jacobs G (1983) Manual for the State-Trait Anxiety Inventory (form Y). Palo Alto, CA: Consulting Psychologists Press.
37. Beck A, Steer R (1993) Manual for the Beck Anxiety Inventory. San Antonio, TX: Psychological Corporation.
38. Beck A, Steer R, Brown G (1996) Manual for Beck Depression Inventory-II. San Antonio, TX: Psychological Corporation.
39. Sullivan MJ, Bishop S, Pivik J (1995) The pain catastrophizing scale: development and validation. Psychological Assessment 7: 524–532.
40. Giamberardino MA, Berkley KJ, Iezzi S, de Bigontina P, Vecchiet L (1997) Pain threshold variations in somatic wall tissues as a function of menstrual cycle, segmental site and tissue depth in non-dysmenorrheic women, dysmenorrheic women and men. Pain 71: 187–197.
41. Granot M, Yarnitsky D, Itskovitz-Eldor J, Granovsky Y, Peer E, et al. (2001) Pain perception in women with dysmenorrhea. Obstet Gynecol 98: 407–411.
42. Bajaj P, Bajaj P, Madsen H, Arendt-Nielsen L (2002) A comparison of modality-specific somatosensory changes during menstruation in dysmenorrheic and nondysmenorrheic women. Clin J Pain 18: 180–190.
43. Amodei N, Nelson-Gray RO (1989) Reactions of dysmenorrheic and nondysmenorrheic women to experimentally induced pain throughout the menstrual cycle. J Behav Med 12: 373–385.
44. Brinkert W, Dimcevski G, Arendt-Nielsen L, Drewes AM, Wilder-Smith OH (2007) Dysmenorrhoea is associated with hypersensitivity in the sigmoid colon and rectum. Pain 132 Suppl 1: S46–51.
45. Rolke R, Magerl W, Campbell KA, Schalber C, Caspari S, et al. (2006) Quantitative sensory testing: a comprehensive protocol for clinical trials. Eur J Pain 10: 77–88.
46. Petryshen TL, Sabeti PC, Aldinger KA, Fry B, Fan JB, et al. (2010) Population genetic study of the brain-derived neurotrophic factor (BDNF) gene. Mol Psychiatry 15: 810–815.
47. Hong CJ, Huo SJ, Yen FC, Tung CL, Pan GM, et al. (2003) Association study of a brain-derived neurotrophic-factor genetic polymorphism and mood disorders, age of onset and suicidal behavior. Neuropsychobiology 48: 186–189.
48. Choi MJ, Kang RH, Lim SW, Oh KS, Lee MS (2006) Brain-derived neurotrophic factor gene polymorphism (Val66Met) and citalopram response in major depressive disorder. Brain Res 1118: 176–182.
49. Obata K, Noguchi K (2006) BDNF in sensory neurons and chronic pain. Neurosci Res 55: 1–10.
50. Ren K, Dubner R (2007) Pain Facilitation and Activity-Dependent Plasticity in Pain Modulatory Circuitry: Role of BDNF-TrkB Signaling and NMDA Receptors. Mol Neurobiol 35: 224–235.
51. Di Lorenzo C, Di Lorenzo G, Daverio A, Pasqualetti P, Coppola G, et al. (2012) The Val66Met Polymorphism of the BDNF Gene Influences Trigeminal Pain-Related Evoked Responses. J Pain 13: 866–873.
52. Berkley KJ, McAllister SL (2011) Don't dismiss dysmenorrhea! Pain 152: 1940–1941.
53. Westling AM, Tu FF, Griffith JW, Hellman KM (2013) The association of dysmenorrhea with noncyclic pelvic pain accounting for psychological factors. Am J Obstet Gynecol 209: 422.e1–422.e10.
54. Giamberardino MA, Costantini R, Affaitati G, Fabrizio A, Lapenna D, et al. (2010) Viscero-visceral hyperalgesia: characterization in different clinical models. Pain 151: 307–322.
55. Yu YB, Zuo XL, Zhao QJ, Chen FX, Yang J, et al. (2012) Brain-derived neurotrophic factor contributes to abdominal pain in irritable bowel syndrome. Gut 61: 685–694.
56. Sarchielli P, Mancini ML, Floridi A, Coppola F, Rossi C, et al. (2007) Increased levels of neurotrophins are not specific for chronic migraine: evidence from primary fibromyalgia syndrome. J Pain 8: 737–745.
57. Haas L, Portela LV, Bohmer AE, Oses JP, Lara DR (2010) Increased plasma levels of brain derived neurotrophic factor (BDNF) in patients with fibromyalgia. Neurochem Res 35: 830–834.
58. Nugraha B, Karst M, Engeli S, Gutenbrunner C (2012) Brain-derived neurotrophic factor and exercise in fibromyalgia syndrome patients: a mini review. Rheumatol Int 32: 2593–2599.
59. Tu C-H, Niddam DM, Chao H-T, Liu R-S, Hwang R-J, et al. (2009) Abnormal cerebral metabolism during menstrual pain in primary dysmenorrhea. Neuroimage 47: 28–35.
60. Vincent K, Warnaby C, Stagg CJ, Moore J, Kennedy S, et al. (2011) Dysmenorrhoea is associated with central changes in otherwise healthy women. Pain 152: 1966–1975.
61. Quartana PJ, Campbell CM, Edwards RR (2009) Pain catastrophizing: a critical review. Expert Rev Neurother 9: 745–758.
62. Groves JO (2007) Is it time to reassess the BDNF hypothesis of depression? Mol Psychiatry 12: 1079–1088.
63. Gatt JM, Nemeroff CB, Dobson-Stone C, Paul RH, Bryant RA, et al. (2009) Interactions between BDNF Val66Met polymorphism and early life stress predict brain and arousal pathways to syndromal depression and anxiety. Mol Psychiatry 14: 681–695.
64. Hapidou EG, De Catanzaro D (1988) Sensitivity to cold pressor pain in dysmenorrheic and non-dysmenorrheic women as a function of menstrual cycle phase. Pain 34: 277–283.
65. Sherman JJ, LeResche L (2006) Does experimental pain response vary across the menstrual cycle? A methodological review. Am J Physiol Regul Integr Comp Physiol 291: R245–256.
66. Hariri AR, Drabant EM, Weinberger DR (2006) Imaging genetics: perspectives from studies of genetically driven variation in serotonin function and corticolimbic affective processing. Biol Psychiatry 59: 888–897.
67. Martinowich K, Lu B (2008) Interaction between BDNF and serotonin: role in mood disorders. Neuropsychopharmacology 33: 73–83.
68. Ignacio ZM, Reus GZ, Abelaira HM, Quevedo J (2014) Epigenetic and epistatic interactions between serotonin transporter and brain-derived neurotrophic factor genetic polymorphism: Insights in depression. Neuroscience 275c: 455–468.
69. Hunnerkopf R, Strobel A, Gutknecht L, Brocke B, Lesch KP (2007) Interaction between BDNF Val66Met and dopamine transporter gene variation influences anxiety-related traits. Neuropsychopharmacology 32: 2552–2560.
70. Zhang H, Ozbay F, Lappalainen J, Kranzler HR, van Dyck CH, et al. (2006) Brain derived neurotrophic factor (BDNF) gene variants and Alzheimer's disease, affective disorders, posttraumatic stress disorder, schizophrenia, and substance dependence. Am J Med Genet B Neuropsychiatr Genet 141B: 387–393.
71. Sun RF, Zhu YS, Kuang WJ, Liu Y, Li SB (2011) The G-712A polymorphism of brain-derived neurotrophic factor is associated with major depression but not schizophrenia. Neurosci Lett 489: 34–37.

16

Naturally Occurring Peer Support through Social Media: The Experiences of Individuals with Severe Mental Illness Using YouTube

John A. Naslund[1]*, Stuart W. Grande[2], Kelly A. Aschbrenner[1,3], Glyn Elwyn[1,2]

1 The Dartmouth Institute for Health Policy and Clinical Practice, Dartmouth College, Hanover, New Hampshire, United States of America, **2** The Dartmouth Center for Health Care Delivery Science, Dartmouth College, Hanover, New Hampshire, United States of America, **3** Department of Psychiatry, Geisel School of Medicine at Dartmouth, Hanover, New Hampshire, United States of America

Abstract

Increasingly, people with diverse health conditions turn to social media to share their illness experiences or seek advice from others with similar health concerns. This unstructured medium may represent a platform on which individuals with severe mental illness naturally provide and receive peer support. Peer support includes a system of mutual giving and receiving where individuals with severe mental illness can offer hope, companionship, and encouragement to others facing similar challenges. In this study we explore the phenomenon of individuals with severe mental illness uploading videos to YouTube, and posting and responding to comments as a form of naturally occurring peer support. We also consider the potential risks and benefits of self-disclosure and interacting with others on YouTube. To address these questions, we used qualitative inquiry informed by emerging techniques in online ethnography. We analyzed n = 3,044 comments posted to 19 videos uploaded by individuals who self-identified as having schizophrenia, schizoaffective disorder, or bipolar disorder. We found peer support across four themes: minimizing a sense of isolation and providing hope; finding support through peer exchange and reciprocity; sharing strategies for coping with day-to-day challenges of severe mental illness; and learning from shared experiences of medication use and seeking mental health care. These broad themes are consistent with accepted notions of peer support in severe mental illness as a voluntary process aimed at inclusion and mutual advancement through shared experience and developing a sense of community. Our data suggest that the lack of anonymity and associated risks of being identified as an individual with severe mental illness on YouTube seem to be overlooked by those who posted comments or uploaded videos. Whether or not this platform can provide benefits for a wider community of individuals with severe mental illness remains uncertain.

Editor: Lieuwe De Haan, Academic Medical Centre Amsterdam, Netherlands

Funding: The authors have no funding to report. The funders had no role in study design, data collection and analysis, decision to publish, or preparation of the manuscript.

Competing Interests: The authors have declared that no competing interests exist.

* Email: John.A.Naslund@gmail.com

Introduction

How might the phenomenon of individuals with severe mental illness (SMI) such as schizophrenia, schizoaffective disorder, or bipolar disorder, who share their illness experiences through video narratives uploaded onto platforms like YouTube constitute the development of a naturally emerging peer support system? Or does this activity represent a risky process of self-exposure, and susceptibility to negative comments, unsolicited content, or exposure to harmful influences of others?

YouTube is a video-sharing website created in 2005 that is currently the third most popular social media website worldwide after Facebook and Google+ [1]. YouTube has videos uploaded in 61 different languages, and reaches more adults ages 18–34 in the United States than any cable network [2]. YouTube is free to use, and any individual with access to the Internet can upload videos, post comments, or share videos with others. While the potential harms and benefits of connecting with others to share health information through social media have been discussed extensively [3–5], diverse patient groups with sensitive health conditions are increasingly turning to social media websites like YouTube to share their illness experiences or seek advice from others with similar conditions [4,6]. As people with diverse health conditions seek greater online connectivity, it is not clear whether YouTube may represent a platform by which individuals with SMI can provide and receive peer support or whether unforeseen risks might prevent such support.

Peer support in SMI includes a system of mutual giving and receiving where individuals who have faced and endured the adversity of mental illness can offer hope, companionship, and encouragement to others facing similar conditions [7,8]. Peer support has been recognized as a promising strategy for mental health recovery and for overcoming limitations of illness [7–10]. However, much of the literature has focused on formal peer support programs delivered within community settings such as mental health centers or psychosocial clubhouses, as well as through Internet support groups, or provided in conjunction with existing evidence-based practices [8,10–12]. Less attention has been given to informal peer-to-peer relationships spanning an individual's community, surroundings, personal life, and social network [13]. Also, with the increasing popularity of social media and its growing importance as a means to connect and interact with others, there is a need to consider whether informal peer support naturally occurs outside of professional services and across a popular social media website such as YouTube.

Evidence suggests individuals with SMI are more likely to share personal views through blogging, build friendships on social media [14], and use the Internet for accessing health information [15] than people without mental illness. This could be in part because social media is perceived as a non-threatening medium that provides opportunities to identify and connect with similar individuals within the safety of one's own home. Yet, uncertainty exists on how social media might be used for online peer support among individuals with SMI [16]. Our search of relevant literature did not identify any studies that characterize or explore types of social interactions or discussion content between peers with SMI on social media websites. Therefore an exploration of these interactions and how they might represent naturally occurring peer support among individuals with SMI is needed.

In the context of YouTube, groups of individuals with diverse health conditions, including multiple sclerosis [17], inflammatory bowel disease [18], or cancer [19], use this platform as a tool for searching for health information [20] and as a forum for sharing personal illness stories or receiving feedback and social support from others. For example, analyses of videos on YouTube generated by people with multiple sclerosis and corresponding comments demonstrate that many individuals frequently disclose personal health information in this online environment [21], and upload videos to provide treatment advice to others and share personal experiences seeking and obtaining medical care [17]. With evidence documenting the widespread use of YouTube among numerous patient groups, in the current study we aim to explore comments posted to YouTube by individuals who self-identify as having a SMI, taking the perspective that naturally occurring peer support through social media may be beneficial. Our objective is to observe how individuals with SMI interact on YouTube with their peers, knowing the risks of disclosure, and whether this might serve as a way to manage their own recovery and provide support to others.

First, to investigate this phenomenon of growing social media use among individuals with SMI, we provide a brief conceptual background to frame peer support and social media within the context of SMI. We then outline our process of exploring the comments associated with uploaded YouTube videos for expressions of peer support. Our analysis details how individuals with SMI use YouTube to interact with each other, and our discussion reflects the value of this popular social media website as a naturally occurring peer support platform.

Peer Support and Severe Mental Illness

Peer support in psychiatry has its roots in the mental health consumer movement of the 1970s, where individuals living with SMI campaigned for basic human rights, mental health care reform, and the right to make their own health care choices [8,22]. These advocacy efforts were in large part a protest against discrimination and injustices, including authoritarian psychiatric practices, compulsory hospitalizations, and coercion to undergo unproven treatments [23]. This activism led to collective action, and to the development of mutual support and self-help activities [8]. Central tenets of peer support in mental health include reciprocity, mutual respect, and shared responsibility [7]. For this highly stigmatized group [24], peer support offers optimism and hope for a better life and acceptance as well as opportunities to relate to one another through common experiences and shared struggles [25]. Relationships between peers are based upon commitment to positive personal growth and wider contribution to community building toward achieving mental health recovery [7].

Recent decades have seen the emergence and demonstrated effectiveness of formal peer provided services [11] including programs targeting mental health recovery [26], medical illness self-management [27,28], and smoking cessation [29]. These programs are often guided by conventional therapeutic boundaries [25], and are delivered in an organized manner involving formal providers or in conjunction with prescribed medical and mental health services [13]. Structured programs fall in between natural and therapeutic relationships, and differ from informal peer support [25].

Informal peer support relationships are considered the foundation of peer support in mental health [30], and occur naturally between individuals who come together through shared experience. Informal peer support creates a sense of belonging and friendship [30], and allows individuals with SMI to feel greater self-worth and self-efficacy by supporting and impacting the life of another peer [25]. However, peers who provide support can also become overwhelmed or frustrated consistent with caregiver distress, or face interpersonal conflicts due to the burden of managing their own symptoms and mental health concerns [25]. As with any informal interactions, recommendations or advice provided by peers are based upon personal experiences, which at times might contradict professional recommendations or the content of structured programs. Despite these concerns, the benefits of informal peer support in SMI are widely accepted [7,8].

Social Media and Peer Support

Social media websites have afforded new opportunities for individuals to connect with others, provide and receive support, and share their illness experiences [4]. There are disease specific support groups on Facebook [31,32], personal video logs posted by patients onto YouTube [21], and entire interactive forums dedicated to sharing illness experiences such as PatientsLikeMe [33]. Despite this widely reported use among the general population, use of popular social media among individuals with SMI has received less attention.

Evidence suggests that individuals with SMI create online relationships at the same rate [34] or higher when compared to individuals without a mental illness [14]. A case study examined the therapeutic benefit of using Facebook to reach an isolated patient with psychiatric comorbidities and foster social relationships [35]. Ethical considerations related to suicidal postings to Facebook among individuals with SMI, including privacy concerns and threats to the therapeutic alliance, have also been explored [36]. However, no prior studies have highlighted any specific risks of social media use among individuals with SMI that extend beyond what would be observed in general patient populations.

Social media may be well suited for peer support among individuals with SMI. These websites facilitate natural community building, where control of entry and exit are independent of social interaction, which allows users to avoid the anxiety and fears associated with face-to-face interactions [34]. With relative anonymity, individuals with SMI can find peers and discuss aspects of living with mental illness in a controlled and personal environment by using the Internet from home [37]. Also, individuals who are stigmatized because of their illness are often highly motivated to seek others with the same condition [38], something that social media can enable.

To date, however, the benefits and understanding the why and motivation of online peer support in SMI have not been established. We know that disclosure of personal information through social media has been linked to individual behavioral control [39] and psychological well-being [40]. One study [16] of unmediated online peer support for individuals with psychiatric disabilities, comparing a listserv and a bulletin board, replicated the spontaneous nature of Internet forums. The authors' found many participants reported both positive experiences and greater distress, suggesting that online peer support may not deliver all intended benefits [16]. The uncertainty of these findings underscores the need to more fully explore the interactions between individuals with SMI on a popular social media website like YouTube to gain insight about informal peer support relationships and to observe whether harms or benefits emerge within an unmonitored and public online platform.

Methods

Recognizing the contribution of social media on health and help seeking behaviors among individuals with SMI we planned an investigation of YouTube. Specifically, we explore uploaded YouTube videos and associated comments for expressions of peer support. We conducted a qualitative analysis of comments detailing how individuals with SMI use YouTube as a platform indicative of naturally occurring peer support.

Online Ethnography for Exploring YouTube

Ethnographic methods in health research focus on expanding our understanding of illness experience and social practices in the context of culture within particular groups [41,42]. Our approach was informed by an online ethnography framework [42,43], where we observed online interactions on YouTube without interfering in natural conversations. Observer interference is typically a limitation of face-to-face observational methods [43]. In contrast to offline ethnographic methods consisting of extensive fieldwork [41], YouTube served as the research field where interactions reflective of peer support among individuals who self-identify as having a SMI were explored.

Study Sample and Data Collection

In June 2013 we searched YouTube for publicly available videos that had been extensively viewed using the following search terms: "*mental illness*", "*schizophrenia*", "*schizoaffective disorder*" or "*bipolar disorder*". To systematically identify a sample of relevant videos, we screened the first 100 videos for each search term. Relevant videos were defined as: posted by an individual, had no advertising, were in the first person, and included our search terms. Also, for each relevant video identified, YouTube generates a page list of 20 recommended videos that describe a similar topic based on our search history and the prior videos we selected and viewed. We reviewed the recommended video lists to identify additional relevant videos.

After viewing relevant videos, we further selected a smaller set of videos based on the following criteria: had a minimum of 5,000 views because videos with more views have more comments [18]; uploaded by an individual who self-identified in the video as having a SMI, either schizophrenia, schizoaffective disorder, or bipolar disorder (these diagnoses are associated with greater disability and stigma [24]); no evidence of involvement of public or private institutions or agencies in the creation of the video; video content detailed experiences living with SMI; and in English. We exported the associated comments for each video, posted by either commenters who self-identified as having a SMI, or video authors (i.e., individuals who uploaded the videos), to a pdf document for thematic analysis.

Ethics

There has been considerable discussion surrounding the ethical concerns of analyzing data retrieved from social media [44,45], including examples where the privacy of users has been at risk [46]. To minimize these concerns, we searched for and included only videos that were publicly available on YouTube. To further protect the identity of commenters and video authors we removed all usernames and did not include video titles or specific demographic characteristics in the results reported here. We also received institutional review board exemption from the Dartmouth College Committee for the Protection of Human Subjects to conduct this study.

Qualitative Analysis

The comments associated with the smaller set of identified videos were then exported as a pdf document into ATLAS.ti software Version 7.0 for thematic analysis. We applied an open coding approach, and developed codes based on the data as they naturally occurred [47]. Informed by grounded theory, we determined concepts and themes related to expressions of peer support based on our analysis where those that were repeated across multiple comments were considered meaningful [48]. This approach has been applied in similarly designed research using online data [49]. We independently coded the comments, and then compared code lists. After combining and reviewing the code lists, we grouped similar codes into categories and resolved code disagreements by consensus. We then condensed the categories into broad themes based on ideas of how peer support exists. Given the exploratory nature of this project, we modeled Patton's (1990) approach for summarizing qualitative results by presenting our data as they appeared on YouTube so that readers may also draw their own interpretations regarding the potential value of YouTube as a platform for informal peer support among individuals with SMI [50].

Results

Our search of YouTube yielded a combined total of approximately 746,200 videos. After screening 400 videos (100 per search term), we followed the recommended other video lists (YouTube) and evaluated 1,100 potential videos. We narrowed this set down to 63 by selecting only videos posted by an individual, without advertising, in the first person. We then applied our strict inclusion criteria and selected 19 videos and their associated 3,044 comments for analysis. The 44 excluded videos did not meet our criteria either because they did not have enough views, did not describe experiences of living with SMI, or appeared to be uploaded by private companies, documentary filmmakers, or academic institutions.

The 19 videos were uploaded by 19 different individuals of which 8 self-identified as being diagnosed with bipolar disorder, 7 with schizoaffective disorder, and 4 with schizophrenia. Common topics included managing illness symptoms, challenges and benefits of seeking treatment, coping strategies for day-to-day concerns, efforts to reach out and help others with similar conditions, and personal stories about life goals, interests and future ambitions. The videos had an average of 19,786 views (range of 5,433 to 88,654) and had been on YouTube between 87 and 1,798 days. Fifteen videos appeared to be posted by young adults (18–35 years) and four by middle-aged adults (36–55 years). We analyzed 3,044 comments posted to the videos, ranging from 27 to 592 for each video, of which 91% were posted by commenters and 9% were posted in response to commenters by video authors. On YouTube, users can rate comments as 'inappropriate', and when a comment receives sufficient 'inappropriate' ratings it is flagged. About 5% (n = 160) of the comments we analyzed were flagged for content viewed as inappropriate such as derogatory or discriminatory statements, advertisements, or spam.

We determined four themes representing key aspects of peer support (see Table 1). The themes are discussed below and examples of unedited comments are cited to provide context.

Minimizing a sense of isolation and providing hope

Efforts to reduce social isolation and achieve a sense of community were expressed in comments posted across all 19 videos. Comments showed appreciation for individuals who shared personal histories and lived experiences. Many commenters acknowledged that having a mental illness is a "lonely road" and were thankful for the videos, conveying reassurance to know that they are not alone with their illness. Individuals who said they felt that they could not talk to anyone about their illness because of fear, embarrassment or simply not having anyone close to them in their lives were particularly positive:

> Thank you soo much for this video it has made me feel a little less alone … i myself have bipolar 2 and have been off meds for about 6 months now and am also feeling the day to day fight i have in my head just to live in the real world …
> *Comment on Video #5: video uploaded by female with bipolar disorder*
> I can relate to almost everything you say … I'm too afraid to talk to people to have someone to relate to and discuss it with. So this video helps me in that I get to listen to your story and what you're going through and feel like I'm not alone …
> *Comment on Video #18: video uploaded by male with schizophrenia*

Peer support also allows individuals with SMI to relate to one another based on shared experiences and perceived membership in a wider supportive network. For some, this sense of belonging came from a sense of normalcy after watching the personal stories shared by others:

> I'm very happy i found you and your videos … Its so good to find people that make me think I'm more "normal" than i think. Thank you and hope alls good!
> *Comment on Video #17: video uploaded by female with schizophrenia*

For some, viewing the videos was a deeply emotional experience, generated by a sense of relief of finding someone to relate to:

> Literally, tears were streaming down my face as I watched this. Thank you so much … your descriptions were so spot on … it felt as if a female version of me from the future made this video … for no other reason but to give helpful advice.
> *Comment on Video #17: video uploaded by female with schizophrenia*

The YouTube videos also served as a source of inspiration, prompting individuals to do the same, and share their own illness stories. The importance of the Internet as a means for reaching others facing similar challenges was frequently cited:

> It's okay, you're not alone, there are many of our kind and we are lost without each other, but now thanks to the internet we can reach out to each other so we can discuss what we hear openly and honestly with no fear of being judged …
> *Comment on Video #3: video uploaded by female with schizoaffective disorder*
> I'm thinking about… making videos about my illness so I can connect with you and others here on youtube …
> *Comment on Video #16: video uploaded by female with schizophrenia*

Comments also reacted to the idea of sensing hope, expressed as optimism for overcoming challenges and moving forward with their lives:

> I can completely relate to your experience. I was diagnosed with Schizophrenia about two years ago and it has been hell for me. Your video was very inspiring to me and it gave me hope that things can get better.
> *Comment on Video #16: video uploaded by female with schizophrenia*

Table 1. Themes representing peer support.

Themes reflecting expressions of naturally occurring peer support on YouTube
1. Minimizing a sense of isolation and providing hope
2. Finding support through peer exchange and reciprocity
3. Coping with the day-to-day challenges of severe mental illness
4. Learning from shared experiences of medication use and seeking mental health care

Finding support through peer exchange and reciprocity

Comments also contained offers of comfort and encouragement. One commenter reassured "hang in there, things can and will get better ... and thank you for sharing your story with us" (*Comment on Video #6: video uploaded by female with schizoaffective disorder*). Another suggested "Together us bipolar people will survive. It's all about support. We will find a cure" (*Comment on Video #1: video uploaded by female with bipolar disorder*).

Insightful dialogues occurred between commenters. In the YouTube environment participants have the opportunity to share their opinions, mirroring the democratic process of giving and receiving that defines informal peer support interactions. For example, discussions emerged about various topics related to SMI, as well as personal anecdotes and common interests like favorite music or art, illustrating the development of forms of social relationships.

> Hey man I can really relate to what you say about being hospitalized and meeting a girl there, and I have schizo affective disorder, and its rough ... The Beatles are my favorite band too man.
> *Comment on Video #18: video uploaded by male with schizophrenia*

Some commenters reached out to video authors to seek additional support for personal concerns outside the public YouTube network. For example, a commenter asks whether the person who uploaded the video would be willing to talk using Skype:

> Would you be opposed to Skyping with someone who wasn't sure about the symptoms they're starting to have? I've just started hearing voices. I don't have anyone to talk to about this.
> *Comment on Video #19: video uploaded by male with schizophrenia*

Commenters rapidly defended individuals who uploaded a video when someone posted a negative comment. This illustrates reciprocity. These negative comments about the video content or the individual elicited strong responses from other commenters overwhelmingly in defense of the video author. One negative commenter stated "bipolar disorder is not real" and that psychiatrists are "evil", claiming that people with mental illness are all "drug addicts":

> You people ... make these vids while your high as a kite to 'prove' you have bipolar. Just shows how fake this fucking disease is ...
> *Comment on Video #3: video uploaded by female with bipolar disorder*

Many comments responded immediately and in strong terms:

> If u actually suffered from bipolar disorder you wouldn't be saying such evil crap it is absolute hell it affects everything and by the way ... i am bipolar ... so u can shove that drug addicted crap up your ass ... keep your hateful insensitive comments to yourself you don't know shit
> *Comment in response to negative comment on Video #3: video uploaded by female with bipolar disorder*

Interactions such as these demonstrate the solidarity created and efforts made to protect the network of those willing to openly share their experience of living with SMI.

Coping with the day-to-day challenges of severe mental illness

YouTube appears to overcome the perceived inability of some people with SMI to learn how to cope, by providing users with the opportunity to share thoughts, struggles, hopes and fears in a receptive network. Commenters admitted to the struggles of living with mental illness and said that posting comments to YouTube may, in itself, serve as a coping mechanism. For some viewers, expressing personal challenges to peers that may be listening appears to be a way to search for validation and elicit supportive responses from others. One commenter wrote:

> I hate being bipolar, it's been the biggest burden by far and it's not the first time I'll say I'm sick of it. I hate having no control over myself ... Stuck in your own head is a good way to put it... I dread knowing it's never going away.
> *Comment on Video #7: video uploaded by male with bipolar disorder*

Others were more graphic in their depiction of living with SMI, and spared no details in illustrating the reality of their condition:

> Sometimes i get anxious as fuck and angry as shit for no reason. i chain smoke two packs worth of cigarettes a day that i handroll myself. The medications made me a fat bastard at 310 pounds and i cant keep up my grooming worth a shit. i still manage to hold down a job and i still live in a group home. there thats my fucking life story. your welcome everyone:)!
> *Comment on Video #2: video uploaded by female with schizoaffective disorder*

Extensive discussions emerged on how to cope with SMI. As individuals described their day-to-day challenges many reflected on the strategies that have helped them to cope and achieve a sense of "normalcy" in their everyday lives. Some commenters recommended coping strategies to each other, or asked for advice for dealing with their disorder. One viewer described how counseling serves as an important coping mechanism, "I go to counseling and that helps more than talking to anyone around me in my life because... the counselors at least have been around more bipolar people" (*Comment on Video #5: video uploaded by female with bipolar disorder*).

Individuals also shared their personal experiences of how to cope, e.g. practicing music:

> Hey man, i wanted to let you know that you have a lot of courage for making this video. You really should find a way to cope with both the manic and depressive episodes. May i suggest an instrument? I picked up the guitar a few years ago to help me cope with my excessive energy during manic states, and it has done wonders, it has helped me more than any drug or any therapy.
> *Comment on Video #3: video uploaded by male with bipolar disorder*

Learning from shared experiences of medication use and seeking mental health care

Commenters helped others better understand what it is like to receive mental health care and even with overcoming fears by sharing lessons learned of using medications and seeking mental health care before or after receiving a mental illness diagnosis. Comments contained detailed accounts of taking medications and filling out prescriptions, and of being hospitalized, visiting mental health providers and medical professionals, and facing difficult diagnoses. There were positive views such as praise for psychiatrists and emphasis on the importance of having a good relationship with mental health providers. One commenter emphasized the importance of taking medications:

> The biggest mistake we can make is to just stop taking your meds. It happens to the best of us. You "think" I'm feeling good I don't need these meds. Not true! I know now that I NEED my meds to be well. It sucks, but it is what it is.
> *Comment on Video #5: video uploaded by female with bipolar disorder*

There were also many examples of frustration with receiving mental health care, describing the negative side effects of taking medications, fear of taking medications, experiences of being hospitalized, and not getting a clear diagnosis from different mental health providers. This individual explains the fear of taking medications:

> This is the best video so far on this topic. Nicely done! I have been going through this battle since I was 11 years old, I am now 23. I currently am not on medication. I'm scared to get back on them. The side effects highten my symptoms …
> *Comment on Video #14: video uploaded by male with schizoaffective disorder*

The following commenter describes the negative consequences of a wrong diagnosis until finally finding the *right* doctor:

> You have only been in the hospital one time? Girl, you really are fortunate. I have been in and out of hospital(s) for the last 12 years. Several attempted suicides due to the fact that it took the "right" doctor to come into my path and finally diagnose me with Bipolar Disorder rather than your standard "Major Clinical Depression"
> *Comment posted to Video #8: video uploaded by female with bipolar disorder*

Comments highlighted individuals' fear of visiting doctors because of the diagnosis that they might get or risk of being institutionalized. Individuals used YouTube to seek advice:

> i have conversations with my self and sometimes only notice what i have done when i stop talking… i also have violent urges out of the blue but i can control them at the moment. i know these are signs of schizerphrnia but im seeing my psychiatrist in 5 days an wondering if i should tell him … i dont want to be put in a mental ward will he put me in there if i tell him these things ???? please respond worried
> *Comment on Video #1: video uploaded by female with schizoaffective disorder*

The video author responded:

> he will DEFINITELY not be able to lock you up in psychiatric unit if you tell him what you've been experiencing. The only way they could send you to the hospital (this is what I've experienced, anyways) is if you tell them that you've been hearing voices telling you to harm yourself or others, or if you have been having suicidal thoughts. … you should really tell your psychiatrist about this, though!!!
> *Response to Comment on Video #1: video uploaded by female with schizoaffective disorder.*

Individuals with SMI appear to use YouTube to seek and share advice about medical related questions and concerns, which might or might not suggest they have been unable to find answers elsewhere. It is also possible that these individuals are looking to validate health information found elsewhere, such as from a recent medical visit or content from health-related websites, which led to their discovering personal accounts from others on YouTube. Whether these individuals feel most comfortable consulting with peers through YouTube, or perhaps use other social media platforms for the same purpose, remains unclear. Regardless, a rich dialogue surrounding shared experiences using medications and seeking mental health care emerged, illustrating another practical reason for engaging in these online peer-to-peer interactions through YouTube.

Discussion

The reciprocal exchange between YouTube commenters in response to content uploaded by individuals who self-identify as having a SMI including schizophrenia, schizoaffective disorder, or bipolar disorder, represents a dynamic, responsive, yet informal, system of peer support. Analysis of the data provided four themes consistent with the central role of peer support in SMI: minimizing a sense of isolation and providing hope; finding support through peer exchange and reciprocity; sharing strategies for coping with the day-to-day challenges of severe mental illness; and learning from shared experiences of medication use and seeking mental health care. We see peer support on YouTube as voluntary–an emergent phenomenon where users are unhindered and have individual autonomy to choose their level of disclosure and engagement, from viewing to commenting to uploading personal videos.

Personal health information was frequently shared and rewarded by positive, encouraging, and insightful viewer responses. These interactions created, what appeared to be, a sense of belonging and means for coping with challenges of SMI. We observed that YouTube served as an environment where individuals with SMI could normalize one's illness and assert their voice and identity by validating shared experiences with peers. That individuals were able to do this suggests the degree of safety they felt in contributing their videos and comments. This "peer exchange" was reinforced by strongly supportive, and at times combative, responses of participants in reaction to negative comments or "outsider" attempts to criticize uploaded videos.

The observation of real world data without researcher interference was a methodological strength because it allowed us to document and analyze naturally occurring interactions. There were also limitations with our methods because we could not obtain data on individual motivation or intention to upload videos, post comments, or publicly disclose personal health information.

This limitation with our data also restricted our ability for more in depth interpretation and analysis of the content posted to YouTube because of increased risk of bias. A previous study of YouTube found viewers were more comfortable commenting on lay videos, citing that the value of interacting with someone with firsthand experience meant it was someone who may be more likely to respond to questions or give advice [18]. Further, we were unable to assess the impact of the videos or comments on the actual individuals with SMI, such as whether the interactions through YouTube offer long-term benefit and genuine support, or whether it was a distraction. There was also no way for us to test out possible harms of using this medium as these were not mentioned by commenters, though we contend that some harms likely do exist. Because of the qualitative nature of this study, we are unable to provide detailed metrics for the included videos and comments, or analysis for patterns within the data, such as between type of comments and number of views, or between positive and negative comments. Lastly, this was an exploratory study and we are unable to generalize our findings to a wider population of individuals with SMI or reach definite conclusions regarding the benefits of naturally occurring peer support on YouTube.

Peer-to-peer interactions and open sharing of personal experiences living with SMI through YouTube exemplify how social media and the Internet are reshaping the way this marginalized group engages their environment and seeks and shares advice related to mental health care. As highlighted in prior research, by sharing illness experiences with others online and through social media, there is potential for improved health and psychosocial outcomes, including benefits such as learning from others, feeling supported, and forming relationships [51]. For example, individuals with depression reported using online support groups to elicit support and empathy from others, express themselves, and serve as a form of community building [52]. Among individuals living with HIV/AIDS, perceived benefits of online peer-to-peer interactions range from seeking informational and emotional support [53,54], to achieving greater empowerment through gathering information, finding positive meaning, receiving social support, and helping others [55].

Then again, other studies found no clear health benefit of peer-to-peer interactions in social media [56]. The presence of promotional material and advertisements may have limited these prior findings [31] by emphasizing awareness and fundraising efforts rather than how individuals share illness experiences and reciprocate peer support [32]. Our findings differed from these prior studies because only a small number of comments from our YouTube sample were flagged as inappropriate or as spam while comments promoting illness awareness or fundraising were not widely visible. This may have occurred because we selected only videos uploaded by individuals who self-identified as having schizophrenia, schizoaffective disorder, or bipolar disorder, as opposed to videos uploaded by foundations, companies, health care organizations or research institutions. While any subsequent exploration using our inclusion criteria would likely find different content, we believe the nature of peer support would be consistent.

As the benefits of social media for individuals with SMI remain unclear, how might sharing experiences and interacting with peers through YouTube specifically support mental health recovery? Listening to the experiences of other individuals with SMI offers value because authentic accounts are easier to understand, can make treatment information more relevant by putting it into a personal context, can help make sense of one's situation, and can help with overcoming fears and feeling more confident in coping with symptoms [51,57]. Also, social media facilitate connections between individuals facing similar health challenges, which creates a sense of community and belonging, helps people feel more "normal", fosters personal empowerment, and provides socially isolated individuals with opportunities to feel connected and less alone [51,58]. Though compelling, future research is needed to better understand whether informal peers openly sharing illness experiences on social media can support mental health recovery in individuals with SMI. In this context, it is "recovery in mental illness" where the emphasis for individuals is on learning to live with their illness while feeling empowered to pursue personal life goals, as opposed to "recovery from mental illness" where amelioration of symptoms and improved daily functioning are the primary focus [59].

Our findings reflect preliminary data that characterize naturally occurring interactions among individuals with SMI through social media and we acknowledge this new medium of communication poses potential risks. For instance, uncertainty remains about what level of information is necessary to determine what an online peer is saying is trustworthy and applicable [60]. On YouTube, perhaps number of video views determines perceived trustworthiness of the content. Alternatively, physical appearance of the person who uploaded the video may contribute to perceived trustworthiness, where an attractive or friendly looking individual may be considered more reliable. Given the largely unregulated nature of YouTube, there is also risk that all sources may be considered equivalent regardless of their trustworthiness [51]. Future research should seek to determine the trustworthiness of the videos as well as the authenticity of the video authors' and commenters' self-identified SMI diagnoses.

Another concern might be that dramatic videos receive more attention through increased views and visibility while routine or unremarkable experiences may receive comparatively little notice [51]. In examining our included videos, we did not observe major differences in tone or content based on the number of views or comments, suggesting such concerns were not present. Yet, consistent with other online networks, clear challenges of balance through YouTube are expected [61]. Additional risks from accessing content on YouTube may include increased anxiety or confusion about one's own symptoms or condition, feeling inferior if others are doing better, unrealistic expectations regarding treatment, and exposure to misleading information. However, these varied risks are not unique to YouTube and could arise in cases where the credentials of the individuals providing advice are not known. As suggested by our data, the potential benefits of interacting with peers online outweigh any potential downsides [51], and the use of YouTube within this vulnerable population group represents an emerging dimension of social life worthy of investigation.

Conclusion

At the time of this study, among the individuals who self-identified as having a SMI and who uploaded videos or posted comments to YouTube, we observed a sense of reward emerging from their interactions, mutual learning, and offered peer support. Of importance is our finding that peer support is happening naturally among individuals with highly stigmatized psychiatric illnesses within an unmonitored and public online platform. The lack of anonymity and associated risks of being identified as an individual with SMI seemed to be overlooked by commenters and video authors. Whether or not this platform can provide benefits for a wider group of individuals with SMI remains uncertain.

Acknowledgments

The authors have no funding to report. The authors wish to thank the Dartmouth College Library for supporting the publication of this work through the Dartmouth Open-Access Publication Equity Fund. The authors also wish to acknowledge the material and technical support provided by The Dartmouth Center for Health Care Delivery Science.

Author Contributions

Conceived and designed the experiments: JAN SWG. Performed the experiments: JAN SWG. Analyzed the data: JAN SWG KAA GE. Contributed reagents/materials/analysis tools: GE. Contributed to the writing of the manuscript: JAN SWG KAA GE. Data collection: JAN SWG. Interpretation of the findings: JAN SWG KAA GE.

References

1. Kosner AW (2013) Watch out Facebook, with Google+ at #2 and YouTube at #3, Google, Inc. could catch up. Forbes. Available: http://www.forbes.com/sites/anthonykosner/2013/01/26/watch-out-facebook-with-google-at-2-and-youtube-at-3-google-inc-could-catch-up/.
2. YouTube (2014) YouTube Statistics. Available: http://www.youtube.com/yt/press/statistics.html.
3. Chou W-YS, Hunt YM, Beckjord EB, Moser RP, Hesse BW (2009) Social media use in the United States: implications for health communication. Journal of Medical Internet Research 11: e48.
4. Vance K, Howe W, Dellavalle RP (2009) Social internet sites as a source of public health information. Dermatologic Clinics 27: 133–136.
5. Moorhead SA, Hazlett DE, Harrison L, Carroll JK, Irwin A, et al. (2013) A new dimension of health care: systematic review of the uses, benefits, and limitations of social media for health communication. Journal of Medical Internet Research 15: e85.
6. Fox S, Jones S (2009) The social life of health information. Washington, DC: Pew Internet & American Life Project: 2009–2012.
7. Mead S, Hilton D, Curtis L (2001) Peer support: a theoretical perspective. Psychiatric Rehabilitation Journal 25: 134–141.
8. Davidson L, Chinman M, Sells D, Rowe M (2006) Peer support among adults with serious mental illness: a report from the field. Schizophrenia Bulletin 32: 443–450.
9. Anthony WA (1993) Recovery from mental illness: the guiding vision of the mental health service system in the 1990s. Psychiatric Rehabilitation Journal 16: 11–23.
10. Solomon P (2004) Peer support/peer provided services underlying processes, benefits, and critical ingredients. Psychiatric Rehabilitation Journal 27: 392–401.
11. Chinman M, George P, Dougherty RH, Daniels AS, Ghose SS, et al. (2014) Peer support services for individuals with serious mental illnesses: assessing the evidence. Psychiatric Services 65: 429–441.
12. Coniglio FD, Hancock N, Ellis LA (2012) Peer support within Clubhouse: A grounded theory study. Community Mental Health Journal 48: 153–160.
13. Davidson L, Chinman M, Kloos B, Weingarten R, Stayner D, et al. (1999) Peer support among individuals with severe mental illness: a review of the evidence. Clinical Psychology: Science and Practice 6: 165–187.
14. Gowen K, Deschaine M, Gruttadara D, Markey D (2012) Young adults with mental health conditions and social networking websites: seeking tools to build community. Psychiatric Rehabilitation Journal 35: 245–250.
15. Berger M, Wagner TH, Baker LC (2005) Internet use and stigmatized illness. Social Science & Medicine 61: 1821–1827.
16. Kaplan K, Salzer MS, Solomon P, Brusilovskiy E, Cousounis P (2011) Internet peer support for individuals with psychiatric disabilities: a randomized controlled trial. Social Science & Medicine 72: 54–62.
17. Mazanderani F, O'Neill B, Powell J (2013) "People power" or "pester power"? YouTube as a forum for the generation of evidence and patient advocacy. Patient Education and Counseling 93: 420–425.
18. Frohlich DO, Zmyslinski-Seelig A (2012) The presence of social support messages on YouTube videos about inflammatory bowel disease and ostomies. Health Communication 27: 421–428.
19. Chou W-YS, Hunt Y, Folkers A, Augustson E (2011) Cancer survivorship in the age of youtube and social media: a narrative analysis. Journal of Medical Internet Research 13: e7.
20. Freeman B, Chapman S (2007) Is "YouTube" telling or selling you something? tobacco content on the YouTube video-sharing website. Tobacco Control 16: 207–210.
21. Fernandez-Luque L, Elahi N, Grajales III FJ (2009) An analysis of personal medical information disclosed in YouTube videos created by patients with multiple sclerosis. In: Adlassnig KP, Blobel B, Mantas J, Masic I, editors. Medical Informatics in a United and Healthy Europe: Proceedings of MIE 2009, the XXII International Congress of the European Federation for Medical Informatics. Amsterdam, The Netherlands: IOS Press. 292–296.
22. Tomes N (2006) The patient as a policy factor: a historical case study of the consumer/survivor movement in mental health. Health Affairs 25: 720–729.
23. Rissmiller D, Rissmiller J (2006) Open forum: evolution of the antipsychiatry movement into mental health consumerism. Psychiatric Services 57: 863–866.
24. Corrigan PW, Thompson V, Lambert D, Sangster Y, Noel JG, et al. (2003) Perceptions of discrimination among persons with serious mental illness. Psychiatric Services 54: 1105–1110.
25. Bracke P, Christiaens W, Verhaeghe M (2008) Self-esteem, self-efficacy, and the balance of peer support among persons with chronic mental health problems. Journal of Applied Social Psychology 38: 436–459.
26. van Gestel-Timmermans H, Brouwers EP, van Assen MA, van Nieuwenhuizen C (2012) Effects of a peer-run course on recovery from serious mental illness: a randomized controlled trial. Psychiatric Services 63: 54–60.
27. Goldberg RW, Dickerson F, Lucksted A, Brown CH, Weber E, et al. (2013) Living Well: an intervention to improve self-management of medical illness for individuals with serious mental illness. Psychiatric Services 64: 51–57.
28. Druss BG, Zhao L, von Esenwein SA, Bona JR, Fricks L, et al. (2010) The Health and Recovery Peer (HARP) Program: a peer-led intervention to improve medical self-management for persons with serious mental illness. Schizophrenia Research 118: 264–270.
29. McKay CE, Dickerson F (2012) Peer supports for tobacco cessation for adults with serious mental illness: a review of the literature. Journal of Dual Diagnosis 8: 104–112.
30. Basset T, Faulkner A, Repper J, Stamou E (2010) Lived experience leading the way: peer support in mental health. London: Together for Mental Wellbeing. Available: http://www.together-uk.org.
31. Greene JA, Choudhry NK, Kilabuk E, Shrank WH (2011) Online social networking by patients with diabetes: a qualitative evaluation of communication with Facebook. Journal of General Internal Medicine 26: 287–292.
32. Bender JL, Jimenez-Marroquin MC, Jadad AR (2011) Seeking support on Facebook: a content analysis of breast cancer groups. Journal of Medical Internet Research 13: e16.
33. Frost JH, Massagli MP (2008) Social uses of personal health information within PatientsLikeMe, an online patient community: what can happen when patients have access to one another's data. Journal of Medical Internet Research 10: e15.
34. Spinzy Y, Nitzan U, Becker G, Bloch Y, Fennig S (2012) Does the Internet offer social opportunities for individuals with schizophrenia? a cross-sectional pilot study. Psychiatry Research 198: 319–320.
35. Veretilo P, Billick SB (2012) Psychiatric illness and Facebook: a case report. Psychiatric Quarterly 83: 385–389.
36. Lehavot K, Ben-Zeev D, Neville RE (2012) Ethical considerations and social media: a case of suicidal postings on Facebook. Journal of Dual Diagnosis 8: 341–346.
37. Bargh JA, McKenna KY (2004) The Internet and social life. Annual Review of Psychology 55: 573–590.
38. Davison KP, Pennebaker JW, Dickerson SS (2000) Who talks? the social psychology of illness support groups. American Psychologist 55: 205–217.
39. Christofides E, Muise A, Desmarais S (2009) Information disclosure and control on Facebook: are they two sides of the same coin or two different processes? CyberPsychology & Behavior 12: 341–345.
40. Ellison NB, Steinfield C, Lampe C (2007) The benefits of Facebook "friends": social capital and college students' use of online social network sites. Journal of Computer-Mediated Communication 12: 1143–1168.
41. Savage J (2000) Ethnography and health care. BMJ 321: 1400–1402.
42. Beneito-Montagut R (2011) Ethnography goes online: towards a user-centred methodology to research interpersonal communication on the Internet. Qualitative Research 11: 716–735.
43. Gatson SN (2011) The methods, politics, and ethics of representation in online ethnography. In: Denzin N, Lincoln Y, editors. Handbook of Qualitative Research. 4 ed. Thousand Oaks, CA: Sage. 513–527.
44. Flicker S, Haans D, Skinner H (2004) Ethical dilemmas in research on Internet communities. Qualitative Health Research 14: 124–134.
45. McKee R (2013) Ethical issues in using social media for health and health care research. Health Policy 110: 298–301.
46. Zimmer M (2010) "But the data is already public": on the ethics of research in Facebook. Ethics and Information Technology 12: 313–325.
47. Charmaz K (2006) Constructing grounded theory: a practical guide through qualitative analysis. London: Sage.
48. Corbin JM, Strauss A (1990) Grounded theory research: procedures, canons, and evaluative criteria. Qualitative Sociology 13: 3–21.
49. Skeels MM, Grudin J (2009) When social networks cross boundaries: a case study of workplace use of Facebook and LinkedIn. Proceedings of the ACM 2009 International Conference on Supporting Group Work: 95–104.
50. Patton MQ (1990) Qualitative evaluation and research methods. Thousand Oaks, CA: Sage.
51. Ziebland S, Wyke S (2012) Health and illness in a connected world: how might sharing experiences on the internet affect people's health? Milbank Quarterly 90: 219–249.
52. Zhu Q (2011) Self-disclosure in online support groups for people living with depression. Singapore: National University of Singapore. 105 p.
53. Coursaris CK, Liu M (2009) An analysis of social support exchanges in online HIV/AIDS self-help groups. Computers in Human Behavior 25: 911–918.

54. Mo PKH, Coulson NS (2008) Exploring the communication of social support within virtual communities: a content analysis of messages posted to an online HIV/AIDS support group. CyberPsychology & Behavior 11: 371–374.
55. Mo PKH, Coulson NS (2012) Developing a model for online support group use, empowering processes and psychosocial outcomes for individuals living with HIV/AIDS. Psychology & Health 27: 445–459.
56. Ellison NB (2007) Social network sites: definition, history, and scholarship. Journal of Computer-Mediated Communication 13: 210–230.
57. Steffen V (1997) Life stories and shared experience. Social Science & Medicine 45: 99–111.
58. Barak A, Boniel-Nissim M, Suler J (2008) Fostering empowerment in online support groups. Computers in Human Behavior 24: 1867–1883.
59. Davidson L, Roe D (2007) Recovery from versus recovery in serious mental illness: One strategy for lessening confusion plaguing recovery. Journal of Mental Health 16: 459–470.
60. Entwistle VA, France EF, Wyke S, Jepson R, Hunt K, et al. (2011) How information about other people's personal experiences can help with healthcare decision-making: a qualitative study. Patient Education and Counseling 85: e291–e298.
61. Entwistle VA (2007) Considering 'balance' in information. Health Expectations 10: 307–308.

Measuring Cognitive Errors Using the Cognitive Distortions Scale (CDS): Psychometric Properties in Clinical and Non-Clinical Samples

Kadir Özdel[1]*, Ibrahim Taymur[2], Seher Olga Guriz[1], Riza Gökcer Tulaci[1], Erkan Kuru[1], Mehmet Hakan Turkcapar[3]

1 Diskapi Yildirim Beyazit Teaching and Research Hospital, Department of Psychiatry, Ankara, Turkey, **2** Sevket Yilmaz Teaching and Research Hospital, Department of Psychiatry, Bursa, Turkey, **3** Hasan Kalyoncu University, Department of Psychology, Istanbul, Turkey

Abstract

The Cognitive Distortions Scale was developed to assess thinking errors using case examples in two domains: interpersonal and personal achievement. Although its validity and reliability has been previously demonstrated in non-clinical samples, its psychometric properties and scoring has not yet been evaluated. The aim of the current study was to evaluate the psychometric properties of the Cognitive Distortions Scale in two Turkish samples and to examine the usefulness of the categorical scoring system. A total of 325 individuals (Sample 1 and Sample 2) were enrolled in this study to assess those psychometric properties. Our Sample 1 consisted of 225 individuals working as interns at the Diskapi Yildirim Beyazit Teaching and Research Hospital and Sample 2 consisted of 100 patients diagnosed with depression presenting to the outpatient unit of the same Hospital. Construct validity was assessed using the Beck Depression Inventory, the State Trait Anxiety Inventory, the Dysfunctional Attitude Scale, and the Automatic Thought Questionnaire. Factor analyses supported a one-factor model in these clinical and non-clinical samples. Cronbach's α values were excellent in both the non-clinical and clinical samples (0.933 and 0.918 respectively). Cognitive Distortions Scale scores showed significant correlation with relevant clinical measures. Study Cognitive Distortions Scale scores were stable over a time span of two weeks. This study showed that the Cognitive Distortions Scale is a valid and reliable measure in clinical and non-clinical populations. In addition, it shows that the categorical exists/does not exist scoring system is relevant and could be used in clinical settings.

Editor: Soraya Seedat, University of Stellenbosch, South Africa

Funding: The authors have no support or funding to report.

Competing Interests: The authors have declared that no competing interests exist.

* Email: kadirozdel@gmail.com

Introduction

Beck's cognitive theory has been one of the most influential contributions in the field of psychotherapy [1]. The main proposal of cognitive theory is that the emotional and behavioral reactions of individuals fundamentally depend upon underlying cognitive structures such as beliefs and thought systems [2–4]. Since one's emotional reactions to events are affected by the mechanisms with which information is processed, negatively biased cognitive processes can lead to maladaptive emotional and behavioral consequences [5].

Cognitive therapy for depression has been demonstrated to be an effective therapeutic modality. It aims to adjust "cognitions" rationally and/or functionally on three levels [6]. First, (Negative) Automatic thoughts emerge at a superficial level and provoke rapid, emotional cognitions. The second level involves intermediate beliefs including rules, attitudes, assumptions and strategies about internal and external events. The third level involves core beliefs that originate at the deepest levels of cognition and create longstanding and unconditional cognitive structures that can affect information processing [7]. For example, a man thinks "she doesn't care about me" when a friend of his doesn't answer his greeting. That man may hold a core belief that "I am unlovable" and may be constantly insecure about his relationships. He may assume "if I let my friends down, they will stop caring about me". He may believe he cannot afford to have any faults. In cognitive therapy for depression, treatment begins with a discussion of the client's experience and the interaction between events, thoughts, emotions and behaviors. Next the therapist urges the client to recognize and adjust his or her automatic thoughts. Repeated evaluations of the automatic thoughts of a depressed patient reveal their biased cognitive style. Going beyond content, negatively biased thought processes are called "*cognitive distortions*" or "*thinking mistakes*" [8]. Core beliefs are considered important risk factors for developing depression [9]. Negative automatic thoughts (NAT's) are not-evidence based and do not reflect reality in functional way, they usually are produced along with cognitive distortions. For instance a NAT of "she doesn't care about me" may accompany a cognitive distortion called *personalization*. Beck et al in their seminal work outlined 7 cognitive distortions that are characteristic of depressed individuals [1]. Burns then expanded this number to 10 (See: reference [10]). Thus, detecting cognitive errors and developing insight about them is an important component of cognitive behavioral therapy for depression.

The literature includes several attempts to measure specific cognitive distortions [11–13]. Covin et al developed a unique two-dimension, 20-item scale to directly measure cognitive distortions [14]. Its contents and dimensions were taken directly from the work of Beck et al and Burns [1,7,10]. The Cognitive Distortions Scale (CDS) seeks to detect cognitive distortions held by a person providing definitions of individual cognitive distortions and illustrating them with one-paragraph case examples for each domain (the interpersonal domain and the personal achievement domain). The subject is asked to estimate how often s/he uses that ***type of thinking***. Covin et al (2011) examined the validity and reliability of the CDS in a non-clinical sample consisting of 318 undergraduates and found it a promising tool with good psychometric properties to measure cognitive distortions [14].

The primary aim of the current study was to evaluate the psychometric properties of the CDS in two Turkish samples, one clinical and one non-clinical. Second, this study aimed to examine whether the CDS's psychometric properties differed across the clinical and non-clinical samples. Third, we wanted to test the usefulness of an alternative categorical scoring system for the CDS.

Material & Methods

Participants

The participants totaled 325 individuals from two samples, non-clinical (sample 1) and clinically depressed (sample 2). Sample 1 consisted of 225 subjects (161 females) from various professions (e.g., medical school students, nursing students, clinical and undergraduate psychology students, and social workers) working as interns at Ankara Diskapi Yildirim Beyazit Teaching and Research Hospital. Sample 2 consisted of 100 patients diagnosed with non-psychotic major depressive disorder (MDD) (71 females), who presented to the Department of Psychiatry out-patient unit of Ankara Diskapi Y.B. Teaching and Research Hospital. Patients with psychotic disorders, bipolar disorder, mental retardation, current substance use disorder, who have less than 8 years of education, or significant cognitive decline, were excluded from the study. Healthy controls screened for active psychopathology using socio-demographic data form, and introductory interview. Healthy controls were excluded from the study if they had any diagnosable psychiatric disorder.

Measures and Assessment Tools

The Cognitive Distortions Scale (CDS; Covin, Dozois, Ogniewicz, & Seeds, 2011). This is a 20-item self-report, Likert type scale instrument developed by Covin et al in 2011 to measure 10 cognitive distortions (*mindreading, catastrophizing, all-or-nothing thinking, emotional reasoning, labeling, mental filter, overgeneralization, personalization, should statements, minimizing the positive*) using a 7-point scale (1 = never, 7 = all the time) [14]. Each cognitive distortion is rated in two domains: interpersonal (IP) and personal achievement (PA). In the original study, the CDS emerged as a one-factor (unitary) scale with good internal consistency (Chronbach's $\alpha = 0.85$).

Assessment of demographic information. All participants completed a demographics and clinical information form assessing age, marital status, education, income, and employment status as well as clinical information such as substance use, suicide attempt history, physical illness, and family history of psychiatric disorders.

The Beck Depression Inventory (BDI; Beck, Ward, Mendelson, Mock, & Erbaugh, 1961). This is a 21-item scale developed and revised by Beck et al. [15] and updated by Beck et al. [16] measuring emotional, cognitive, somatic and motivational symptoms. It is based on data obtained from clinical observations [17]. In the Turkish version of this test (BDI-II), a score of 17 is considered the cut off point for validity and reliability [18,19].

The State Trait Anxiety Inventory (STAI; Spielberger, Gorsuch, & Lushene, 1970). This scale was developed by Spielberger et al. [20]. The STAI consists of two sub-scales, each composed of 20-items, measuring state and trait anxiety. The STAI state sub-scale (STAI-S) asks respondents to rate how they feel 'right now... at this moment' using a 4-point scale (1 = not at all, 4 = very much so) in response to a series of self-descriptive statements. The STAI trait subscale (STAI-T) asks respondents to rate how they feel 'in general' using a 4-point scale (1 = almost never, 4 = almost always) in response to relevant statements (Chronbach's α = 0.90). The Turkish version of the STAI has been demonstrated to be valid and reliable (Chronbach's α = 0.94) [21].

Dysfunctional Attitudes Scale-Form A (DAS; Weissman and Beck, 1978). In its original form, the DAS was developed by Weissman and Beck [22]. The 40-item short form of the DAS (Form A) was used in the current study. The DAS is a self-report questionnaire containing statements such as "It is difficult to be happy unless one is good looking, intelligent, rich and creative". These statements are expressions of various dysfunctional attitudes frequently found in psychiatric patients and associated with vulnerability to depression. Statements are rated on a 7-point scale ranging from 1 (totally disagree with that statement) to 7 (totally agree with that statement). Its validity and reliability have been shown in many different populations [23–25] including the Turkish population [26]. The internal consistency of the Turkish version is good (Cronbach's $\alpha = 0.79$) and has four factors: *"perfectionism", "need for approval", "independent attitudes" and "mixed attitudes"*. All sub-scales except the *independent attitudes* subscale discriminated between depressive and non-depressive individuals in a Turkish population [27].

Automatic Thought Questionnaire (ATQ; Hollon & Kendall, 1980). The ATQ was created by Hollon and Kendall (1980) to identify and measure the frequency of automatic thoughts associated with depression [28]. This is a 30-item self-report instrument that measures the frequency of the occurrence of negative automatic thoughts, or self-statements. Each item represents a thought and respondents rate the frequency of this thought on a 5-point scale ranging from 1 (not at all) to 5 (all the time), for the past week. The Turkish version of the ATQ has been shown to be valid and reliable with very good internal consistency (Chronbach's Alfas 0.89 to 0.91) [29].

The Structured Clinical Interview for DSM-IV Axis I Disorders (SCID-I; First, Spitzer, Gibbon, & Williams, 1997). This is a structured clinical interview form developed by First et al. (1997) to diagnose DSM-IV Axis I disorders. Validity and reliability was established for the Turkish test by Özkürkçü-kigil, Aydemir, Yıldız, Danaca, & Köroğlu (1999) [30,31].

Procedures

All participants were instructed to complete the following paper-and-pencil tests. Individuals from Sample 1 filled out the measures individually in a testing room routinely used for psychological assessment. Forms and questionnaires were administered in four different orders. The socio-demographic information form and CDS were administered first for all subjects but the order of administration of the DAS, ATQ, BDI, and STAI was changed throughout the sample. In addition to this process Sample 2 subjects completed a clinical interview using The Structured Clinical Interview for DSM-IV Axis I Disorders (SCID-I). No compensation of any kind was given to the participants. All participants from Sample 1 filled out the questionnaires anonymously. However, the first 30 participants who re-took the tests two weeks later wrote down the last 4 digits of their cell phone numbers to allow pairing. A written informed consent was obtained from all participants. Since all participants including the individuals from the non-clinical group and depressed group were older than 18 years of age and not having any condition that could interfere with their capacity (e.g., psychosis, intellectual disability, or illiteracy) all the consent papers were obtained from the participants themselves and no surrogate consent procedure was conducted. This study was conducted in accord with the Helsinki Declaration and was approved by the Ethics Committee of the Diskapi Y. B. Teaching and Research Hospital.

Translation of the CDS. The Turkish translation of the CDS was used in the current project. When creating the Turkish version guidelines widely used in cross-cultural research were followed [32]. Accordingly, three cognitive behavioral therapists separately translated the CDS into Turkish. A consensus version was translated into back into English and reviewed a second time. The final version was then approved by the same three clinicians in addition to the authors of this paper.

Statistical Analyses. All analyses were conducted using SPSS for Windows. Spearman correlation coefficients were calculated for convergent validity, comparing CDS scores and subscale scores with BDI, DAS, ATQ, and STAI scores. Internal consistency was evaluated using Cronbach's α and item/total correlations (and also "if item deleted" co-efficient") using the Spearman correlation coefficient. For parametric variables, student t tests were used to compare means. Frequencies were analyzed using a Chi-Square test. To evaluate the adequacy of the samples to construct validity analyses, Kaiser-Meyer-Olkin and Barlett tests were used. Principal component analysis with relevant rotation technique was used when evaluating the factor structure of the CDS. When determining the components of the scale, the following criteria were used: 1) Eigen values should be greater than one according to Kaiser Criterion (1961) 2) A Scree plot test was evaluated 3) all interpretations were derived from the theoretical background of the tests.

Results

Demographic & Clinical Properties

Sample 1 and sample 2 were similar in terms of gender (71.6% and 71% respectively were women). Sample 1 was younger and had more education (24.24±4.94 years versus 26.54±7.91 years, $p<0.05$; 15.56±2.2 versus 13.21±3.55 educational years, $p<0.001$). The two groups were made up mostly of single people (81.3% and 67%, respectively). Sample 1 had higher incomes as compared with Sample 2 (69.7% of Sample 1 had ≥ 2000 Turkish Liras whereas 45% of Sample 2 had ≥ 2000 Turkish Liras). The presence of family psychiatric history was similar in both groups (14.2% and 14% respectively).

In the clinical sample, 46% of the patients were having another DSM-IV Axis-I disorder diagnosis. MDD past episode was the commonest DSM-IV diagnosis with a proportion of 23%. It was followed by Generalized Anxiety Disorder (GAD) and Specific Phobia (SP) with 12%, Dysthymic Disorder (DD) with 11%. When the two groups (i.e., non-clinical sample and depressed individuals) were compared in relation to their levels of depression, state & trait anxiety, cognitive distortions and dysfunctional attitudes, they differed significantly on many items (please see Table 1).

Validity Measurements

Factor Analysis. A principal component analysis with Varimax rotation was performed for the full 20 items of the CDS. This procedure revealed four factors with eigenvalues greater than one (8.90, 1.67, 1.17, 1.05) in the Sample 1. Sixty four point three percent (64.03%) of the total variance was accounted for by four factors. CDS *catastrophizing* item of interpersonal domain (CDS-2IP), CDS *labeling* item of interpersonal domain (CDS-5IP), CDS *personalization* items of both interpersonal and personal achievement domains (CDS-8IP and CDS-8PA), CDS *should statements* items of both interpersonal and personal achievement domains (CDS-9IP and CDS9PA), CDS *minimizing or disqualifying the positive* items of interpersonal and personal achievement domains (CDS-10IP and CDS-10PA) were cross-loaded for the two different factors. Further examination of the data using Cattell's scree test and considering high rates of cross-loading indicated that it is more logical to consider these items on a unitary scale with one factor. According to this approach all items except mind reading items were loaded at a value greater than 0.10 and factor loadings were greater than 0.30 for all 10 items. On the current form 44.50% of the variance was accounted by one factor only.

The same procedure was repeated for Sample 2. This analysis revealed six factors with eigenvalues greater than one (7.91, 1.78, 1.45, 1.28, 1.15, 1.01) in Sample 2. Seventy two point ninety eight percent (72.98%) of the total variance was accounted for by those six factors. However CDS-6IP, CDS-7IP, CDS-2IP, CDS-4IP, CDS-4PA, CDS-3PA, CDS-6PA, and CDS-7PA were cross-loaded under, at least, two different factors. A Cattell's scree test consideration of very high cross-loadings indicated a one factor solution would be more reasonable for Sample 2 as well as for Sample 1. In the clinical sample factor loading was under 0.10 for six items including CDS-10PA, CDS-5IP, CDS-8PA, CDS-3PA and CDS-7PA. One factor accounted for 39.55% of the total variance.

Construct validity. To examine the construct validity of the CDS and its subscales, we computed correlations between CDS scores and the clinical measures included in the current study. The results of these analyses conducted both on the data from Sample 1 and Sample 2 are presented in Table 2. In addition, calculations were made for the correlations between CDS scores and scores on the DAS, its subscales, and the ATQ which measure similar cognitive tendencies in depression. These results are in Table 3. In the non-clinical group each item of the CDS was significantly correlated with BDI scores (weak to moderate correlations as indicated by correlation coefficients $r=0.158$ to $r=0.338$) as well as STAI-S and STAI-T scores. In the non-clinical sample every item of the CDS was correlated in some way with primary affect measures (i.e., BDI, STAI-S, and STAI-T).

However, in the clinical sample only *catastrophizing* (personal achievement domain), *emotional reasoning* (interpersonal domain), *overgeneralization* (interpersonal domain), *and disqualifying the positive* (interpersonal domain) were significantly correlated with total BDI scores. In the clinical group STAI-T scores were correlated to ten CDS items whereas BDI scores were correlated to only four items of the CDS (See Table 2).

One of the questions raised by the original study was whether there was a difference between errors made in interpersonal contexts and achievement contexts. Since the intention of creating a two-domain scale (e.g., interpersonal context and achievement context) was to test if some thinking errors occur in one context rather than in the other. Ten dependent *t* tests were conducted for each thinking mistake with a corrected p value of $p<0.01$. Both in the non-clinical sample and the clinical sample *mind-reading*

Table 1. The means, standard deviations and comparisons of BDI, STAI, CDS, and DAS scales' scores between the clinical and non-clinical samples.

Measure	Non-clinical sample (Sample 1) N = 225		Depressive Patients (Sample 2) N = 100		P values
	Mean	SD	Mean	SD	
Beck Depression Inventory*	4.83	4.68	28.96	9.43	0.000
STAI-State Anxiety*	34.12	9.12	50.92	11.01	0.000
STAI-Trait Anxiety *	38.03	7.99	56.50	8.71	0.000
Cognitive Distortion Scale-IP*	29.92	10.70	42.70	12.36	0.000
Cognitive Distortion Scale-PA*	28.62	10.48	40.15	11.70	0.000
Cognitive Distortion Scale-Total *	58.54	20.64	82.85	22.72	0.000
DAS-Perfectionism*	44.57	15.08	60.29	19.05	0.000
DAS-Need for Approval*	38.22	10.02	49	10.91	0.000
DAS-Independent Attitudes	18.62	5.50	23.41	5.96	0.017
DAS-Mixed Attitudes	19.30	4.05	20.54	4.72	0.025

STAI = State Trait Anxiety Inventory, IP = Interpersonal subscale of CDS, PA = Personal Achievement subscale of CDS, DAS = Dysfunctional Attitudes Scale.
T tests were performed using Bonferroni correction. Accordingly p value was set $p<0.005$.
*Statistically significant differences between the two groups.

($p = 0.001$; $p = 0.009$), *emotional reasoning* ($p = 0.00$; $p = 0.001$), and *overgeneralization* ($p = 0.00$; $p = 0.001$) occurred more frequently in the interpersonal domain.

Discriminant Validity. Table 1 shows the mean scores of the CDS and its subscales in the clinical and non-clinical samples. The CDS and its subscales' scores were significantly statistically different between the two groups.

Reliability Measurements

Internal consistency was computed using Cronbach's α. For the sample 1, Cronbach's α values were 0.933 for the CDS total, 0.871 for the interpersonal subscale, 0.874 for the personal achievement subscale. Item total score correlations varied 0.495 to 0.711. No significant change was observed if any item was deleted out of the 20 items. For the sample 2, Cronbach's α values were 0.918 for the CDS total, 0.868 for the interpersonal subscale, 0.847 for the personal achievement subscale. Item total score correlations varied from 0.478 to 0.703 for the 20-item CDS. Once again, no significant change was observed if any item was deleted out of the 20 items in sample 2. To assess Test-retest Reliability, 30 individuals from Sample 1 were re-administered the CDS two weeks later. CDS score totals were strongly correlated between the two assessment times ($r = 0.783$, $p<0.001$). The interpersonal and the individual achievement subscale scores showed similar correlations ($r = 0.735$, $p<0.001$ and $r = 0.809$, $p<0.001$).

Results for the CDS using alternative scoring procedure

Although no other scoring system was offered in the original paper, raw scores were used in previous statistics as recommended in the original study. However, an alternative scoring procedure was also used. In this procedure an item was rated as "1-exists" if a participant marked 6 or 7 on the Likert type scale and "0-doesn't exist" if a participant marked below the 6. A similar approach was used to score the Young Schema Questionnaire, developed for assessing early maladaptive schemas (see: Young, Klosko, & Weishaar, 2003, p. 75) [33]. Every participants' number of cognitive distortions were calculated. The number of cognitive distortions endorsed by each individual participant showed a difference between the two groups ($p<0.001$). In the non-clinical sample the mean number of cognitive distortion was 1.66 ± 2.87 whereas for the clinical sample the mean was 5.69 ± 4.65. The total numbers of cognitive distortions were significantly correlated with STAI-state, STAI-trait, and BDI scores in non-clinical ($r = 0.233$, $p<0.01$; $r = 0.418$, $p<0.01$; $r = 0.326$, $p<0.01$ respectively) and clinical samples ($r = 0.187$, $p>0.05$; $r = 0.343$, $p<0.01$; $r = 0.299$, $p<0.01$ respectively).

Conclusions

The aim of the current study was twofold. First, to examine the psychometric properties, reliability, and validity of the CDS. Second, to test an alternative scoring method evaluating cognitive distortions as categorical entities (exists or doesn't exist). The Psychometric properties that appeared in the current study were mostly similar to the results of the original study. We suggest that the CDS is a valid and reliable measure of cognitive distortions in both clinical and non-clinical samples with some caution about its use for clinical and experimental purposes. In addition, a categorical approach in scoring the CDS appeared more relevant especially in the clinical sample.

The two-factor structure was not supported in this study, in accord with to the original study that created the CDS [14]. This was the case for both clinical and non-clinical groups, again in accord with the previous studies [14,34]. Although our factor analytic work supports a one-factor model it doesn't necessarily imply that a two-factor model is clinically not useful. In the current study cognitive distortions including mind-reading, emotional reasoning and overgeneralization consistently appeared more frequently in the interpersonal domain. Again this is partially in accord with Covin et al.'s study. In addition, they found that *mental filtering* was reported more frequently in one of the two non-clinical samples of the study. These findings suggest that CDS scores endorsed in interpersonal and personal achievement contexts may not be related to given cognitive errors, but rather may be related to an individual's deeper cognitive structures, like assumptions or core beliefs [5]. Since the CDS items are based on two different vignettes for each cognitive distortion it might give us more opportunities to find cognitive distortions in two main contexts (i.e., interpersonal and personal achievement) [35].

Table 2. The correlations between the individual items of CDS and BDI, STAI-S, and STAI-T.

Individual items of CDS		Non-clinical sample (Sample 1) N = 225			Depressive Patients (Sample 2) N = 100		
		BDI	STAI-S	STAI-T	BDI	STAI-S	STAI-T
1-Mind reading	IP	,192**	,166*	,253**	,039	,080	,331**
	PA	,277**	,273**	,305**	,013	,123	,193
2-Catastrophizing	IP	,268**	,235**	,384**	,143	,208*	,355**
	PA	,245**	,262**	,388**	,237*	,113	,284**
3-All-or Nothing Thinking	IP	,154*	,211**	,248**	,092	,134	,118
	PA	,218**	,334**	,327**	−,002	,014	,022
4-Emotional Reasoning	IP	,231**	,207**	,260**	,249*	,085	,168
	PA	,273**	,274**	,353**	,062	,164	,120
5-Labeling	IP	,307**	,165*	,333**	,052	,058	,120
	PA	,274**	,262**	,386**	,069	,087	,176
6-Mental Filter	IP	,298**	,214**	,398**	,033	,086	,240*
	PA	,247**	,224**	,348**	,102	,135	,159
7-Overgenaralization	IP	,329**	,275**	,441**	,266**	,201*	,293**
	PA	,329**	,275**	,441**	,171	,095	,152
8-Personalization	IP	,175**	,213**	,337**	,125	,064	,237*
	PA	,220**	,356**	,203**	,127	,071	,209*
9-Should statements	IP	,279**	,363**	,201**	,075	,157	,341**
	PA	,338**	,385**	,243**	,041	,096	,216*
10-Minimizing or Disqualifying the Positive	IP	,228**	,400**	,237**	,267**	,179	,322**
	PA	,219**	,240**	,420**	,152	−,030	,130

Pearson correlation coefficients were calculated between the variables.
*Statistically significant at the level of $p<0.05$.
**Statistically significant at the level of $p<0.001$.

Table 3. Correlations between CDS scores and DAS & ATQ scores in two samples.

	Non-clinical sample (Sample 1) N = 225					Depressive Patients (Sample 2) N = 100				
	DAS-P	**DAS-NA**	**DAS-IA**	**DAS-MA**	**ATQ**	**DAS-P**	**DAS-NA**	**DAS-IA**	**DAS-MA**	**ATQ**
Cognitive Distortion Scale-IP	,380**	,433**	,269**	,209**	,371**	,324**	,239*	,132	,130	,391**
Cognitive Distortion Scale-PA	,399**	,424**	,272**	,177**	,404**	,364**	,262**	,170	,183	,305**
Cognitive Distortion Scale-Total	,400**	,440**	,278**	,198**	,397**	,364**	,265**	,160	,165	,370**

DAS-P: Dysfunctional Attitude Scale-Perfectionism subscale; DAS-NA: Dysfunctional Attitude Scale-Need for Approval subscale; DAS-IA: Dysfunctional Attitude Scale-Independent Attitudes subscale; DAS-MA: Dysfunctional Attitude Scale-Mixed Attitudes Subscale. ATQ: Automatic Thought Questionnaire. IP = Interpersonal subscale of CDS, PA = Personal Achievement subscale of CDS.
Pearson correlation coefficients were calculated between the variables.
*Statistically significant at the level of $p<0.05$.
**Statistically significant at the level of $p<0.001$.

Accordingly, using the CDS as it is has a potential in clinical settings despite the lack of statistical evidence in this regard.

Validity findings along with very good reliability coefficients across the two samples indicate that the CDS is a valid and reliable measure in clinical and non-clinical groups. The CDS also differentiated the depressive and non-depressive groups.

Despite good internal consistency and validity findings some unexpected results appeared. In the non-clinical sample, like in the study of Covin et al., each item of the CDS was correlated to depression, and anxiety scores. The correlations between the trait anxiety measures and cognitive distortions were usually stronger than those between the depression scores and cognitive distortions' scores. In the non-clinical sample negative affective states were generally concurrent with cognitive distortions. However, in the clinical (depressed) group some cognitive distortions (i.e., catastrophizing, emotional reasoning, overgeneralization, and Minimizing or Disqualifying the Positive) had more concurrent predictive values for depressive affect while some cognitive distortions (i.e., mind reading, catastrophizing, mental filter, overgeneralization, personalization, should statements, and Minimizing or Disqualifying the Positive) had more concurrent predictive values for trait anxiety features. It is very interesting that cognitive errors had stronger correlations for the trait anxiety measure. This finding when combined with those from Covin et al.'s study suggests that cognitive distortions are not specific to depressive symptoms but rather related to general distress or negative affect.

When we look at the correlations between the CDS and the scores of the measures that assess similar but not identical cognitive functions (i.e., dysfunctional attitudes and negative automatic thoughts) we observe stronger correlations. However, correlation analyses does not support the two-dimension structure of the CDS since DAS-NA scores had stronger correlations to CDS total and subscales scores in the non-clinical group whereas the DAS-P scores had stronger correlations to the same scores. Negative automatic thoughts showed similar correlations across the two samples and to CDS, CDS-PA, CDS-IP scale scores. These findings support that the cognitive distortions are more related to automatic thoughts and dysfunctional attitudes than to depressive symptoms.

In addition to psychometric analyses of the CDS we assessed the usefulness of an alternative approach in scoring CDS in this study. Since cognitive distortions seen in depression rarely appear individually but instead appear concurrently with one another [1,36] we rated each cognitive distortion item either to exist or not to exist and counted the number of cognitive distortions endorsed. The number of cognitive distortions distinguished the depressive and non-depressive groups. In addition, those scores were correlated more strongly to depressive symptom severity while correlations between the cognitive distortions and trait anxiety scores were similar. These findings suggest that a categorical approach to cognitive distortions may be more relevant to understanding the relationship between cognitive distortions and severity of depression.

An obvious limitation of this study is that the individuals in clinical sample filled out the questionnaires when they were depressed. Since current mood effects the endorsement of dysfunctional beliefs [37] clinical data should be considered with caution. The CDS has the same limitations as other self-report measures. A "perceived bias" cannot be ruled out due to the absence of a structured attempt to measure the actual demonstration of errors. Finally, these results cannot be generalized to all clinical and non-clinical populations because being a volunteer in a study reflects special attitudes linked to self selection biases.

In sum, the CDS is a valid and reliable scale measuring cognitive distortions effectively in clinical and non-clinical populations. Although its subscales may be used in clinical settings it seems that a unitary scale could measure cognitive distortions in interpersonal and personal achievement contexts. Further, a categorical scoring of the scale may be more useful in clinical settings.

Acknowledgments

We thank Dr. S. U. Kilic, S. Sahinöz, and Ö. Y. Alkar for their help in data collection.

Author Contributions

Conceived and designed the experiments: KÖ MHT SOG IT RGT EK. Performed the experiments: KÖ EK RGT MHT. Analyzed the data: KÖ MHT IT. Contributed reagents/materials/analysis tools: KÖ IT EK RGT. Contributed to the writing of the manuscript: KÖ SOG IT MHT RGT EK. Conducted statistical analyses: KÖ. Critically reviewed the manuscript: MHT SOG IT RGT EK. Gave final approval of the version to be submitted: KÖ MHT SOG IT RGT EK.

References

1. Beck AT, Rush A, Shaw B, Emery G (1979) Cognitive therapy of depression. New York: Guilford Press.
2. Dryden W, DiGuiseppe R, Neenan M (2003) A Primer on Rational Emotive Behavior Therapy. Illinois: Research Press.
3. Akkoyunlu S, Türkçapar MH (2012) A Technique: Examining the Evidence. JCBPR 1: 184–190.
4. Akkoyunlu S, Türkçapar MH (2013) Bir Teknik: Alternatif Düşünce Oluşturulması. JCBPR 2: 53–59.
5. Dozois DJA, Beck AT (2008) Cognitive schemas, beliefs and assumptions. In: Dobson KS, Dozois DJA, editors. Risk factors in depression. Oxford, England: Elsevier/Academic Press. pp. 121–143.
6. Beck JS (2011) Cognitive Behavior Therapy Basics and Beyond. Second Edi. New York: The Guilford Press.
7. Beck AT (1983) Cognitive therapy of depression: New perspectives. In: Clayton PJ, Barrett JE, editors. Treatment of Depression: Old controversies and new approaches. New York: Raven Press. pp. 265–284.
8. Türkçapar MH (2009) Klinik Uygulamada Bilişsel Davranışçı Terapi: Depresyon. Ankara: Hekimler Yayın Birliği.
9. Alloy LB, Riskind JH, editors (2006) Cognitive Vulnerability to Emotional Disorders. Hillsdale, NJ: Lawrence Erlbaum.
10. Burns DD (1980) Feeling good: The new mood therapy. New York: Signet.
11. Krantz SE, Hammen CL (1979) Assessment of cognitive bias in depression. J Abnorm Psychol 88: 611–619.
12. Frost RO, MacInnis DJ (1983) The Cognitive Bias Questionnaire: further evidence. J Pers Assess 47: 173–177. doi:10.1207/s15327752jpa4702_12.
13. Lefebvre MF (1981) Cognitive distortion and cognitive errors in depressed psychiatric and low back pain patients. J Consult Clin Psychol 49: 517–525.
14. Covin R, Dozois DJA, Ogniewicz A, Seeds PM (2011) Measuring Cognitive Errors: Initial Development of the Cognitive Distortions Scale (CDS). Int J Cogn Ther 4: 297–322. Available: http://guilfordjournals.com/doi/abs/10.1521/ijct.2011.4.3.297.
15. Beck AT, Ward CH, Mendelson M, Mock J, Erbaugh J (1961) An inventory for measuring depression. Arch Gen Psychiatry 4: 561–571.
16. Beck AT, Steer RA, Brown GK (1996) Manual for the Beck Depression Inventory. Second. San Antonio, TX: The Psychological Corporation.
17. Beck AT, Steer RA, Carbin MG (1988) Psychometric properties of the Beck Depression Inventory: Twenty-five years of evaluation. Clin Psychol Rev 8: 77–100. Available: http://linkinghub.elsevier.com/retrieve/pii/0272735888900505.
18. Hisli N (1988) A study on the validity of Beck Depression Inventory. Turkish J Psychol 6: 118–123.
19. Kapci EG, Uslu R, Turkcapar H, Karaoglan A (2008) Beck Depression Inventory II: evaluation of the psychometric properties and cut-off points in a Turkish adult population. Depress Anxiety 25: 104–110. Available: http://www.ncbi.nlm.nih.gov/pubmed/17876817.
20. Spielberger CD, Gorsuch RL, Lushene RE (1970) Manual for State-Trait Anxiety Inventory. California: Consulting Psychologist Pres.
21. Öner N, Le Compte A (1988) Durumluk Sürekli Anksiyete Envanteri el kitabı. Boğaziçi Üniversitesi Yayınları. Istanbul: Boğaziçi Üniversitesi Yayinlari.
22. Weissman AN, Beck AT (1978) Development and validation of the Dysfunctional Attitude Scale: A preliminary investigation Paper presented at the annual meeting of the American Educational Research Association, Toronto, Ontario, Canada.
23. Chioqueta AP, Stiles TC (2004) Psychometric properties of the Norwegian version of the Dysfunctional Attitude Scale (Form A). Cogn Behav Ther 33: 83–86. Available: http://www.tandfonline.com/doi/abs/10.1080/16506070410023951. Accessed 23 October 2013.
24. Mukhtar F, Oei TPS (2010) Exploratory and confirmatory factor validation of the Dysfunctional Attitude Scale for Malays (DAS-Malay) in Malaysia. Asian J Psychiatr 3: 145–151. Available: http://www.ncbi.nlm.nih.gov/pubmed/23051574. Accessed 23 October 2013.
25. Floyd M, Scogin F, Chaplin WF (2004) The Dysfunctional Attitudes Scale: factor structure, reliability, and validity with older adults. Aging Ment Health 8: 153–160. Available: http://www.ncbi.nlm.nih.gov/pubmed/14982720. Accessed 2 February 2014.
26. Savaşır I, Şahin NH (1997) Bilişsel-Davranışçı Terapilerde Değerlendirme: Sık Kullanılan Ölçekler. Savaşır I, Şahin NH, editors Ankara: Türk Psikologlar Derneği Yayinlari.
27. Sahin NH, Sahin N (1992) How dysfunctional are the dysfunctional attitudes in another culture? Br J Med Psychol 65 (Pt 1): 17–26.
28. Hollon SD, Kendall PC (1980) Cognitive self-statements in depression: Development of an automatic thoughts questionnaire. Cognit Ther Res 4: 383–395. doi:10.1007/BF01178214.
29. Şahin NH, Şahin N (1992) Reliability and validity of the Turkish version of the automatic thoughts questionnaire. J Clin Psychol 48: 334–340.
30. First MB, Spitzer RL, Gibbon M, Williams JBW (1997) Structured clinical interview for DSM-IV axis I disorders, clinician version (SCID-CV). Washington, DC: American Psychiatric Association.
31. Özkürkçükigil A, Aydemir Ö, Yıldız M, Danaca EA, Köroğlu HE (1999) DSM-IV Eksen I bozuklukları için yapılandırılmış klinik görüşmenin Türkçe'ye uyarlanması ve güvenirlik çalışması. İlaç Tedavi Derg 12: 233–236.
32. Brislin RW (1970) Back-Translation for Cross-Cultural Research. J Cross Cult Psychol 1: 185–216. doi:10.1177/135910457000100301.
33. Young JE, Klosko JS, Weishaar ME (2003) Schema Therapy A Practitioner's Guide.
34. Messer SC, Kempton T, Hasselt VB Van, Null JA, Bukstein OG (1994) Cognitive distortions and adolescent affective disorder. Validity of the CNCEQ in an inpatient sample. Children's Negative Cognitive Error Questionnaire. Behav Modif 18: 339–351.
35. Nietzel MT, Harris MJ (1990) Relationship of dependency and achievement/autonomy to depression. Clin Psychol Rev 10: 279–297.
36. Norman WH, Klee SH, Miller IW (1983) Assessment of cognitive distortion in a clinically depressed population. Cognit Ther Res 7: 133–140. doi:10.1007/BF01190066.
37. Miranda J, Persons JB, Byers CN (1990) Endorsement of dysfunctional beliefs depends on current mood state. J Abnorm Psychol 99: 237–241. Available: http://www.ncbi.nlm.nih.gov/pubmed/2212273.

18

The Efficacy of Mindfulness-Based Cognitive Therapy as a Public Mental Health Intervention for Adults with Mild to Moderate Depressive Symptomatology

Wendy T. M. Pots[1,2]*, Peter A. M. Meulenbeek[1,3], Martine M. Veehof[1], Jorinde Klungers[3], Ernst T. Bohlmeijer[1]

1 University of Twente, Department of Psychology, Health & Technology, Enschede, the Netherlands, **2** Dimence, Community Mental Health Center, Almelo, the Netherlands, **3** GGNET, Community Mental Health Center, Warnsveld, the Netherlands

Abstract

Objective: Although there has been growing evidence for the efficacy of mindfulness-based cognitive therapy (MBCT) for different clinical populations, its effectiveness as a public mental health intervention has not been studied. The present study evaluates a community-based MBCT intervention for adults with mild to moderate depressive symptomatology in a large multi-site, pragmatic randomized controlled trial.

Method: The participants with mild to moderate depressive symptomatology were recruited from the general population and randomized to the MBCT intervention ($n = 76$) or to a waiting list control group ($n = 75$). Participants completed measures before and after the intervention. Participants in the experimental condition also completed these measures at a 3-month follow-up.

Results: In the experimental condition significant reductions in depression, anxiety, and experiential avoidance, and improvements in mindfulness and emotional- and psychological mental health were found, compared to the waiting list (effect sizes Cohen's $d = 0.31$–0.56). These effects were sustained at the 3-month follow-up. The likelihood of a clinically significant change in depressive symptoms was significantly higher for the MBCT group [odds ratio (OR) 3.026, $p < 0.01$ at post-treatment; NNT = 5.10].

Discussion: MBCT as a public mental health intervention for adults with mild to moderate depressive symptoms seems effective and applicable in a natural setting.

Editor: Gabriel S. Dichter, UNC Chapel Hill, United States of America

Funding: The study was funded by University of Twente (www.utwente.nl). The funder had no role in study design, data collection and analysis, decision to publish, or preparation of the manuscript.

Competing Interests: The authors have declared that no competing interests exist.

* Email: w.t.m.pots@utwente.nl

Introduction

Minor depression is a highly prevalent disorder with a large negative impact on quality of life and yielding high economic costs [1]. Offering interventions for people with depressive symptomatology is a necessary public mental health strategy complementary to the treatment of depression in inpatient and outpatient settings [2]. One such effective strategy is to pro-actively offer treatments for people with mild to moderate symptoms of depression [3,4]. However, a public mental health intervention needs to be attractive for people who don't suffer from severe symptoms of depression yet [5]. Using a positive framework and promoting positive mental health as well as reducing psychological distress offers opportunities to attract more people [6–8]. Mindfulness-based cognitive therapy (MBCT) may be such an intervention, as it focuses on promoting positive mental health instead of only focusing on the reduction of psychological distress. MBCT is an 8-week group-based training that combines meditation exercises with cognitive techniques. It was originally designed for prevention of relapse in people with recurrent depression [9]. In patients with three or more previous episodes of depression, MBCT significantly reduced the risk of relapse compared to the treatment as usual [10–12]. Moreover, in a recently published randomized controlled trial Williams et al. [13] found evidence that the number of episodes is a marker for those with greater vulnerability due to a history of childhood trauma and adversity. Strauss et al. [14] conducted a meta-analysis on mindfulness based interventions for people diagnosed with a current episode of an anxiety or depressive disorder and found that MBCT can also be effective for people who are currently depressed. MBCT targets processes such as avoidance of negative emotions and engaging with maladaptive thinking and rumination, that maintain depressive symptomatology in general [15,16]. Mindfulness is often referred to as intentionally paying attention to present moment experiences in a non-judgemental way [17]. Awareness and acceptance of negative experiences will reduce experiential avoidance (EA) [15]. EA has been defined as the unwillingness to remain in contact with experiences such as feelings, thoughts, and bodily sensations, as an attempted means of behavioral regulation [15]. Psychological flexibility is the counterpart of experiential avoidance. As EA could be seen as an important factor that maintains depressive symptomatology, MBCT may also be effective as a public mental health intervention for people with depressive symptomatology. This fits with a growing interest in adapting MBCT to other psychiatric disorders, such as anxiety disorders, and bipolar disorder, but also treatment-resistant major depressive disorder (for a recent review see Chiesa & Serretti [18]). Research into the potential mechanisms of action in MBCT is in its infancy. In a recent review Chiesa and Serretti [19] suggested that mindfulness-based interventions may enhance positive emotion regulation strategies, as well as self-compassion levels, and decrease rumination and experiential avoidance. They suggested that these changes are associated with several clinical benefits, including the reduction of stress and depression levels, as well as the enhancement of positive emotions. Recently, Kaviani et al. [20] found that MBCT can be effective in a non-clinical population of female students in Iran. Also, Cavanagh et al. [21] adapted MBCT as a brief online intervention and found it to be effective in a non-clinical population of students. To our knowledge, there is no research on the effectiveness of a community-based MBCT intervention for adults with depressive symptomatology. In order to modify the original MBCT as a public mental health intervention a few changes were made in time-investment. We expected a community-based MBCT with a reduced weekly time-investment to be more acceptable for the target group.

The aim of this study was to evaluate the effect of mindfulness-based cognitive therapy modified as a public mental health intervention for depressive symptomatology, in a sample of self-referred adults with mild to moderate depressive symptomatology, and offered by community mental health centers. We evaluated the effect with respect to various psychological variables, such as depression, anxiety and positive mental health. We hypothesized that changes in depressive symptoms would be mediated by psychological flexibility and mindfulness. To strengthen the trial's external validity, the intervention was studied in its natural setting.

Method

The protocol for this trial and supporting CONSORT checklist are available as supporting information; see Checklist S1 and Protocol S1. This study was approved by the METiGG, a medical ethics committee for research in mental health settings in the Netherlands. In addition, this study has been registered in the Nederlands Trial Register, the Primary Dutch register for clinical trials (NTR2096).

Design

A pragmatic, multi-site, randomized controlled trial was conducted comparing MBCT with a control condition. Participants were randomly assigned after receiving their written consent, either to MBCT or to the waiting list control, by means of a centrally conducted randomization process executed by an independent researcher. The randomization was carried out for the two groups with stratification on gender, using a computer generated random sequence of numbers. The control condition consisted of a waiting list, where wait-listed people were free to use other kinds of care. The wait-listed participants knew that they could start the training after the experimental condition had completed the intervention, i.e. after 3 months. The study is pragmatic as it mimics the Dutch health care system as closely as possible in terms of patient recruitment, conducting intake, offering interventions, and monitoring outcomes.

Participants and procedure

Participants were recruited from November 2009 until October 2010, through advertisements in regional newspapers, information booklets and general practitioners. Four Dutch community mental health centers, from both urban and rural areas, participated in the study. In the advertisements, distributed within the regions of the participating community mental health services, the target group was described as adults who were hindered by depressive symptoms. Applicants were referred to a specifically developed website, where they could find detailed information about the study. When interested, they were sent an information letter and an informed consent form. For screening, the standard procedures employed by the mental health institutions were used. The community mental health centers were responsible for the procedure, and the in- and exclusion criteria were examined by experienced mental health nurses on the basis of a checklist, under supervision of a clinical psychologist. The inclusion criteria were: adults of 18 years and over, presenting depressive symptoms. Applicants were excluded if diagnosed with a current severe major depressive episode (MDE; eight or nine out of a total of nine symptoms) or when having a moderate to high suicide risk, according to the Dutch version of the Mini International Neuropsychiatric Interview (MINI) [22,23]. Other exclusion criteria were: receiving psychological or pharmacological treatment for mental complaints within the last three months, and presence of other severe mental or social problems warranting treatment or likely to interfere with participation in the group course. People meeting one of the exclusion criteria were advised to seek regular treatment.

Power analysis

A sample of 60 participants per condition at post-intervention was needed to detect an effect size of 0.50 (Cohen's d) for the primary outcome with a statistical power of $(1-\beta) = 0.80$ in a two-tailed test ($p<0.05$). Taking into account a drop-out rate of 20%, 150 eligible participants were needed.

Measures

Measurements were taken at baseline (T0), and at post-treatment after 3 months (T1). In order to study the stability of the effect of MBCT, the patients in the experimental group received a follow-up measurement (T2) at 6 months after baseline. For the control condition, the measurement at 6 months is a post-treatment measurement. All measurements had good psychometric properties and are frequently applied in international studies.

The primary outcome measure was depressive symptomatology, measured by the Dutch version of the Center of Epidemiological Studies - Depression Scale (CES-D; 20 items, score 0–60) [24]. Higher scores mean more depressive symptoms [24,25].

Secondary outcome measures were anxiety symptoms and positive mental health. Anxiety was measured by the Hospital

Anxiety and Depression Scale - Anxiety subscale (HADS-A; 7 items, score 0–21) [26] for assessing the presence and severity of anxiety symptoms. Higher scores mean more anxiety symptoms [26,27]. Positive mental health was measured by the Mental Health Continuum - Short Form (MHC-SF) [28], that measures emotional well-being (3 items; score 0–15), social well-being (5 items; score 0–25) and psychological well-being (6 items; score 0–30). Higher scores indicate greater emotional, social, and psychological well-being [28,29].

Measures of proposed processes of change included measures of EA and mindfulness. The Acceptance and Action Questionnaire-II (AAQ-II; 10 items, score 10–70) [30] was used to measure the willingness to be in contact with aversive internal experiences, to accept these events, and to pursue values in the presence of the experiences. Higher scores indicate lower levels of EA or higher levels of psychological flexibility [30,31]. The Five Facet Mindfulness Questionnaire (FFMQ) [32] was used to measure mindfulness in five sub-dimensions: (1) observing (8 items), defined in terms of noticing or attending to internal and external experiences; (2) describing (8 items), defined in terms of labelling internal experiences with words; (3) acting with awareness (8 items), defined in terms of attending to one's activities of the moment (opposite of acting on automatic pilot); (4) non-judging of inner experience (8 items), defined in terms of taking a non-evaluative stance toward thoughts and feelings; and (5) and non-reactivity to inner experience (7 items), defined in terms of allowing thoughts and feelings to come and go, without getting caught up in or carried away by them. Facet scores range from 8 to 40 (except for the non-reactivity, which ranges from 7 to 35), with higher scores indicating more mindfulness [32,33].

To evaluate the level of satisfaction of the participants after the intervention, a self-developed evaluation questionnaire was used, including a question on how the participants evaluated the program using a scale from 1(very poor) to 10 (excellent).

Waiting list control

Participants in the control condition participated in the MBCT training after a 3-month waiting list period. Participants were instructed to seek help from their general practitioner, family or other sources, as they normally would, should they encounter symptomatic deterioration or other difficulties during the waiting list period.

Intervention

In this study MBCT was delivered according to the guidelines of Segal et al. [9]. The original training was adapted to suit a public mental health approach. The intervention was aimed at people with mild to moderate symptoms of depression. In order to lower the threshold for people without severe distress to participate in MBCT, the participants were asked to practice meditations for 15 minutes a day instead of the original 45 minutes a day, and the sessions were limited to 1, 5 hours instead of the original 2, 5 hours. To ensure that all of the elements of the original course were preserved, the eight-session training was extended to 11 sessions. Key themes of the sessions included awareness (sessions 1, 2, 3), acceptance (sessions 5, 7, 9, 10) and disengaging from thoughts (sessions 4, 6, 8), with the last session (session 11) focusing on evaluation and integration. The training teaches skills to become more aware of, and to relate differently to thoughts, feelings and bodily sensations. A core feature of the training is to learn to become aware of, and disengage from habitual dysfunctional (cognitive) routines, to stop reacting automatically to internal experiences, and to act more 'mindfully'. During the period of the training, the program consisted of daily homework exercises. The exercises were aimed at increasing attention to present moment experiences in a non-judgmental way, together with exercises designed to integrate application of awareness skills into daily life. To support homework assignments, participants received weekly homework registration forms, guided (taped) and unguided meditations, and information in a booklet. Group sizes varied between eight and 15 participants.

Therapists

The MBCT instructors were all experienced psychologists and mental health nurses, with extensive former training in the original MBCT protocol by Segal [9] and Group psychotherapy. The trainers were also experienced meditators, with meditation experience ranging from 2 to 15 years.

Statistical analyses

The statistical analyses were performed using SPSS 18. The data was analyzed on an intention-to-treat (ITT) basis. Missing values at baseline, post-intervention and follow-up were imputed with the use of SPSS Missing Value Analysis on the continuous measures with the expectation-maximization (EM) method. This method computes missing values based on maximum likelihood estimates using observed data in an iterative process [34]. The total percentage of missing data (T0-T1-T2) was 5%, due to unanswered items (0,6%) and incomplete assessments (4,4%). A comparison of results based on the imputed intention-to-treat sample versus the observed data revealed similar outcomes. Therefore, only the results from the intention-to-treat analyses are reported.

Independent sample t-tests and chi-square tests were conducted to examine differences between the two groups at baseline on sociodemographic variables and outcome measures. Analysis of covariance (ANCOVA) was conducted with depressive symptoms post-treatment as the dependent variable, treatment group as the independent variable, and five covariates consisting of pre-treatment depression score and four dummy-coded variables for each treatment site. The same analyses were conducted for the secondary measures. Analysis of variance (ANOVA) was conducted with process measures post-treatment as the dependent variable and treatment group as the independent variable. Assumptions for performing parametric analysis of (co)variance were all met. To investigate whether the effects in the intervention condition were maintained at follow-up paired-sample t-tests were carried out, comparing the scores on the follow-up (T2) with those at baseline (T0). Also, paired-sample t-tests were carried out for the control group, to measure the effect of the MBCT intervention after the waiting time period, comparing scores at post-treatment (T2 for the control group) with those at pre-treatment (T1 for the control group).

Effect sizes at post-treatment (T0-T1) were calculated with Cohen's d using the means and the pooled standard deviations of the measurements in the conditions. For the effect sizes at follow-up (T0-T2) the Cohen's d was corrected for dependence among means by using the correlation between the two means [35]. To interpret Cohen's d an effect size of less than 0.33 is considered small, while 0.33 to 0.55 is considered moderate and effect sizes of 0.56 to 1.2 are considered large [36]. Comparisons were two-tailed and interpreted with a significance value of $p<0.05$.

With the Jacobson and Truax methodology, the proportion of participants was determined who made a clinically significant change on the CES-D from baseline to post-treatment [37]. First, the reliable change was calculated with the reliable change index (RCI). Jacobson and Truax suggest that subjects can be considered to have improved when they shift from a dysfunctional distribution to a functional one, and the reliable change scores exceed measurement error (calculated by dividing the difference between the pretest and posttest scores by the standard error of the measurement). Second, the recovery criterion was defined as a post-treatment score below the cut-off value of 16 for clinically relevant depressive symptoms [38,39]. Because we studied a population with a mild to moderate symptomatology, the mean score at baseline was already at the recovery criterion (M = 16.04; range 1–43; S.D. = 8.08). A clinically significant change on the CES-D is thus defined as having a reliable change between the measurements, which required a post-treatment score below the cut-off of 16. Participants that had a clinically significant change were either coded 1 (implying a favorable treatment response, 'success') or 0 ('failure'). The binary outcome was used to calculate the odds ratio (OR) using logistic regression. Based on the clinically significant change proportions, the number needed to treat (NNT) was calculated [40]. To provide a more complete representation of the effects of the intervention, the outcomes were also analyzed for intervention completers only (somewhat arbitrarily defined as participants that attended at least 9 sessions).

The process measures were expected to be mediators between the MBCT intervention and post-treatment levels of depressive symptomatology (CES-D). Mediation was performed for all process measures that were significantly different between the intervention and control condition in the ANOVA. Then, all steps outlined by Baron and Kenny [41] were used. In the first step linear regression analysis was performed, with treatment group as independent variable and depressive symptoms post-treatment as the dependent variable. In the second step we tested the effect of the independent variable on the proposed mediators with linear regression analyses, with treatment group as independent variable and the residual change scores of the proposed mediators as the dependent variables. The third step tested the effect of the proposed mediator on the dependent variable. The indirect effect of the mediator on the outcome was assessed to examine whether an increase in psychological flexibility and mindfulness during the intervention would mediate the effects of the intervention on depressive symptomatology at post-intervention. Simple mediational analyses with bootstrapping procedures (n = 5000 bootstrap resamples) were used to assess the indirect effect of the mediator on the outcome [42]. An indirect effect was considered significant in the case zero was not contained in the 95% confidence interval.

Results

Enrollment, treatment adherence, satisfaction and drop-out

Figure 1 provides an overview of the flow of participants. A total of 251 persons were interested in the training. During telephone screening, 43 persons presented other psychiatric symptoms or practical restraints that precluded them from participation in the trial. The remaining 208 applicants were assessed for eligibility. Through interviewing, a further 57 were excluded. After signing the informed consent form, the included 151 participants were randomly assigned to the MBCT intervention (n = 76) and the waiting list condition (n = 75).

After randomization, two participants decided not to start with the intervention due to time constraints (n = 1) and health problems (n = 1). Four other participants in the MBCT (8%) group did not complete the intervention (attendance of at least 9 sessions). The reasons given for non-completion were that the intervention was too time consuming (n = 1), practicality reasons (n = 1), insufficient concentration (n = 1), and an unknown reason (n = 1). Two of the four community mental health centers evaluated the course resulting in anonymous evaluation forms of all participants, including those who did not participate in the study. Based on these results overall the intervention was evaluated as positive on a scale from 1 to 10 (m = 7.98, sd = 0.72, n = 130).

At T1 (post-treatment for the MBCT group and pre-treatment for the waiting list group), data was available for 143 participants (drop-out rate 5.3%) and at T2 (follow-up for the MBCT group and post-treatment for the waiting list group), data was available for 139 participants (drop-out rate 7.9%). There were no significant differences at baseline on all the measurements between participants who completed the assessments and those who did not complete all measures.

Baseline characteristics

Table 1 shows an overview of the participants' characteristics. Participants had a mean age of 48 years (SD = 11.29, range 20–81) and were predominantly female (78.1%). The majority was of Dutch origin (96%), had a paid job (66.9%), and were living with a partner (75.5%). The level of education was high for 65.5% of the participants and intermediate for 30.5%. At the entry of the study, 2.6% met the criteria of mild MDE and 4% were diagnosed with moderate MDE. There were no significant differences at baseline between the MBCT group and the control group for any of the demographic variables or outcome measurements. Also, there were no significant changes in the waiting time period for the control group, comparing scores at baseline (T0) with pre-treatment measurement (T1), on any of the outcome measures.

Treatment effects

Primary outcome

The means and standard deviations for the primary outcome measure, the results of the ANCOVA and the effect sizes are presented in Table 2. Compared to the control condition, participants in the intervention condition reported significantly decreased depressive symptoms at post-treatment (Table 2). The effects of the intervention condition on depressive symptoms were maintained at follow-up compared to baseline measurement [$t(75) = -3.46$, $p<0.01$]. Moderate effect sizes were found at post-treatment ($d = 0.50$) and follow-up ($d = 0.40$). The control group also showed significant reductions in depression after they received the intervention at T2 [$t(74) = -3.03$, $p<0.01$].

Clinically significant change

The reliable change on the CES-D appeared to be a pre-post difference of at least 7 scale points. Clinically significant change was thus defined as a recovery condition of a score ≤16 points on the CES-D (n = 138) and a RCI of 7 points. The proportion of participants with a score of ≥7 at T0 that reached a clinically significant change was 24/70 (34%) in the intervention group, versus 10/68 (15%) in the control condition [OR 3.026, 95% confidence interval (CI) 1.316–6.961, $p<0.01$, NNT = 5.10, under an intention-to-treat analysis]. These results compare well with completers-only findings: OR 2.916, 95% CI 1.252–6.795, $p< 0.01$, NNT = 5.26.

Secondary outcome measures

The means and standard deviations for the secondary outcome measures, the results of the ANCOVA and the effect sizes are presented in Table 2. Compared to the control condition, participants in the intervention condition reported significantly decreased anxiety symptoms after the intervention. At follow-up, the effects of the intervention condition on anxiety symptoms were maintained compared to baseline measurement [$t(75) = -8.40$,

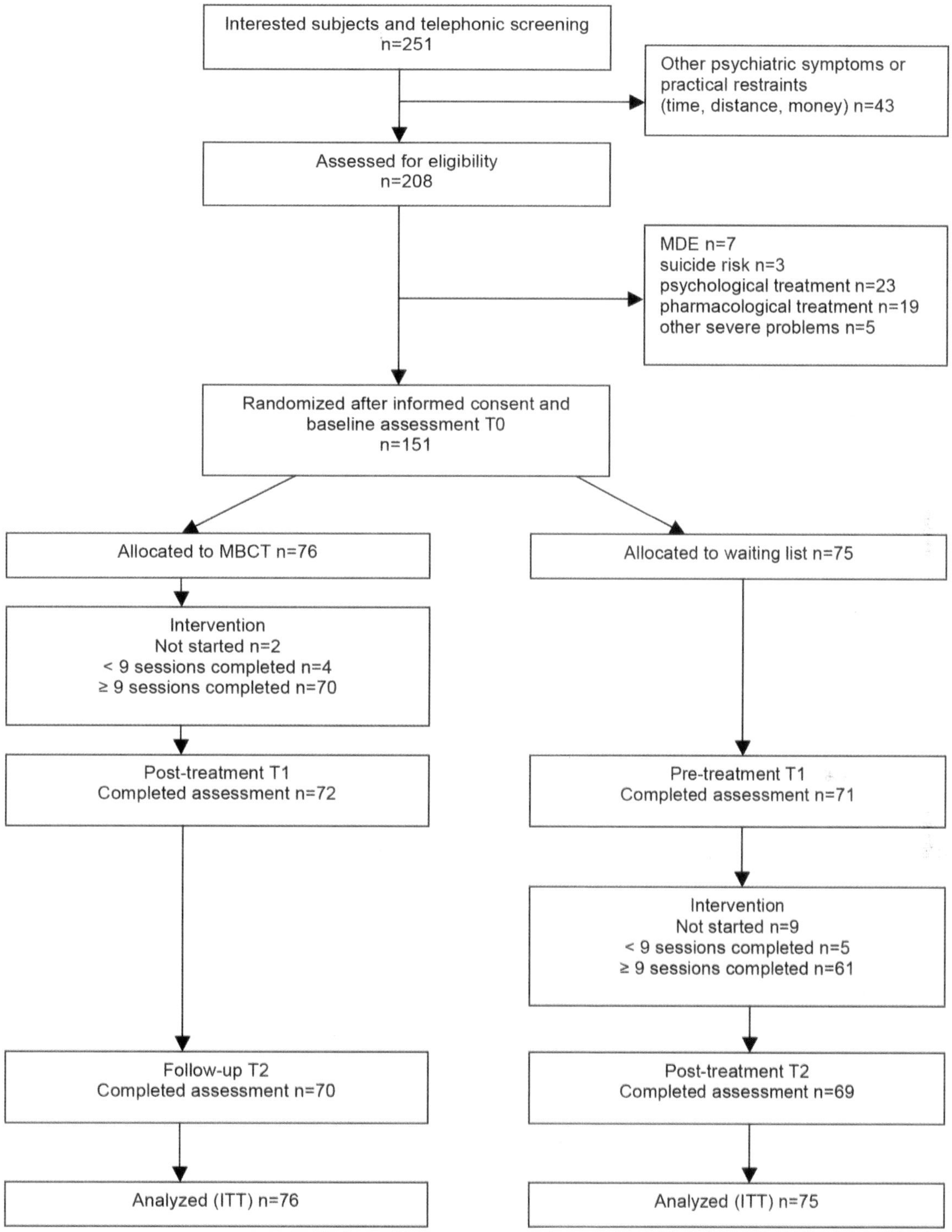

Figure 1. Participant flow. MDE = major depressive episode.

$p<0.001$]. The effect sizes for anxiety symptoms at post-treatment ($d = 0.56$) and at follow-up ($d = 0.97$) were large. The control group also showed significant reductions in anxiety after they received the intervention at T2 [$t(74) = -5.15$, $p<0.001$].

At post treatment, significant improvements in emotional well-being and psychological well-being were found. The effects of the intervention condition on emotional and psychological well-being were maintained at follow-up compared to baseline measurement [emotional well-being $t(75) = 4.13$, $p<0.001$; psychological well-being $t(75) = 5.20$, $p<0.001$]. Effect sizes at post-treatment were small (emotional well-being, $d = 0.31$) to moderate (psychological well-being, $d = 0.34$). The effect sizes at follow-up were moderate (emotional well-being, $d = 0.50$) to large (psychological well-being, $d = 0.56$). No significant effects were found at post-treatment for social well-being, with a small effect size ($d = 0.22$). At follow-up, there was a significant increase in social well-being compared to

Table 1. Baseline characteristics of the total sample, MBCT intervention and waiting list control condition.

		MBCT (n = 76)		Waiting list (n = 75)		Total (n = 151)	
		n	%	n	%	n	%
Age[a]	Mean (SD)	47.99 (10.59)		47.88 (12.02)		47.93 (11.29)	
	Range	24–74		20–81		20–81	
Gender[b]	Female	59	77,6	59	78,7	118	78,1
	Male	17	22,4	16	21,3	33	21,9
Marital status[b]	Single	17	22,4	20	26,7	37	24,5
	Living with partner	59	77,6	55	73,3	114	75,5
Race[b]	Dutch	71	93,4	74	98,7	145	96,0
	Other	5	6,6	1	1,3	6	4,0
Education[b]	Low	2	2,6	4	5,3	6	4,0
	Middle	21	27,6	25	33,3	46	30,5
	High	53	69,7	46	61,3	99	65,5
Employment[b]	Paid	53	69,7	48	64,0	101	66,9
	No paid	23	30,3	27	36,0	50	33,1
Diagnosis[b]	Mild MDE	3	3,9	1	1,3	4	2,6
	Moderate MDE	0	0,0	6	8,0	6	4,0

Note. MDE, major depressive episode.
[a] No significant differences between intervention and control condition (t-test with $P<0.05$).
[b] No significant differences between intervention and control condition (chi-square-test with $P<0.05$).

Table 2. Means and standard deviations for outcome measures and results of ANCOVA for intervention effects, and Cohen's d.

Measures	MBCT		Waiting list				
	(n = 76)		(n = 75)				
	M[a]	SD[a]	M[a]	SD[a]	F(df)[b]	*P*	*d*
Primary outcome							
CES-D baseline	15.62	7.86	16.46	8.32			
CES-D post-treatment	11.79	8.76	16.43	9.94	10.91(1)	0.001	0.50
CES-D follow-up[c]	11.77	8.25	13.60	8.88			
Secondary outcomes							
HADS-A baseline	7.96	3.40	8.57	3.58			
HADS-A post-treatment	6.14	3.52	8.22	3.89	12.42(1)	0.001	0.56
HADS-A follow-up[c]	4.88	2.88	6.54	3.84			
MHC-SF-EM baseline	3.15	0.95	3.15	0.78			
MHC-SF-EM post-treatment	3.46	0.85	3.19	0.88	5.32(1)	0.023	0.31
MHC-SF-EM follow-up[c]	3.54	0.95	3.61	0.78			
MHC-SF-SOC baseline	2.38	1.04	2.28	0.96			
MHC-SF-SOC post-treatment	2.72	1.08	2.49	1.05	1.62(1)	0.206	0.22
MHC-SF-SOC follow-up[c]	2.91	1.12	2.85	0.86			
MHC-SF-PSY baseline	2.92	0.89	2.96	1.00			
MHC-SF-PSY post-treatment	3.26	0.98	2.90	1.11	8.60(1)	0.004	0.34
MHC-SF-PSY follow-up[c]	3.37	0.93	3.41	0.89			

Note. ANCOVA, Analysis of covariance; CES-D, Center for Epidemiologic Studies - Depression.
Scale; HADS-A, Hospital Anxiety and Depression Scale - Anxiety subscale; MHC-SF, Mental Health Continuum - Short form; EM, emotional; SOC, social; PSY, psychological.
[a] Unadjusted condition means and standard deviations (SD).
[b] F-value, corrected for baseline values.
[c] Follow-up for intervention group and post-treatment for waiting list group.

baseline measurement [$t(75) = 5.58$, $p<0.001$], with a large effect size ($d = 0.63$).

The control group showed significant reductions on positive mental health after they received the intervention at T2 [social well-being $t(74) = 4.79$, $p<0.001$; emotional well-being $t(74) = 5.47$, $p<0.001$; psychological well-being $t(74) = 6.21$, $p< 0.001$].

Process measures

Table 3 shows all process measurements, the results of the ANOVA, and the effect-sizes. Compared to the control condition, participants in the intervention condition showed significant improvement in psychological flexibility and all mindfulness facets (except for FFMQ-Describe). The effects of the intervention condition on all process measures were maintained at follow-up compared to baseline measurement [psychological flexibility, $t(75) = 6.17$, $p<0.001$; FFMQ observing, $t(75) = 7.67$, $p<0.001$; FFMQ describing, $t(75) = 6.82$, $p<0.001$; FFMQ acting with awareness, $t(75) = 6.20$, $p<0.001$; FFMQ non-judging of inner experience, $t(75) = 6.46$, $p<0.001$; FFMQ non-reactivity to inner experience, $t(75) = 8.97$, $p<0.001$]. The effect sizes post-treatment were small to large ($d = 0.13$–0.84) and large at follow-up ($d = 0.71$–1.03).

Mediational analyses

Figure 2 shows the results of the first three steps of mediation. The FFMQ-Describe was excluded from the mediational analyses, having no significantly different effect in the ANOVA. The first step shows that the intervention condition had significantly decreased depressive symptoms at post-treatment, compared to the control condition. Step two shows that the intervention condition was significantly improved in psychological flexibility and mindfulness compared to the control condition. In step 3, all change scores of the process measures were significantly associated with the scores on the CES-D at post-treatment. In the last step of the mediational analysis, following Preacher & Hayes [42], results showed that the effect of the intervention on depressive symptoms was mediated by all process measures. Full mediation was found for improvement of psychological flexibility (direct effect $\beta = .145$, $p = 0.057$; indirect effect $\beta = -.387$, 95% CI 0.89–3.45), and mindfulness facets Observing (direct effect $\beta = 0.132$, $p = 0.106$; indirect effect $\beta = -.308$, 95% CI 0.98–3.60), and Non-reactivity to inner experience (direct effect $\beta = .135$, $p = 0.108$; indirect effect $\beta = -.275$, 95% CI 0.83–3.73). Partial mediation was found for improvement of mindfulness facets Acting with awareness (direct effect $\beta = .176$, $p = 0.044$; indirect effect $\beta = -.160$, 95% CI 0.18–2.84), and Non-judging of inner experience (direct effect $\beta = .208$, $p = .011$; indirect effect $\beta = -.158$, 95% CI 0.06–1.74).

Discussion

Main findings

To our best knowledge, this is the first study that evaluated MBCT as a public health intervention for adults with mild to moderate depressive symptomatology within a large pragmatic multi-site trial. The potential of offering MBCT to the community as a public mental health intervention is of importance, as the idea that MBCT is only effective in patients suffering from recurrent depression is superseded. In the present study the participants suffered from mild to moderate depressive symptoms but differed from severe clinical samples, as indicated by the substantially lower mean degree of severity of depressive symptoms as measured by the CES-D and the MINI. This corresponds to the nature and structure of the community-based MBCT, offered in our study. The results from this study indicate that MBCT as a public mental health intervention is effective in reducing depressive symptoms. We found a moderate effect size for depressive symptoms at post-treatment in comparison with the control group ($d = 0.50$). This effect size is comparable to the effect size of 0.42 that was found for psychological treatments on subthreshold depression [43]. The only studies of MBCT in community-based samples to our knowledge are from Kaviani et al. [20] and Cavanagh et al. [21]. Both conducted a randomized controlled trial in a sample of students comparing MBCT to a waiting list control group. They showed significant reductions of depressive and anxiety symptoms over time, with effect limited by low generalizability. Our study corroborates with these findings, further showing that MBCT seems to be effective in a population of adults with mild to moderate depressive symptomatology, and that MBCT can be used as a public mental health intervention in the community. Our finding that the results are maintained at 3 months follow-up is promising, but needs to be substantiated by longer follow-up measurements under controlled conditions. Offering a public mental health intervention in a positive framework might be less stigmatizing for participants with depressive symptomatology or minor depression [5]. MBCT focuses on the enhancement of promoting positive skills and therefore has the potential to offer an alternative to stigmatization.

The likelihood of a clinically significant change in depressive symptomatology in our study was substantially higher in the intervention condition compared to the waiting-list control group. As the presence of clinically relevant depressive symptoms is known to be an important risk factor for clinical depression [44], this outcome suggests that MBCT implemented as a public mental health intervention for adults with mild to moderate depressive symptomatology may decrease the risk of developing a MDE. It is shown that the effects on clinical cases of interventions for people with sub-clinical symptomatology are most prominently found after longer periods of time [45]. However this result needs to be corroborated with longer follow-up measurement and the use of diagnostic instruments as outcome measures.

Moreover, the MBCT intervention resulted in significant reductions in anxiety symptoms with large effect sizes post-treatment and at the 3-month follow-up. The effect of MBCT on anxiety symptoms are consistent with the meta-analysis by Vøllestad et al. [46], which found a large effect size ($g = 0.83$) for controlled studies of mindfulness and acceptance-based interventions for patients with anxiety symptoms. Strauss et al. [14] found no effects on anxiety symptom severity in their meta-analysis, applying a more stringent definition and excluding trials with interventions based on Acceptance and Commitment Therapy. Our study supports the findings of Vøllestad et al. [46], indicating that MBCT as a public mental health intervention could be effective in not only reducing depressive symptoms, but also in significantly reducing anxiety symptoms post-treatment and, even more substantially, at the 3-month follow-up. As anxiety symptoms often coexist with depression and may precipitate depression [47], these findings could indicate that the application of MBCT has the potential to further decrease the incidence of depression. However, this needs to be substantiated by further research.

The results also show a significant effect on positive mental health. It thus seems that MBCT has the potential not only to reduce psychological distress, but also to improve emotional, psychological, and social (only at follow-up) well-being as well. This finding confirms earlier studies that show that MBCT can promote well-being in patients with anxiety or depression [20,48]. The effects of MBCT on positive mental health are of importance.

Table 3. Means and standard deviations for process measures, results of ANOVA and Cohen's d for intervention effects.

Measures	MBCT		Waiting list				
	(n = 76)		(n = 75)				
Process outcomes	**M**	**SD**	**M**	**SD**	**F(df)**	*P*	*d*
AAQ-II baseline	44.28	8.42	43.03	7.86			
AAQ-II post-treatment	49.59	8.80	44.36	10.01	11.62(1)	0.001	0.56
AAQ-II follow-up[a]	50.93	9.04	48.91	8.89			
FFMQ - Observe baseline	24.77	5.58	25.21	5.77			
FFMQ - Observe post-treatment	27.98	5.15	25.28	6.29	8.34(1)	0.004	0.47
FFMQ - Observe follow-up[a]	28.46	4.54	29.07	4.74			
FFMQ - Describe baseline	26.39	6.14	27.43	6.89			
FFMQ - Describe post-treatment	28.60	5.56	27.80	6.35	0.68(1)	0.410	0.13
FFMQ - Describe follow-up[a]	29.24	6.03	29.77	6.76			
FFMQ - ActAware baseline	20.92	5.45	22.61	5.48			
FFMQ - ActAware post-treatment	25.31	5.53	22.67	6.05	7.86(1)	0.006	0.46
FFMQ - ActAware follow-up[a]	25.08	5.51	26.31	5.30			
FFMQ - NonJudge baseline	23.64	6.04	22.87	5.48			
FFMQ - NonJudge post-treatment	27.68	5.16	24.72	5.66	11.28(1)	0.001	0.55
FFMQ - NonJudge follow-up[a]	28.16	5.57	28.05	5.52			
FFMQ - NonReact baseline	19.73	4.29	19.31	4.29			
FFMQ - NonReact post-treatment	23.86	4.27	20.24	4.32	26.82(1)	0.000	0.84
FFMQ - NonReact follow-up[a]	24.24	4.04	23.54	4.22			

Note. AAQ-II, Acceptance and Action Questionnaire-II; ANOVA, Analysis of variance; FFMQ, Five Facet Mindfulness Questionnaire; Observe, observing; Describe, describing; ActAware, acting with awareness; NonJudge, non-judging of inner experience; NonReact, non-reactivity to inner experience.

[a] Follow-up for intervention group and post-treatment for waiting list group.

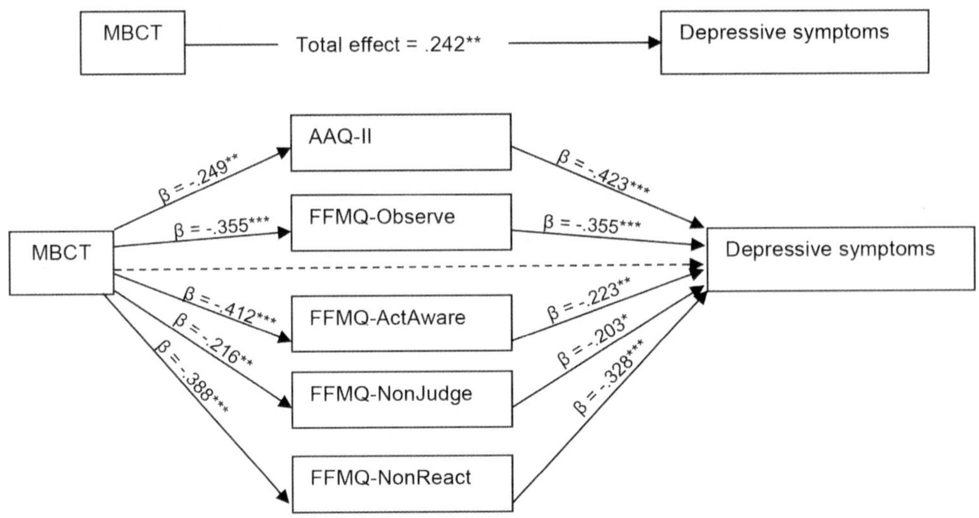

Figure 2. Mediation model of psychological flexibility and mindfulness as mediators. *Note.* AAQ-II, Acceptance and Action Questionnaire-II; FFMQ, Five Facet Mindfulness Questionnaire; Observe, observing; ActAware, acting with awareness; NonJudge, non-judging of inner experience; NonReact, non-reactivity to inner experience. *$P<0.05$; **$P<0.01$; ***$P<0.001$.

There is growing evidence that positive mental health and psychopathology are related but different dimensions of mental health [49], and that positive mental health is a protective factor against mental illnesses [6,7]. Several researchers suggest that aspects of psychological well-being (e.g. meaning, mastery, autonomy, goals) increase personal resilience [50–52]. The findings of this study suggest that adults with mild to moderate depressive symptomatology that participated in this public mental health intervention will be able to better cope with life adversity in the future. Moreover, offering a public mental health intervention in a positive framework might be less stigmatizing for participants with depressive symptomatology [5].

Mediational analyses show that the efficacy of MBCT compared to the control group on reducing post-treatment depressive symptoms is mediated by an increase in psychological flexibility and all mindfulness skills, except for the subscale 'describe'. Our results are in line with Kuyken et al. [53], which showed that 15-month follow-up level of depression were mediated by mindfulness skills and self-compassion. Developing a compassionate attitude toward one's own negative thoughts and feelings mediated the effect of MBCT on depressive symptoms and relapse. These findings are also in line with earlier studies that demonstrated the association between low psychological flexibility (i.e. experiential avoidance) and mindfulness and psychopathology [15,54,55]. The increase of psychological flexibility and mindfulness that mediated the effects of MBCT on depressive symptomatology suggests that participants have gained additional adaptive emotion regulation skills in response to negative affect-producing stressors [19,54].

The original MBCT training was designed for people with a history of depression and requires participants to commit to a 2.5-hour group session and to 45 to 60 minutes of mindfulness practice each day for 8 weeks [9]. The current study suggests that mindfulness exercises of a total of 15 minutes a day may be effective for adults with mild to moderate depressive symptomatology. Much of the research on the effects of MBCT is conducted based on a clinical population. For the non-clinical population, mostly still working and active socially, the required time commitment on a weekly and daily basis may be a barrier to effectively integrate exercises into daily life. Carmody and Baer [56] concluded in their review that the correlation between mean effect size and number of in-class hours was non-significant for both clinical and non-clinical samples. They suggested that adaptations that include less class time may be worthwhile for populations for whom reduction of psychological distress is an important goal and for whom longer time commitment may be a barrier to their ability or willingness to participate. Our findings are in line with a number of studies which have shown that short-term meditation can lead to more tolerance, and a lower distress of pain and perceived stress (e.g. [57,58]). For example, Klatt et al. [57] showed that a 60-minute training together with 20 minutes of daily practice of meditation can have a significant positive effect on levels of perceived stress in healthy working adults ($p = .0025$). Also, Cavanagh et al. [21] effectively adapted their online MBCT to a brief intervention with daily mindfulness meditation practices of 10 minutes. Our finding that an 11-week MBCT training with 15 minutes of daily mindfulness meditation practice can sufficiently and significantly reduce depressive symptomatology seems promising from a public mental health perspective and is in line with Carmody and Baer [56]. The finding that the community-based MBCT intervention was very positively evaluated by the participants (scoring 7.98 out of 10), and that very few people dropped out of the intervention or dropped out of the study, underscores the feasibility and the attractiveness of the intervention.

Limitations

Some limitations must also be acknowledged. First, for the design of the study as a waiting-list compared RCT, controlling for the influence of possible non-specific factors, such as attention and social interaction, was unlikely. Future research should use an active control intervention or an attention placebo controlled design to overcome this limitation. Secondly, the study used a short follow-up period of 3 months for which the follow-up was limited to a within group analysis. For ethical reasons, the time until the control group could receive the intervention was limited to 3 months. For future research, a longer follow-up (e.g. 1-year follow-up) is recommended to study the impact of MBCT on the incidence of depression. Third, the design was a pragmatic randomized controlled trial with self-referred participants, so the results of the study may have been influenced by a selection bias. All measures were self-report: no psychiatric diagnoses were available because participants were recruited from the general public. Generalizability of the findings to patients seeking treatment cannot be assumed. On the other hand, no restrictions were made to the level of depressive symptoms, as is customary to the procedures applied in community mental health centers. In this regard, the study was representative for standard general practice.

Conclusion

This study shows that MBCT as a public mental health intervention for adults with mild to moderate depressive symptomatology is effective by not only reducing depressive symptoms and anxiety symptoms, but also enhancing positive mental health and psychological flexibility. Furthermore, this study shows that the intervention is applicable and effective in a natural setting.

Supporting Information

Checklist S1 CONSORT Checklist.

File S1 Metadata file.

Protocol S1 Trial protocol English translation.

Protocol S2 Trial protocol original Dutch language.

Acknowledgments

The authors wish to thank the therapists and participants that took part in this study.

Author Contributions

Conceived and designed the experiments: WTP PAM MMV JJK ETB. Performed the experiments: JJK. Analyzed the data: WTP PAM MMV. Contributed reagents/materials/analysis tools: WTP PAM MMV JJK ETB. Wrote the paper: WTP PAM MMV JJK ETB.

References

1. Cuijpers P, Smit F, Oostenbrink J, De Graaf R, Ten Have M, et al. (2007) Economic costs of minor depression: A population-based study. Acta Psychiatr Scand 115: 229–236.
2. Muñoz RF, Cuijpers P, Smit F, Barrera AZ, Leykin Y (2010) Prevention of major depression. Annu Rev Clin Psychol 6: 181–212.
3. Jané-Llopis E, Barry M, Hosman C, Patel V (2005) Mental health promotion works: a review. Promot Educ Suppl 2: 9–25, 61, 67.
4. Cuijpers P, Beekman ATF, Reynolds CF (2012) Preventing depression: A global priority. JAMA 307: 1033–1034.
5. Cuijpers P, Van Straten A, Warmerdam L, Van Rooy MJ (2010) Recruiting participants for interventions to prevent the onset of depressive disorders: Possibile ways to increase participation rates. BMC Health Serv Res 10: 181.
6. Keyes CLM, Dhingra SS, Simoes EJ (2010) Change in level of positive mental health as a predictor of future risk of mental Illness. Am J Public Health 100: 2366–2371.
7. Wood AM, Joseph S (2010) The absence of positive psychological (eudemonic) well-being as a risk factor for depression: A ten year cohort study. J Affect Disord 122: 213–217.
8. Fledderus M, Bohlmeijer ET, Smit F, Westerhof GJ (2010) Mental health promotion as a new goal in public mental health care: A randomized controlled trial of an intervention enhancing psychological flexibility. Am J Public Health 100: 2372–2378.
9. Segal ZV, Williams JMG, Teasdale JD (2002) Mindfulness-based Cognitive Therapy for Depression: A New Approach to Preventing Relapse. New York: The Guilford Press.
10. Ma SH, Teasdale JD (2004) Mindfulness-Based Cognitive Therapy for Depression: Replication and Exploration of Differential Relapse Prevention Effects. J Consult Clin Psychol 72: 31–40.
11. Teasdale JD, Segal ZV, Williams JMG, Ridgewaya VA, Soulsby JM, et al. (2000) Prevention of relapse/recurrence in major depression by mindfulness-based cognitive therapy. J Consult Clin Psychol 68: 615–623.
12. Piet J & Hougaard E (2011) The effect of mindfulness-based cognitive therapy for prevention of relapse in recurrent major depressive disorder: A systematic review and meta-analysis. Clin Psychol Rev, 31: 1032–1040.
13. Williams JMG, Crane C, Barnhofer T, Brennan K, Duggan DS, et al. (2014) Mindfulness-based cognitive therapy for preventing relapse in recurrent depression: A randomized dismantling trial. J Consult Clin Psychol 82: 275–286.
14. Strauss C, Cavanagh K, Oliver A, Pettman D (2014) Mindfulness-based interventions for people diagnosed with a current episode of an anxiety or depressive disorder: A meta-analysis of randomised controlled trails. PLOS ONE 9:e96110. doi: 10.1371/journal.pone.0096110
15. Hayes SC, Luoma JB, Bond FW, Masuda A, Lillis J (2006) Acceptance and Commitment Therapy: Model, processes and outcomes. Behav Res Ther 44: 1–25.
16. Aldao A, Nolen-Hoeksema S (2010) Specificity of cognitive emotion regulation strategies: A transdiagnostic examination. Behav Res Ther 48: 974–983.
17. Kabat-Zinn J (1990) Full catastrophe living: Using the wisdom of your body and mind to face stress, pain and illness. New York: Delacorte.
18. Chiesa A, Serretti A (2011) Mindfulness based cognitive therapy for psychiatric disorders: A systematic review and meta-analysis. Psychiatry Res 187: 441–453.
19. Chiesa A, Anselmi R, Serretti A (2014) Psychological mechanisms of mindfulness-based interventions: What do we know? Holist Nurs Pract 28: 124–148.
20. Kaviani H, Hatami N, Javaheri F (2012) The impact of Mindfulness-based Cognitive Therapy (MBCT) on mental health and quality of life in a sub-clinically depressed population. Arch Gen Psychiatry 14: 21–28.
21. Cavanagh K, Strauss C, Cicconi F, Griffiths N, Wyper A, et al. (2012) A randomised controlled trial of a brief online mindfulness-based intervention. Behav Res Ther 51: 573–578.
22. Sheehan DV, Lecrubier Y, Sheehan KH, Amorim P, Janavs J, et al. (1998) The Mini-International Neuropsychiatric Interview (M.I.N.I.): the development and validation of a structured diagnostic psychiatric interview for DSM-IV and ICD-10. J Clin Psychiatry 59: 22–33.
23. Van Vliet IM, De Beurs E (2007) The MINI-International Neuropsychiatric Interview (M.I.N.I.). A brief structured diagnostic psychiatric interview for DSM-IV and ICD-10 psychiatric disorders [in Dutch]. Tijdschr Psychiatr 49: 393–397.
24. Radloff LS (1977) The CES-D scale, a self report depression scale for research in the general population. Appl Psychol Meas 1: 385–401.
25. Haringsma R, Engels GI, Beekman ATF, Spinhoven P (2004) The criterion validity of the Center for Epidemiological Studies Depression Scale (CES-D) in a sample of self-referred elders with depressive symptomatology. Int J Geriatr Psychiatry 19: 558–563.
26. Zigmond AS, Snaith RP (1983) The hospital anxiety and depression scale. Acta Psychiatr Scand 67: 361–370.
27. Spinhoven P, Ormel J, Sloekers PPA, Kempen GIJM, Speckens AEM, et al. (1997) A validation study of the hospital anxiety and depression scale (HADS) in different groups of Dutch subjects. Psychol Med 27: 363–370.
28. Keyes CLM, Wissing M, Potgieter JP, Temane M, Kruger A, et al. (2008) Evaluation of the mental health continuum-short form (MHC-SF) in Setswana-speaking South Africans. Clin Psychol Psychother 15: 181–192.
29. Lamers SMA, Westerhof GJ, Bohlmeijer ET, Ten Klooster PM, Keyes CLM (2011) Evaluating the psychometric properties of the mental health Continuum-Short Form (MHC-SF). J Clin Psychol 67: 99–110.
30. Bond FW, Hayes SC, Baer RA, Carpenter KM, Guenole N, et al. (2011) Preliminary Psychometric Properties of the Acceptance and Action Questionnaire-II: A Revised Measure of Psychological Inflexibility and Experiential Avoidance. Behav Ther 42: 676–688.
31. Fledderus M, Oude Voshaar MAH, ten Klooster PM, Bohlmeijer ET (2012) Further evaluation of the psychometric properties of the acceptance and action questionnaire-II. Psychol Assess 24: 925–936.
32. Baer RA, Smith GT, Hopkins J, Krietemeyer J, Toney L (2006) Using self-report assessment methods to explore facets of mindfulness. Assessment 13: 27–45.
33. Bohlmeijer E, Klooster PM, Fledderus M, Veehof M, Baer R (2011) Psychometric properties of the five facet mindfulness questionnaire in depressed adults and development of a short form. Assessment 18: 308–320.
34. Dempster AP, Laird NM, Rubin DB (1977) Maximum likelihood from incomplete data via the EM algorithm. J R Stat Soc Series B Stat Methodol 39: 1–38.

35. Morris SB, DeShon RP (2002) Combining effect size estimates in meta-analysis with repeated measures and independent-groups designs. Psychol Methods 7: 105–125.
36. Lipsey MW, Wilson DB (1993) The efficacy of psychological, educational, and behavioral treatment: Confirmation from meta-analysis. Am Psychol 48: 1181–1209.
37. Jacobson NS, Truax P (1991) Clinical significance: A statistical approach to defining meaningful change in psychotherapy research. J Consult Clin Psychol 59: 12–19.
38. Beekman ATF, Deeg DJH, Van Limbeek J, Braam AW, De Vries MZ, et al. (1997) Criterion validity of the Center for Epidemiologic Studies Depression scale (CES-D): Results from a community-based sample of older subjects in the Netherlands. Psychol Med 27: 231–235.
39. Smit F, Ederveen A, Cuijpers P, Deeg D, Beekman A (2006) Opportunities for cost-effective prevention of late-life depression: An epidemiological approach. Arch Gen Psychiatry 63: 290–296.
40. Cook RJ, Sackett DL (1995) The number needed to treat: A clinically useful measure of treatment effect. Br Med J 310: 452–454.
41. Baron RM, Kenny DA (1986) The moderator-mediator variable distinction in social psychological research: conceptual, strategic, and statistical considerations. J Pers Soc Psychol 51: 1173–1182.
42. Preacher KJ, Hayes AF (2008) Asymptotic and resampling strategies for assessing and comparing indirect effects in multiple mediator models. Behav Res Methods 40: 879–891.
43. Cuijpers P, Smit F, Van Straten A (2007) Psychological treatments of subthreshold depression: A meta-analytic review. Acta Psychiatr Scand 115: 434–441.
44. Cuijpers P, Smit F (2004) Subthreshold depression as a risk indicator for major depressive disorder: A systematic review of prospective studies. Acta Psychiatr Scand 109: 325–331.
45. Cuijpers P, Van Straten A, Smit F, Mihalopoulos C, Beekman A (2008) Preventing the onset of depressive disorders: A meta-analytic review of psychological interventions. Am J Psychiatry 165: 1272–1280.
46. Vøllestad J, Nielsen MB, Nielsen GH (2012) Mindfulness- and acceptance-based interventions for anxiety disorders: A systematic review and meta-analysis. Br J Clin Psychol 51: 239–260.
47. Horn PJ, Wuyek LA (2010) Anxiety disorders as a risk factor for subsequent depression. Int J Psychiatry Clin Pract 14: 244–247.
48. Kuyken W, Byford S, Taylor RS, Watkins E, Holden E, et al. (2008) Mindfulness-Based Cognitive Therapy to Prevent Relapse in Recurrent Depression. J Consult Clin Psychol 76: 966–978.
49. Lamers SMA, Westerhof GJ, Kovács V, Bohlmeijer ET (2012) Differential relationships in the association of the Big Five personality traits with positive mental health and psychopathology. J Res Pers 46: 517–524.
50. Fava GA, Tomba E (2009) Increasing psychological well-being and resilience by psychotherapeutic methods. J Pers 77: 1903–1934.
51. Ruini C, Fava GA (2012) Role of Well-Being Therapy in Achieving a Balanced and Individualized Path to Optimal Functioning. Clin Psychol Psychother 19: 291–304.
52. Ryff CD, Friedman EM, Morozink JA, Tsenkova V (2012) Psychological resilience in adulthood and later life: Implications for health. Annu Rev Gerontol Geriatr 32: 73–92.
53. Kuyken W, Watkins E, Holden E, White K, Taylor RS, et al. (2010) How does mindfulness-based cognitive therapy work? Behav Res Ther 48: 1105–1112.
54. Kashdan TB, Rottenberg J (2010) Psychological flexibility as a fundamental aspect of health. Clin Psychol Rev 30: 865–878.
55. McCarney RW, Schulz J, Grey AR (2012) Effectiveness of mindfulness-based therapies in reducing symptoms of depression: A meta-analysis. European Journal of Psychotherapy and Counselling 14: 279–299.
56. Carmody J, Baer RA (2009) How long does a mindfulness-based stress reduction program need to be? A review of class contact hours and effect sizes for psychological distress. J Clin Psychol 65: 627–638.
57. Klatt MD, Buckworth J, Malarkey WB (2009) Effects of low-dose mindfulness-based stress reduction (MBSR-ld) on working adults. Health Educ Behav 36: 601–614.
58. Liu X, Wang S, Chang S, Chen W, Si M (2012) Effect of Brief Mindfulness Intervention on Tolerance and Distress of Pain Induced by Cold-Pressor Task. Stress Health 29: 199–204.

Risk of Developing Depressive Disorders following Rheumatoid Arthritis: A Nationwide Population-Based Study

Shu-Li Wang[2]✤, Cheng-Ho Chang[1]✤, Li-Yu Hu[1], Shih-Jen Tsai[3,4], Albert C. Yang[3,4,5], Zi-Hong You[6,7]*

1 Department of Psychiatry, Kaohsiung Veterans General Hospital, Kaohsiung, Taiwan, **2** Department of Dental Laboratory Technology, Central Taiwan University of Science and Technology, Taichung, Taiwan, **3** Department of Psychiatry, Taipei Veterans General Hospital, Taipei, Taiwan, **4** School of Medicine, National Yang-Ming University, Taipei, Taiwan, **5** Center for Dynamical Biomarkers and Translational Medicine, National Central University, Chungli, Taiwan, **6** Division of Nephrology, Department of Internal Medicine, Taichung Veterans General Hospital, Chia-Yi Branch, Chia-Yi, Taiwan, **7** Institute of Medicine, Chung Shan Medical University, Taichung, Taiwan

Abstract

Background & Aims: To evaluate the risk of depressive disorders among rheumatoid arthritis (RA) by using the Taiwan National Health Insurance Research Database (NHIRD).

Methods: We conducted a retrospective study of a matched cohort of 18 285 participants (3 657 RA patients and 14 628 control patients) who were selected from the NHIRD. Patients were observed for a maximum of 10 years to determine the rates of newly diagnosed depressive disorders, and Cox regression was used to identify the risk factors associated with depressive disorders in RA patients.

Results: During the 10-year follow-up period, 205 (11.2 per 1000 person-years) RA patients and 384 (5.1 per 1000 person-years) control patients were diagnosed with depressive disorders. In RA patients, most depressive disorders (n = 163, 80%) developed with five years of being diagnosed with RA. The incidence risk ratio of depressive disorders between RA patients and control patients was 2.20 (95% confidence interval [CI], 1.84–2.61, $P<.001$). After adjusting for age, sex, and comorbidities, RA patients were 2.06 times more likely to develop depressive disorders (95% CI, 1.73–2.44, $P<.001$) compared with the control patients. Hyperthyroidism (HR = 1.67) was an independent risk factor for depressive disorders in patients with RA.

Conclusions: The likelihood of developing depressive disorders is greater among RA patients than among patients without RA. Symptoms of depression should be sought in patients with RA.

Editor: Melvin G. McInnis, University of Michigan, United States of America

Funding: This study was supported by a grant from the Taipei Veterans General Hospital (V101D-001-2) and SJT received the funding. The funder had no role in study design, data collection and analysis, decision to publish, or preparation of the manuscript.

Competing Interests: The authors have declared that no competing interests exist.

* Email: zihongyou@gmail.com

✤ These authors contributed equally to this work.

Introduction

Rheumatoid arthritis (RA) is a systemic chronic autoimmune disorder affecting primarily cartilage and bone. In addition, several organs such as lung, vessels, and kidney may be involved. In general, RA affects 0.5–1% of the population [1]. Despite of substantial advances in medical treatment, chronic pain, fatigue, and functional disability causes much psychosocial burden for these patients with RA [2,3].

Therefore, interest in the psychiatric aspects of rheumatoid arthritis has grown. Several studies have reported a high depression prevalence rate in patients with RA [4–12], and a significant correlation was observed among depression and increased pain levels in patients with RA [13]. Comorbid depression has been also shown to independently increase disability and a low quality of life in patients with RA [14–18]. In addition, depression has been demonstrated to be an independent risk factor for non-suicide mortality in patients with RA [19]. Hence, the depression symptoms should be examined in patients with RA because depression is a modifiable illness that is amenable to treatment.

However, in previous studies focusing on depression among patients with RA, depression was often evaluated by using rating scales, such as the Beck Depression Inventory or the Epidemiological Studies Depression Scale, rather than diagnosis by a psychiatrist [5–12]. The real prevalence rate of clinical depressive disorders in patients with RA remains unknown. In addition, the design of former studies prevented the temporal causal relationship between RA and depressive disorders from being clarified because the designs of these studies were almost cross-sectional studies [4–12]. Furthermore, whether there is an independent risk factor for newly diagnosed depressive disorders in patients with RA has never been studied.

We performed a population-based retrospective cohort study using data derived from the National Health Insurance (NHI) system in Taiwan. The purpose of our study was to determine whether RA was associated with an increased risk of clinical depressive disorders. Independent risk factors for newly diagnosed depressive disorders among the patients with RA were also identified.

Materials and Methods

Data Sources

Instituted in 1995, the NHI program is a mandatory health insurance program that offers comprehensive medical care coverage, including outpatient, inpatient, emergency, and traditional Chinese medicine, to all residents of Taiwan; the coverage rate is as high as 99% [20]. The NHI research database (NHIRD) contains comprehensive information regarding clinical visits, including prescription details and diagnostic codes based on the International Classification of Diseases, ninth revision, Clinical Modification (ICD-9-CM). The NHIRD is managed by the National Health Research Institutes (NHRI) and confidentiality is maintained according to the directives of the Bureau of the NHI. The data source for our study was the Longitudinal Health Insurance Database 2005 (LHID 2005), which is a dataset of NHIRD. Data for the LHID was collected by systematically and randomly sampling from the NHIRD; the database included the data of one million individuals. The NHRI of Taiwan reports that there were no significant differences in gender distribution, age distribution, or average insured payroll-related amount between the patients in the LHID and those in the original NHIRD [21]. Detailed information about the data source is provided on the NHRI website (http://nhird.nhri.org.tw). Comments, problems or requests about the data application could be sent to e-mail address at the NHRI (e-mail: nhird@nhri.org.tw).

Ethics Statement

The Institutional Review Board of the Taipei Veterans General Hospital approved this study (2013-03-035AC). Written consent from study patients was not obtained because the NHI dataset consists of de-identified secondary data for research purposes, and the Institutional Review Board of Taipei Veterans General Hospital issued a formal written waiver for the need for consent.

Study Population

Using data extracted from the LHID 2005, we conducted a retrospective cohort study of patients aged 20 years and older who were newly diagnosed with RA by a rheumatologist between January 1, 2000 and December 31, 2008. RA was defined as ICD-9-CM code: 714. We excluded patients who were diagnosed with depressive disorders (ICD-9-CM code: 296.2X-296.3X, 300.4, and 311.X) before enrollment. Insurance premiums, calculated according to the beneficiary's total income, were used to estimate monthly income. Monthly income was grouped into low income (monthly income <20,000 New Taiwan Dollar [NTD]), median income (20,000 NTD≤monthly income <40,000 NTD), and high income (monthly income ≥40,000 NTD). Urbanization was divided into three groups: urban, suburban, and rural. Urbanization and monthly income levels were used to represent socioeconomic status. For each cirrhotic patient included in the final cohort, 4 age-, sex-, and enrolment-date-matched control patients who were not diagnosed with rheumatoid arthritis or depressive disorder were randomly selected from the LHID 2005. All RA and control patients were observed until diagnosed with a depressive disorder by a psychiatrist, death, withdrawal from the NHI system, or December 31, 2009. The primary clinical outcome assessed was psychiatrist-diagnosed depressive disorder.

Statistical Analyses

The incidence of newly diagnosed depressive disorders in the RA and control patients, stratified by gender and age (equal or older than 60 years old or younger than 60 years old) was calculated. Independent *t*-tests and chi-squared tests were used to examine the differences in the demographic characteristics between the RA and control patients.

A Cox proportional-hazards regression model was used to identify variables that predicted depressive disorder in the RA and control patients, and in the RA patients only. Control variables, such as age; sex; common comorbidities, including hypertension, diabetes mellitus, dyslipidemia, coronary artery disease, congestive heart failure, cirrhosis, hyperthyroidism, hypothyroidism, cerebrovascular disease, and malignancy; urbanization; and monthly income were included as covariates in the univariate model. Factors that demonstrated a moderately significant statistical relationship in the univariate analysis ($P<.1$) were entered by forward selection in a multivariate Cox proportional-hazards regression model [22].

The Perl programming language (version 5.12.2) was used to extract and compute data. The Microsoft SQL Server 2005 (Microsoft Corp., Redmond, WA, USA) was used for data linkage, processing, and control sampling. IBM SPSS (version 19.0 for Windows; IBM Corp., New York, NY, USA) and SAS statistical software (version 9.2; SAS Institute Inc., Cary, NC, USA) were used to perform all statistical analyses. The comparisons resulting in a P-value of less than .05 were considered to indicate a statistically significant relationship.

Results

Participant Selection (Figure 1)

The sample comprised 3657 RA patients and 14 628 control patients without depression, among whom 72.8% were female. The median age at enrollment was 51 years (interquartile range [IQR], 41–61 years), and the median follow-up period was 4.72 years (IQR, 2.59–7.42 years) for RA patients and 4.92 years (IQR, 2.69.21–7.55 years) for control patients. The comorbidities, including hypertension, diabetes mellitus, dyslipidemia, congestive heart failure, hyperthyroidism, hypothyroidism, and cerebrovascular disease were more common in RA patients than control patients. The comparisons of the demographic and clinical variables between the RA and control patients are presented in Table 1.

Incidence Rate of Depressive Disorders

During the study period, 205 (11.2 per 1000 person-years) RA patients and 384 (5.1 per 1000 person-years) control patients were diagnosed with depressive disorders. The incidence risk ratio (IRR)

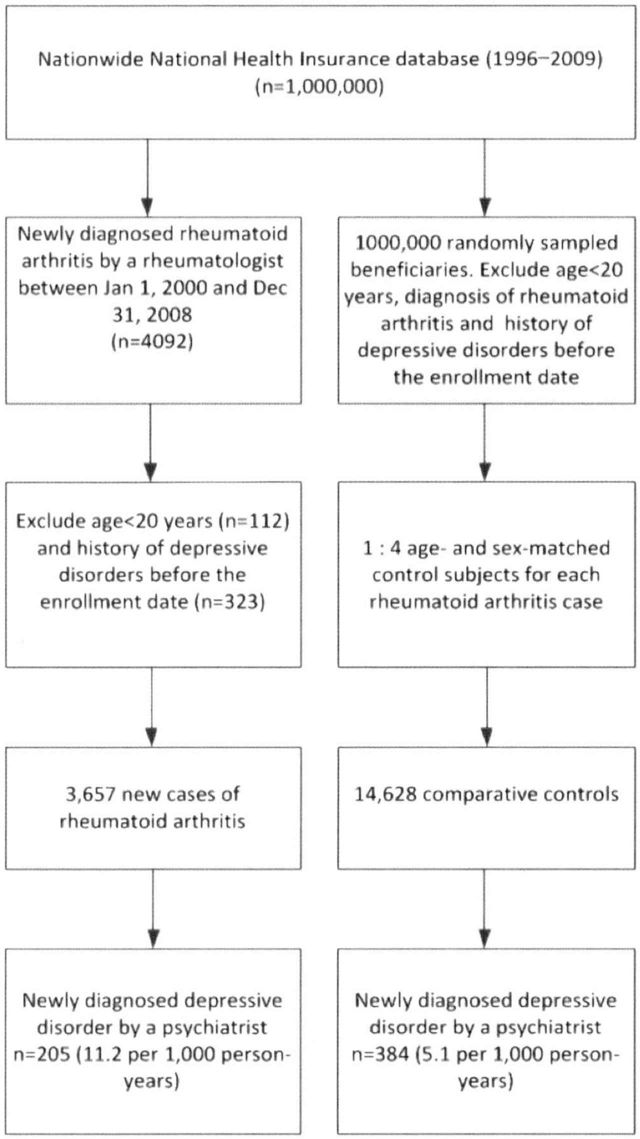

Figure 1. Flow chart of sample selection criteria.

of depressive disorders between RA patients and control patients was 2.20 (95% CI, 1.84–2.61, $P<.001$). When stratified by gender and age, the IRR of depressive disorders was still higher in the RA patients than in the control patients. The results are shown in Table 2. In RA patients, most depressive disorders (n = 163, 80%) developed with five years of being diagnosed with RA.

Rheumatoid arthritis on Risks of Clinical Depression

After adjusting for age, sex, comorbidities, urbanization, and monthly income, the hazard ratio (HR) for developing depressive disorders during the follow-up period was 2.06 times (95% CI, 1.73–2.44, $P<.001$) greater for the RA patients than for the control patients (Table 3 and figure 2).

Risks Factors for Depression in Rheumatoid arthritis Patients

In Table 4, we applied univariate analysis to predict the development of depressive disorders in the RA cohort, and the results demonstrated that the female sex (HR = 1.37, 95% CI, 0.98–1.90, $P = .063$), diabetes mellitus (HR = 1.39, 95% CI, 1.00–1.94, $P = .051$), hyperthyroidism (HR = 1.79, 95% CI, 1.09–2.94, $P = .022$), cerebrovascular disease (HR = 1.55, 95% CI, 0.99–2.41, $P = .054$) and high income (HR = 0.56, 95% CI, 0.34–0.94, $P = .028$) are significant prognostic factors. The multivariate analysis confirmed that hyperthyroidism (HR = 1.67, 95% CI, 1.01–2.76, $P = .045$) was an independent risk factor for depressive disorder in the patients with RA.

Discussion

The key findings of our study are that (1) the incidence rate of depressive disorders in patients with RA was 11.2 per 1000 person-year; (2) the risk of clinical depressive disorders was higher when patients with RA (HR = 2.06) and most depressive disorders (n = 163, 80%) developed within five years of being diagnosed with RA; (3) hyperthyroidism (HR = 1.67) might be an independent risk factor for depressive disorders among patients with RA.

The strengths of this study are the large sample size, the long follow-up period, and the diagnosis of clinical depressive disorders and rheumatoid arthritis by specialists. In addition, our study design involved an unbiased participant selection process. Because participation in the NHI is mandatory and all residents of Taiwan can access low-cost health care, referral bias is low and follow-up compliance is high.

Consistent with the results of previous studies [4–11], we found that the risk of depression in RA patients was higher than that in the non-RA control patients. Chronic inflammation is one of the possible causes. RA is a chronic inflammatory disease, and accumulating evidence implicates inflammation as a critical mediator in the pathophysiology of depressive disorders [23–26]. In the Cardiovascular Health Study of 4 268 patients, a significant association was noted between high levels of C-reactive protein and depression symptoms, even after adjusting for confounding factors [27]. Administration of cytokines including tumor necrosis factor-α in animal and human studies has been shown to induce depressive symptoms, including sleep disturbance, anorexia, loss of interest and mood disturbances [28]. Potential involved mechanisms include direct effects of pro-inflammatory cytokines on monoamine, dysregulation of the hypothalamic-pituitary-adrenal axis, impaired neuroplasticity and structural and functional brain changes [29].

The symptoms of RA such as pain and fatigue may be another possible cause for higher risk of depression in RA patients than that in the non-RA control patients. Symptoms of RA such as pain and fatigue may impair patients' function and quality of life and influence patients' perception of health status, and make the patients more prone to develop depressive symptoms [12,30]. RA patients often suffered pain and pain intensity was more clearly related to disability in RA patients [31]. Several studies have shown that chronic pain was an important risk factor for depression and suicidal behavior [32–34]. Previous study has shown that the degree of depression in RA patients varies in proportion to the level of pain [31].

Furthermore, physical comorbidities might be another possible cause for a higher prevalence of depressive disorder in RA patients. Our findings are consistent with the results of previous studies that found that a higher percentage of many physical comorbidities in RA patients, such as hypertension [35], diabetes mellitus [36], congestive heart failure [37], hypothyroidism [38], and cerebrovascular disease [39]. All of above diseases had been proposed to be related with increased the risk of depression [40–43].

Table 1. Baseline Characteristics of Patients with and without Rheumatoid Arthritis.

Demographic data	Patients with rheumatoid arthritis		Patients without rheumatoid arthritis		P-value
	n=3,657		n=14,628		
	n	%	n	%	
Age (years) (interquartile range)	51 (41–61)		51 (41–61)		
≥60	961	26.3	3,851	26.3	.966
<60	2,696	73.7	10,777	73.7	.
Sex					
Male	993	27.2	3972	27.2	.999
Female	2,664	72.8	10,656	72.8	.
Comorbidities					
Hypertension	1,186	32.4	4,032	27.6	<.001
Diabetes mellitus	687	18.8	2,305	15.8	<.001
Dyslipidemia	1,098	30.0	3,002	20.5	<.001
Coronary artery disease	45	1.2	168	1.1	.673
Congestive heart failure	172	4.7	533	3.6	.004
Cirrhosis	62	1.0	198	1.4	.117
Hyperthyroidism	219	6.0	477	3.3	<.001
Hypothyroidism	107	2.9	178	1.2	<.001
Cerebrovascular disease	316	8.6	929	6.4	<.001
Malignant neoplasms	96	2.6	338	2.3	.274
Degree of urbanization					
urban	2,238	61.2	8,787	60.1	.435
suburban	1,040	28.4	4,268	29.2	
rural	326	8.9	1,362	9.3	
Income group					
low income	1,731	47.3	7,151	48.9	.001
median income	1,430	39.1	5,820	39.8	
high income	496	13.6	1,657	11.3	
Follow-up years (median)	4.72 (2.59–7.42)		4.92 (2.69–7.55)		.004

Finally, long-term drug use in RA patients and inevitable side effects of various medications might also impaired quality of life in RA patients and increased the risk of depression in RA patients [44,45]. Previous study showed that disease-modifying drugs used for RA patients had been related to higher rates of depression, and suicidal ideation among RA patients, serving as an alert to the importance of considering also this factors in therapeutic decisions [46].

Table 2. Incidence of Depressive Disorders in Patients with and without Rheumatoid Arthritis.

	Patients with rheumatoid arthritis		Patients without rheumatoid arthritis		Risk ratio (95% CI)	P value
	No. of Depressive disorders	Per 1 000 person-years	No. of Depressive disorders	Per 1 000 person-years		
Total	205	11.2	384	5.1	2.20 (1.84–2.61)	<.001
Age						
≥60	49	2.8	109	1.4	1.85 (1.29–2.61)	<.001
<60	156	8.5	275	3.7	2.33 (1.91–2.85)	<.001
Sex						
Male	45	2.5	88	1.2	2.10 (1.44–3.05)	<.001
Female	160	8.7	296	3.9	2.22 (1.82–2.70)	<.001

CI indicates confidence interval.

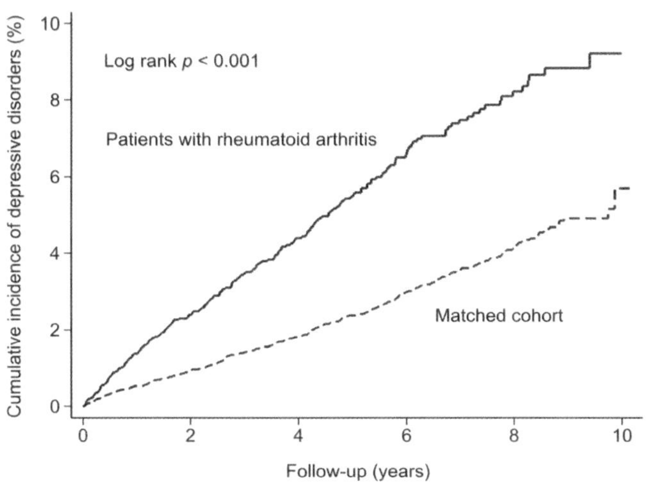

Figure 2. Cumulative incidence of depressive disorders in patients with rheumatoid arthritis (RA) and matched cohort.

According to previous studies, conservative estimates of the prevalence of depressive disorder among patients with RA ranged between 13 and 20% [13,45,47]. This prevalence rate was much higher than the rate calculated in this study. The possible reason for these two discrete findings might be partly due to difference in the methods of assessing depression [13]. In the most previous studies regarding RA and depression [5–12], rating scales, such as the Beck depression inventory, rather than diagnosis by a psychiatrist, were used for evaluation of depression in those studies. People who were recorded as depressed on rating scales may not meet the diagnostic criteria for clinical depressive disorders. However, depressive disorders in RA patients may be underdiagnosed in our study because symptoms of depressive disorders may mimic symptoms of RA, such as easily fatigue, sleep disturbance, and loss of interests with multiple somatic complaints. Physicians may have viewed RA patients' depressive symptoms as physical discomforts caused by RA and overlooked these symptoms, rather than viewing these symptoms as warning signs of depressive disorder.

There has been some discussion in the literature regarding the factors that influence the development of depression in patients with RA [48–50]. However, whether there is certain physical comorbidity as an independent risk factor for new-onset depressive disorders following a RA diagnosis has never been studied. In our study, we found that hyperthyroidism was an independent risk factor for depressive disorders in patients with RA. Studies have shown that mood disturbance, especially depressive disorders, often accompanies hyperthyroidism patients [51–54]. Alterations in components of the hypothalamic-pituitary-thyroid axis have been documented for the development of depressive disorder among patients with hyperthyroidism [53]. In addition, functional impairment caused by hyperthyroidism might play a vital role in causing psychological distresses including depressive disorders among patients with hyperthyroidism [55].

Table 3. Analyses of Risk Factors for Depressive Disorders in Patients with and without Rheumatoid Arthritis.

Predictive variables	Univariate analysis		Multivariate analysis	
	HR (95% CI)	*P* value	HR (95% CI)	*P* value
Rheumatoid arthritis	2.20 (1.86–2.60)	<.001	2.06 (1.73–2.44)	<.001
Age (<60 = 1, ≥60 = 0)	0.91 (0.76–1.10)	.327		
Sex (female = 1, male = 0)	1.34 (1.10–1.62)	.003	1.29 (1.06–1.57)	.011
Comorbidities				
Hypertension	1.39 (1.17–1.65)	<.001	1.00 (0.82–1.21)	.957
Diabetes mellitus	1.63 (1.34–1.99)	<.001	1.20 (0.96–1.50)	.116
Dyslipidemia	1.77 (1.48–2.12)	<.001	1.39 (1.14–1.71)	.001
Coronary artery disease	1.32 (0.62–2.77)	<.001	1.00 (0.47–2.13)	.995
Congestive heart failure	1.16 (0.75–1.79)	.505		
Cirrhosis	2.33 (1.39–3.89)	.001	1.91 (1.14–3.20)	.014
Hyperthyroidism	2.24 (1.61–3.12)	<.001	1.79 (1.27–2.52)	.001
Hypothyroidism	1.75 (1.01–1.76)	<.001	1.01 (0.57–1.78)	.973
Cerebrovascular disease	2.13 (1.65–2.76)	<.001	1.78 (1.36–2.33)	<.001
Malignant neoplasms	1.16 (0.65–2.05)	.622		
Degree of urbanization				
urban	Reference			
suburban	0.91 (0.76–1.10)	.319		
rural	0.85 (0.63–1.14)	.286		
Income group				
low income	Reference		Reference	
median income	0.94 (0.79–1.12)	.484	0.98 (0.83–1.17)	.847
high income	0.69 (0.51–0.92)	.013	0.75 (0.56–1.02)	.063

HR indicates hazard ratio; CI indicates confidence interval.

Table 4. Analyses of Risk factors for Depressive Disorders in Rheumatoid Arthritis Patients.

Predictive variables	Univariate analysis		Multivariate analysis	
	HR (95% CI)	*P* value	HR (95% CI)	*P* value
Age (<60 = 1, ≥60 = 0)	1.07 (0.77–1.47)	.701		
Sex (female = 1, male = 0)	1.37 (0.98–1.90)	.063	1.28 (0.92–1.79)	.146
Comorbidities				
Hypertension	1.13 (0.84–1.51)	.429		
Diabetes mellitus	1.39 (1.00–1.94)	.051	1.27 (0.90–1.78)	.171
Dyslipidemia	1.23 (0.91–1.66)	.174		
Coronary artery disease	0.97 (0.24–3.92)	.968		
Congestive heart failure	1.11 (0.57–2.16)	.766		
Cirrhosis	1.90 (0.85–4.29)	.120		
Hyperthyroidism	1.79 (1.09–2.94)	.022	1.67 (1.01–2.76)	.045
Hypothyroidism	1.34 (0.63–2.84)	.452		
Cerebrovascular disease	1.55 (0.99–2.41)	.054	1.46 (0.93–2.29)	.098
Malignant neoplasms	1.04 (0.43–2.54)	.925		
Degree of urbanization				
urban	Reference			
suburban	0.96 (0.71–1.31)	.793		
rural	0.78 (0.46–1.33)	.365		
Income group				
low income	reference		reference	
median income	1.04 (0.78–1.38)	.808	1.08 (0.81–1.44)	.603
high income	0.56 (0.34–0.94)	.028	0.62 (0.37–1.04)	.068

HR indicates hazard ratio; CI indicates confidence interval.

Our findings have certain limitations. Information regarding the family history of psychiatric disorders [56,57], lifestyle factors [58], self-perceived health, disability [59], and environmental factors (life stresses, such as recent major life event, domestic violence, childhood trauma, and social support) [60–63] are not included in the NHIRD, and all of which might be associated with the risk of development of depressive disorders. In addition, the severity of RA could not be ascertained. Whether the severity of RA influences the risk of developing depressive disorders warrants further study, despite previous studies indicating that disease activity of RA alone does not equate with depressive symptoms in RA patients reliably [47]. Furthermore, physicians may view RA patients' depressive symptoms as physical discomforts caused by RA and overlook these symptoms. Therefore, in our study, the incidence of clinical depressive disorders may be underestimated.

This population-based retrospective cohort study demonstrated that the risk of developing depressive disorders is higher among RA patients than those without RA, and that RA is an independent risk factor for depressive disorders. Hyperthyroidism is an independent risk factor for developing depressive disorders among patients with RA. Because depression was related to impairing the quality of life of RA patients, and depressive disorder is modifiable illness that is amenable to treatment, symptoms of depression should be sought in patients with RA. Future population-based prospective studies are needed to further investigate the association between RA and the risk of developing depressive disorders.

Acknowledgments

We thank Stephen Chow, Huei-Sing Chang, Cheng-Fang Hong, Chun-Hsin Hu, and Ai-Ling Hu for technical assistance. The study is based in part on data from the National Health Insurance Research Database, provided by the Bureau of National Health Insurance, Department of Health and managed by National Health Research Institutes. The interpretation and conclusions contained herein do not represent those of the Bureau of National Health Insurance, Department of Health or National Health Research Institutes.

Author Contributions

Conceived and designed the experiments: SLW LYH ZHY. Performed the experiments: SLW LYH SJT ACY. Analyzed the data: SLW LYH CHC. Contributed reagents/materials/analysis tools: SJT ACY. Contributed to the writing of the manuscript: SLW LYH ZHY.

References

1. Scott DL, Wolfe F, Huizinga TW (2010) Rheumatoid arthritis. Lancet 376: 1094–1108.
2. Rezvani A, Ayture L, Arslan M, Kurt E, Eroglu Demir S, et al. (2014) Affective temperaments in patients with rheumatoid arthritis. Int J Rheum Dis 17: 34–38.
3. Cross M, Smith E, Hoy D, Carmona L, Wolfe F, et al. (2014) The global burden of rheumatoid arthritis: estimates from the Global Burden of Disease 2010 study. Ann Rheum Dis.
4. Ahles TA, Khan SA, Yunus MB, Spiegel DA, Masi AT (1991) Psychiatric status of patients with primary fibromyalgia, patients with rheumatoid arthritis, and

subjects without pain: a blind comparison of DSM-III diagnoses. Am J Psychiatry 148: 1721–1726.
5. Callahan LF, Kaplan MR, Pincus T (1991) The Beck Depression Inventory, Center for Epidemiological Studies Depression Scale (CES-D), and General Well-Being Schedule depression subscale in rheumatoid arthritis. Criterion contamination of responses. Arthritis Care Res 4: 3–11.
6. Belza BL (1995) Comparison of self-reported fatigue in rheumatoid arthritis and controls. J Rheumatol 22: 639–643.
7. Serbo B, Jajic I (1991) Relationship of the functional status, duration of the disease and pain intensity and some psychological variables in patients with rheumatoid arthritis. Clin Rheumatol 10: 419–422.
8. Kasl SV, Cobb S (1969) The intrafamilial transmission of rheumatoid arthritis. V. Differences between rheumatoid arthritics and controls on selected personality variables. J Chronic Dis 22: 239–258.
9. Scheidt CE, Mueller-Becsangele J, Hiller K, Hartmann A, Goldacker S, et al. (2014) Self-reported symptoms of pain and depression in primary fibromyalgia syndrome and rheumatoid arthritis. Nord J Psychiatry 68: 88–92.
10. Allaire SH, Meenan RF, Anderson JJ (1991) The impact of rheumatoid arthritis on the household work performance of women. Arthritis Rheum 34: 669–678.
11. Lisitsyna TA, Zeltyn AE, Vel'tishchev D, Kovalevskaia OB, Seravina OF, et al. (2012) [Cognitive impairment and anxiety-depressive disorders in patients with rheumatoid arthritis]. Zh Nevrol Psikhiatr Im S S Korsakova 112: 96–103.
12. Coskun B, Coskun BN, Atis G, Ergenekon E, Dilek K (2014) Evaluation of sexual function in women with rheumatoid arthritis. Urol J 10: 1081–1087.
13. Dickens C, McGowan L, Clark-Carter D, Creed F (2002) Depression in rheumatoid arthritis: a systematic review of the literature with meta-analysis. Psychosom Med 64: 52–60.
14. Lowe B, Willand L, Eich W, Zipfel S, Ho AD, et al. (2004) Psychiatric comorbidity and work disability in patients with inflammatory rheumatic diseases. Psychosom Med 66: 395–402.
15. Lisitsyna TA, Veltishchev DY, Gerasimov AN, Seravina OF, Kovalevskaya OB, et al. (2013) [The magnitude of fatigue and its association with depression, pain, and inflammatory activity in rheumatoid arthritis]. Ter Arkh 85: 8–15.
16. van den Hoek J, Roorda LD, Boshuizen HC, van Hees J, Rupp I, et al. (2013) Long-term physical functioning and its association with somatic comorbidity and comorbid depression in patients with established rheumatoid arthritis: a longitudinal study. Arthritis Care Res (Hoboken) 65: 1157–1165.
17. Katz PP, Yelin EH (1994) Life activities of persons with rheumatoid arthritis with and without depressive symptoms. Arthritis Care Res 7: 69–77.
18. Wolfe F, Hawley DJ (1993) The relationship between clinical activity and depression in rheumatoid arthritis. J Rheumatol 20: 2032–2037.
19. Ang DC, Choi H, Kroenke K, Wolfe F (2005) Comorbid depression is an independent risk factor for mortality in patients with rheumatoid arthritis. J Rheumatol 32: 1013–1019.
20. Wu CY, Chen YJ, Ho HJ, Hsu YC, Kuo KN, et al. (2012) Association between nucleoside analogues and risk of hepatitis B virus-related hepatocellular carcinoma recurrence following liver resection. JAMA 308: 1906–1914.
21. Database. NHIR National Health Research Institutes.
22. Bednarek PH, Creinin MD, Reeves MF, Cwiak C, Espey E, et al. (2011) Immediate versus delayed IUD insertion after uterine aspiration. N Engl J Med 364: 2208–2217.
23. Lu Y, Feng L, Feng L, Nyunt MS, Yap KB, et al. (2013) Systemic inflammation, depression and obstructive pulmonary function: a population-based study. Respir Res 14: 53.
24. Pasco JA, Nicholson GC, Williams LJ, Jacka FN, Henry MJ, et al. (2010) Association of high-sensitivity C-reactive protein with de novo major depression. Br J Psychiatry 197: 372–377.
25. D'Mello C, Swain MG (2011) Liver-brain inflammation axis. Am J Physiol Gastrointest Liver Physiol 301: G749–761.
26. Madeeh Hashmi A, Awais Aftab M, Mazhar N, Umair M, Butt Z (2013) The fiery landscape of depression: A review of the inflammatory hypothesis. Pak J Med Sci 29: 877–884.
27. Kop WJ, Gottdiener JS, Tangen CM, Fried LP, McBurnie MA, et al. (2002) Inflammation and coagulation factors in persons >65 years of age with symptoms of depression but without evidence of myocardial ischemia. Am J Cardiol 89: 419–424.
28. Shimbo D, Chaplin W, Crossman D, Haas D, Davidson KW (2005) Role of depression and inflammation in incident coronary heart disease events. Am J Cardiol 96: 1016–1021.
29. Rosenblat JD, Cha DS, Mansur RB, McIntyre RS (2014) Inflamed moods: A review of the interactions between inflammation and mood disorders. Prog Neuropsychopharmacol Biol Psychiatry.
30. Katz PP, Yelin EH (2001) Activity loss and the onset of depressive symptoms: do some activities matter more than others? Arthritis Rheum 44: 1194–1202.
31. Peck JR, Smith TW, Ward JR, Milano R (1989) Disability and depression in rheumatoid arthritis. A multi-trait, multi-method investigation. Arthritis Rheum 32: 1100–1106.
32. Hassett AL, Aquino JK, Ilgen MA (2014) The risk of suicide mortality in chronic pain patients. Curr Pain Headache Rep 18: 436.
33. Hooley JM, Franklin JC, Nock MK (2014) Chronic pain and suicide: understanding the association. Curr Pain Headache Rep 18: 435.
34. Li JX (2014) Pain and depression comorbidity: A preclinical perspective. Behav Brain Res.
35. Manavathongchai S, Bian A, Rho YH, Oeser A, Solus JF, et al. (2013) Inflammation and hypertension in rheumatoid arthritis. J Rheumatol 40: 1806–1811.
36. Su CC, Chen Ie C, Young FN, Lian Ie B (2013) Risk of diabetes in patients with rheumatoid arthritis: a 12-year retrospective cohort study. J Rheumatol 40: 1513–1518.
37. Nicola PJ, Maradit-Kremers H, Roger VL, Jacobsen SJ, Crowson CS, et al. (2005) The risk of congestive heart failure in rheumatoid arthritis: a population-based study over 46 years. Arthritis Rheum 52: 412–420.
38. Raterman HG, van Halm VP, Voskuyl AE, Simsek S, Dijkmans BA, et al. (2008) Rheumatoid arthritis is associated with a high prevalence of hypothyroidism that amplifies its cardiovascular risk. Ann Rheum Dis 67: 229–232.
39. Wolfe F, Freundlich B, Straus WL (2003) Increase in cardiovascular and cerebrovascular disease prevalence in rheumatoid arthritis. J Rheumatol 30: 36–40.
40. Johansen A, Holmen J, Stewart R, Bjerkeset O (2012) Anxiety and depression symptoms in arterial hypertension: the influence of antihypertensive treatment. the HUNT study, Norway. Eur J Epidemiol 27: 63–72.
41. Freedland KE, Rich MW, Skala JA, Carney RM, Davila-Roman VG, et al. (2003) Prevalence of depression in hospitalized patients with congestive heart failure. Psychosom Med 65: 119–128.
42. Gothe F, Enache D, Wahlund LO, Winblad B, Crisby M, et al. (2012) Cerebrovascular diseases and depression: epidemiology, mechanisms and treatment. Panminerva Med 54: 161–170.
43. Guimaraes JM, de Souza Lopes C, Baima J, Sichieri R (2009) Depression symptoms and hypothyroidism in a population-based study of middle-aged Brazilian women. J Affect Disord 117: 120–123.
44. Pollard L, Choy EH, Scott DL (2005) The consequences of rheumatoid arthritis: quality of life measures in the individual patient. Clin Exp Rheumatol 23: S43–52.
45. Sheehy C, Murphy E, Barry M (2006) Depression in rheumatoid arthritis–underscoring the problem. Rheumatology (Oxford) 45: 1325–1327.
46. Pinho de Oliveira Ribeiro N, Rafael de Mello Schier A, Ornelas AC, Pinho de Oliveira CM, Nardi AE, et al. (2013) Anxiety, depression and suicidal ideation in patients with rheumatoid arthritis in use of methotrexate, hydroxychloroquine, leflunomide and biological drugs. Compr Psychiatry 54: 1185–1189.
47. Dickens C, Creed F (2001) The burden of depression in patients with rheumatoid arthritis. Rheumatology (Oxford) 40: 1327–1330.
48. Ramjeet J, Koutantji M, Barrett EM, Scott DG (2005) Coping and psychological adjustment in recent-onset inflammatory polyarthritis: the role of gender and age. Rheumatology (Oxford) 44: 1166–1168.
49. Covic T, Adamson B, Spencer D, Howe G (2003) A biopsychosocial model of pain and depression in rheumatoid arthritis: a 12-month longitudinal study. Rheumatology (Oxford) 42: 1287–1294.
50. Curtis R, Groarke A, Coughlan R, Gsel A (2005) Psychological stress as a predictor of psychological adjustment and health status in patients with rheumatoid arthritis. Patient Educ Couns 59: 192–198.
51. Placidi GP, Boldrini M, Patronelli A, Fiore E, Chiovato L, et al. (1998) Prevalence of psychiatric disorders in thyroid diseased patients. Neuropsychobiology 38: 222–225.
52. Kathol RG, Turner R, Delahunt J (1986) Depression and anxiety associated with hyperthyroidism: response to antithyroid therapy. Psychosomatics 27: 501–505.
53. Musselman DL, Nemeroff CB (1996) Depression and endocrine disorders: focus on the thyroid and adrenal system. Br J Psychiatry Suppl: 123–128.
54. Demet MM, Ozmen B, Deveci A, Boyvada S, Adiguzel H, et al. (2002) Depression and anxiety in hyperthyroidism. Arch Med Res 33: 552–556.
55. Lee H, Roh HS, Yoon JS, Lee SY (2010) Assessment of quality of life and depression in Korean patients with Graves' ophthalmopathy. Korean - J Ophthalmol 24: 65–72.
56. Kaur G, Tee GH, Ariaratnam S, Krishnapillai AS, China K (2013) Depression, anxiety and stress symptoms among diabetics in Malaysia: a cross sectional study in an urban primary care setting. BMC Fam Pract 14: 69.
57. Tenev VT, Robinson RG, Jorge RE (2009) Is family history of depression a risk factor for poststroke depression? Meta-analysis. Am J Geriatr Psychiatry 17: 276–280.
58. Psaltopoulou T, Sergentanis TN, Panagiotakos DB, Sergentanis IN, Kosti R, et al. (2013) Mediterranean diet and stroke, cognitive impairment, depression: A meta-analysis. Ann Neurol.
59. Becofsky K, Baruth M, Wilcox S (2013) Physical functioning, perceived disability, and depressive symptoms in adults with arthritis. Arthritis 2013: 525761.
60. Monroe SM, Slavich GM, Gotlib IH (2013) Life stress and family history for depression: The moderating role of past depressive episodes. J Psychiatr Res.
61. Chuang CH, Cattoi AL, McCall-Hosenfeld JS, Camacho F, Dyer AM, et al. (2012) Longitudinal association of intimate partner violence and depressive symptoms. Ment Health Fam Med 9: 107–114.
62. Heim C, Newport DJ, Mletzko T, Miller AH, Nemeroff CB (2008) The link between childhood trauma and depression: insights from HPA axis studies in humans. Psychoneuroendocrinology 33: 693–710.
63. Vilhjalmsson R (1993) Life stress, social support and clinical depression: a reanalysis of the literature. Soc Sci Med 37: 331–342.

Overexpression of Human GATA-1 and GATA-2 Interferes with Spine Formation and Produces Depressive Behavior in Rats

Miyeon Choi[1]❡, Sung Eun Wang[2]❡, Seung Yeon Ko[2]❡, Hyo Jung Kang[3]❡, Seung Yeun Chae[2], Seung Hoon Lee[2], Yong-Seok Kim[1,2], Ronald S. Duman[4], Hyeon Son[1,2]*

1 Department of Biochemistry and Molecular Biology, College of Medicine, Hanyang University, Seoul, Korea, **2** Graduate School of Biomedical Science and Engineering, Hanyang University, Seoul, Korea, **3** Department of Life Science, Chung-Ang University, Seoul, Korea, **4** Laboratory of Molecular Psychiatry, Center for Genes and Behavior, Departments of Psychiatry, Neurobiology, and Laboratory Medicine, Yale University School of Medicine, New Haven, Connecticut, United States of America

Abstract

Functional consequences to which vertebrate GATA transcription factors contribute in the adult brain remain largely an open question. The present study examines how human GATA-1 and GATA-2 (hGATA-1 and hGATA-2) are linked to neuronal differentiation and depressive behaviors in rats. We investigated the effects of adeno-associated viral expression of hGATA-1 and hGATA-2 (AAV-hGATA1 and AAV-hGATA2) in the dentate gyrus (DG) of the dorsal hippocampus on dendrite branching and spine number. We also examined the influence of AAV-hGATA1 and AAV-hGATA2 infusions into the dorsal hippocampus on rodent behavior in models of depression. Viral expression of hGATA-1 and hGATA-2 cDNA in rat hippocampal neurons impaired dendritic outgrowth and spine formation. Moreover, viral-mediated expression of hGATA-1 and hGATA-2 in the dorsal hippocampus caused depressive-like deficits in the forced swim test and learned helplessness models of depression, and decreased the expression of several synapse-related genes as well as spine number in hippocampal neurons. Conversely, shRNA knockdown of GATA-2 increased synapse-related gene expression, spine number, and dendrite branching. The results demonstrate that hGATA-1 and hGATA-2 expression in hippocampus is sufficient to cause depressive like behaviors that are associated with reduction in spine synapse density and expression of synapse-related genes.

Editor: Shashank M. Dravid, Creighton University, United States of America

Funding: This research was supported by National Research Foundation grant of Korea (No. 2011-0028317) funded by Korea government awarded to HS. The funders had no role in study design, data collection and analysis, decision to publish, or preparation of the manuscript.

Competing Interests: The authors have declared that no competing interests exist.

* Email: hyeonson@hanyang.ac.kr

❡ These authors contributed equally to this work.

Introduction

There is a rich cross-talk between transcription factors and signaling pathways that regulate neuronal growth and synapse formation [1,2], and there is extensive evidence that changes in spine morphology couple with synaptic function in neurons [3]. These functional and structural changes in dendritic spines are thought to be the basis for learning and memory in the brain [4,5]. Consistent with this idea, changes in spine density are seen in several psychiatric disorders that are associated with deficits in social interaction, cognition and memory function [6]. However, how transcriptional regulation ultimately leads to specific alteration of brain function is not fully understood.

GATA-1 is a member of a family of six zinc-finger proteins, which bind to the (T/A)GATA(G/A) consensus sequence and play important roles in cellular differentiation and proliferation [7]. GATA transcription factors were first described for their role in the proliferation of progenitors and in lineage specification during early hematopoiesis [8,9]. Recently, GATA-1 was shown to exert repressive effects on spine formation in rat cortical neurons [10] and has been implicated in major depressive disorder (MDD) based on evidence that GATA-1 levels are increased postmortem prefrontal cortex and hippocampus of MDD subjects [11].

GATA-1 is expressed at relatively low levels in brain, but another member of the family GATA-2 is expressed at higher levels in mature neurons in mouse and rats [12–14]. GATA-2 plays a role in development of the mouse brain [15,16]. Phylogenic comparison reveals that GATA-1 protein and two of the DNA binding zinc finger domains are fully conserved between human, mouse and rat [17,18] (see also www.ihop-net.org/UniPub/iHOP). Human GATA-2 shares 98% amino acid sequence similarity to rats and mouse [7,19,20] and has identical zinc finger homology among these species. The zinc finger domains of hGATA-1 and hGATA-2 also have high sequence homology of ~98% (www.ihop-net.org/UniPub/iHOP). These findings indicate that the GATA-1 and GATA-2 are conserved in vertebrates. However, the influence of GATA transcription factors on adult brain, particularly the hippocampus, remains unclear. In addition, the role of GATA-2 in the actions of stress and in depression-like behaviors has not been examined.

In the current study we examined the influence of stress on the expression of GATA-2, and investigated and compared the effects of hGATA-1 and hGATA-2 transcription factors on neurite outgrowth, spine formation, and synapse-related genes that are regulated by these GATA transcription factor members in rat hippocampal neurons. We also examined the influence of hGATA-1 and hGATA-2 on depressive behaviors in rodent models. The studies aim to elucidate the functional relevance of the GATA transcription factors in hippocampal neurons and how these synaptic changes translate to alterations of depressive behaviors.

Materials and Methods

Culture of hippocampal primary neurons

Primary hippocampal neurons were prepared and processed as described previously [21]. Hippocampi from embryo day 16.5 Sprague–Dawley rat (Harlan Sprague Dawley, Indianapolis, IN, USA) embryos were used.

Construction of adeno-associated viral plasmids and viral production

To construct human GATA expression vector, human GATA cDNA was cloned from human cDNA library (Human Fetus Marathon-Ready cDNA, Clontech, Mountain View, CA, USA) by PCR. The following primer pairs were used for GATA cDNA cloning: for GATA-1 cloning, 5′-GCCACCATGGAGTTCCCT-GGCCTG-3′, which includes underlined Kozak sequence and spans nucleotides 1–18 of the human GATA-1 cDNA coding sequence (NM002049.3 GI: 183227689); and 5′-TCATGAGCT-GAGCGGAGC-3′, which is complementary to nucleotides 1225–1242 of the human GATA-1 cDNA coding sequence. For GATA-2 cloning, 5′-GCCACCATGGAGGTGGCGCCC-3′, which includes underlined Kozak sequence and spans nucleotides 1–15 of the human GATA-2 cDNA coding sequence (NM001145661.1 GI: 224611698); and 5′-CTAGCCCATGGCGGTCA-3′, which is complementary to nucleotides 1427–1443 of the human GATA-2 cDNA coding sequence.

PCR amplifications were performed in 50 μl reaction volumes with 1 μl (10–100 ng fetal cDNA), 4 U Pyrobest DNA polymerase (TAKARA, Tokyo, Japan), 200 μM each dNTP, 0.6 μM each primer, and 1.3 M betaine on a Thermal cycler (TECHNE, Staffordshire, UK). PCR reactions began with a denaturation step at 94°C for 5 min and 10 cycles of Touchdown (TD) PCR followed by 30 cycles of standard PCR were performed. TD PCR conditions were as follows: 10 s at 98°C, 30 s at annealing temperature stepdowns every cycles of 0.5°C (from +68°C to +63°C), and 2 min at 72°C. The annealing temperature for the final 30 cycles of standard PCR was 62°C with denaturation and extension phases as above. Human GATA cDNA obtained from human fetus cDNA library (Clontech, Mountain View, CA, USA) by PCR was subcloned into pGEM-T-Easy vector (Promega, Madison, WI, USA). After confirmation of its sequence by DNA sequencing, cDNA clone was digested by *Eco*RI. The *Eco*RI fragments were blunt-ended with Klenow DNA polymerase (New England Biolabs, Ipswich, MA, USA) and ligated into the *Eco*RV site of modified adeno-associated viral vector encoding enhanced GFP (AAV-eGFP), generating AAV-eGFP-hGATA1 and AAV-eGFP-hGATA2. The virus was generated using a triple-transfection, helper-free method and was purified with a modified version of a published protocol [22].

Transfection with small hairpin RNA (shRNA)

Rat shRNAs of GATA2 and a control vector were purchased from GeneCopoeia (Rockville, MD, USA). Transfection of shRNAs (100 nM; target sequence, GGATGGCGTCAAGTAT-CAA) was performed using a Lipofectamine 2000 reagent according to the manufacturer's instructions (Invitrogen, Carlsbad, CA, USA).

RT-PCR analysis

Total RNA was prepared from cells with Trizol reagent (Life-technologies, Rockville, MD, USA). Reverse-transcription was conducted as previously described [21]. For quantitative real-time PCR (qRT-PCR), PCR was performed on an iCycler iQ Multi-Color Real-Time PCR Detection System (Bio-Rad Laboratories, Hercules, CA, USA). The housekeeping gene GAPDH was used as a control. Expression of each gene was normalized to the amount of GAPDH to calculate relative transcript levels. Normalized expression values were averaged, and average fold changes were calculated. The primer sequences are as follows: GAPDH, forward: 5′- CTCGTCCCATAGACAAAATGGT-GAAG-3′, reverse: 5′- AGACTCCACGACATACTCAG-CACC-3′; hGATA-1, forward: 5′-CTTGTAGTAGAGGCCG-CAGG-3′, reverse: 5′-GCTCTACCCTGCCTCAACTG-3′; hGATA-2, forward: 5′-TACCACAAGATGAATGGGCA-3′, reverse: 5′-TCTCCTGCATGCACTTTGAC-3′; rGATA1, forward: 5′- GATGGAATCCAGACGAGGAA -3′, reverse: 5′-CTCTCCGCAATTCCCACTAC -3′; rGATA2, forward: 5′-CAG CCT CCA GCT TCA CCC CT-3′ reverse 5′-TGA TGA GCG GCC GAT TCT GT-3′; PSD-95, forward: 5′-GACAAC-CAAGAAATACCGCT-3′, reverse: 5′-GCTTCTAGGGTGTC-CGTGTT-3′; GAP-43, forward: 5′-GGCTCTGCTACTACC-GATGC-3′, reverse: 5′-CTGTCGGGCACTTTCCTTAG-3′; RAB4B, forward: 5′-AGCCGGGAGACATACAACTC-3′, reverse: 5′-CCATCCTCTCCGGATCTAGT-3′; MAP2, forward: 5′-GCAAAGTAAGCCTGGTGA-3′, reverse, 5′-ATCTAAGG-GAAGAGTGAAAC-3′. GAD1, forward: 5′-CAGAAGTGAA-AACAAAAGGC-3′, reverse: 5′-AAACGCTCCATAAACAG-TCG-3′; vGluT1, forward: 5′-GGCAGTTTCCAGGACCTC-CACTC-3′, reverse: 5′-GCAAGAGGCAGTTGAGAAGGAGA-GAG-3′.

Immunocytochemistry and Immunohistochemistry

Cells were fixed as described before [23]. The following primary antibodies were used: mouse monoclonal anti-green fluorescent protein (GFP) (1:400, Roche Applied Sciences, Mannheim, Germany) and mouse monoclonal microtubule-associated protein-2 (MAP2) (1:500, Sigma-Aldrich, Saint Louis, MO, USA) antibodies. Cells were placed in goat anti-mouse secondary antibody conjugated to Alexa488 (1:400, Invitrogen, Carlsbad, CA, USA) or Cy3 (1:400, Roche Applied Sciences, Mannheim, Germany). Cells were photographed with a confocal microscope (Leica Microsystems, Wetzlar, Germany). Immunohistochemistry in rat brain was conducted as described previously [21].

Western blot analysis

Protein extracts were prepared as described previously [23]. The blot was probed with mouse monoclonal β-actin (1:1000, Santa Cruz, CA, USA), rabbit monoclonal anti-GATA-1 (1:500, Cell Signaling, Danvers, MA, USA), rabbit monoclonal anti-GATA-2 (1:500, Abcam, Cambridge, UK), rabbit polyclonal anti-postsynaptic density protein 95 (PSD-95) (1:1000, Abcam, Cambridge, UK), rabbit polyclonal anti-GAP43 (1:1000, Abcam, Cambridge, UK), mouse monoclonal anti-Tuj1 (1:1000, Covance,

Berkeley, CA, USA), rabbit polyclonal anti-lamin B1 (1:1000, Abcam, Cambridge, UK), mouse monoclonal anti-GFP (1:500, Santa Cruz, CA, USA) followed by treatment goat with anti-mouse or anti-rabbit IgG conjugated with peroxidase (1:1000, Santa Cruz, CA, USA). Bands were visualized with an ECL detection kit (GenDEPOT, TX, USA).

Spine density and dendritic arborization analysis

Images were acquired through Z-stacks, which typically consisted of 10 scans at high zoom at 1-µm steps in the z axis. For analysis of spine density in cultured hippocampal neurons, dendrite segments 40 µm in length, from 3 to 5 dendrites per neuron, were sampled from the cell body (proximal) and from end of dendrites (distal). In the hippocampal DG, we focused on second- or third-order dendrites from cells localized in one half of outer molecular layer. For each cell, 3 or more dendritic segments were used for spine analysis. Spine counting was conducted with a 60× objective using the Leica TCS SP5 (Leica Microsystems, Wetzlar, Germany). The number of spines was counted in a 10 µm segment. The final value was averaged from three rats per group and expressed as the number of spines/10 µm. Dendritic branching was investigated by Sholl analysis [24]. A transparent grid showing concentric circles was placed over the dendritic image, the smallest circle was centered in the soma and the distance between each circle was equivalent to 10 µm. Total dendritic length was estimated by counting the total number of circle intersections, and the density of dendrites was defined by counting the number of intersections on each circle. The confocal images of neurons were analyzed using Image J software (http://rsbweb.nih.gov/ij/) and the Sholl analysis plug-in.

Transcription factor binding motif search

The TFSEARCH (http://www.cbrc.jp/research/db/TFSEARCH.html) was used for the binding motif search in the promoter regions of candidate genes. The transcription factor binding sites were determined in the set of promoters with the parameter of exact matches of core sequences (threshold score = 90.0 as default value cut off) in the vertebrate matrix.

Animals, stereotaxic surgery and infusions

Male Sprague-Dawley rats (175–250 g) were pair-housed and maintained in standard conditions with a 12-hour light-dark cycle and ad libitum access to food and water. All animal experiments were approved by the Institutional Animal Care and Use Committee of Hanyang University and were performed in accordance with relevant guidelines and regulations. Stereotaxic surgery and infusions were conducted as previously described [21]. Rats were anesthetized with xylazine (6 mg/kg, i.m., Lloyd laboratories, Shenandoar, IA) and ketamine (80 mg/kg i.m., Fort Dodge Animal Health, Overland Park, KS). Bilateral viral injections were performed with coordinates −4.1 mm (anterior/posterior), ±2.4 mm (lateral), and −4.1 mm (dorsal/ventral) relative to the bregma.

Acute and chronic unpredictable stress (CUS) procedure

For acute stress, rats were individually restrained for a 2 h session in hemicylindrical (20.5×9×6 cm), well-ventilated, Plexiglas tubes. Animals were subsequently killed by rapid decapitation at 2 h after the onset of stress [25]. Ketamine was injected 30 min prior to the onset of stress. Control animals were decapitated immediately after removal from their home cages (total time lapse from removal from cage to decapitation: 1–3 min). CUS is an experimental procedure in which animals are exposed to a variable sequence of mild and unpredictable stressors. Our CUS procedure has been successfully used in the laboratory to produce behavioral changes. The CUS animals were subjected to the same 10 stressors (2 per day) described in Li *et al* [26], for a total of 21 days. Rats were then were treated with vehicle or ketamine (10 mg/kg, i.p.) on day 21 of CUS treatment 24 prior to sacrifice.

Forced swim test

A forced swim test (FST) was conducted as previously described [21]. Behavioral tests were analyzed by an experimenter blinded to the study code.

Learned helplessness paradigm

The learned helplessness procedure was performed in commercial shuttle boxes divided into two equal compartments by a central barrier (Gemini Avoidance System, San Diego Instruments, San Diego, CA, USA), as previously described [27]. A computer-operated guillotine door built into the central barrier allowed passage between compartments. On day 1, inescapable footshock (IES) was administered at one side of the shuttle box with the guillotine door closed (60 footshocks, 0.85 mA intensity, 15 sec average duration, 60 sec average intershock interval). Active avoidance testing consisted of 30 trials of escapable footshock (0.65 mA intensity, 35 sec maximum duration, 90 sec average intertribal interval) with the guillotine door open. Each trial used a fixed-ratio 1 schedule, during which one shuttle crossing by rats terminated the shock. Shock was terminated automatically if rats did not escape after 35 sec. A computer automatically recorded the number of escape failures.

Novelty suppressed feeding test and sucrose preference test

A novelty suppressed feeding test (NSFT) and sucrose preference test (SPT) were conducted as previously described [21].

Locomotor activity test (LMA)

The general locomotor activity of the rats in the open field test was measured by an automatic video tracking system (SmarTrack, Smartech, Madison, WI, USA). Rats were placed in the central part of the square-shaped arena (77 cm×77 cm×25 cm) and allowed to explore it for 10 min. Total distance traveled (locomotion activity) were recorded for 10 min.

Statistical analysis

Statistical significance was determined by Student's *t*-test. For behavioral results, statistical differences were determined by analysis of the variance (ANOVA; StatView 5, SAS Software). The *F* values and experimental degrees of freedom are included in the legends of the figures. All data were expressed as mean ± s.e.m.

Results

Expression of hGATA-1 and hGATA-2 in cultured rat hippocampal neurons

We first analyzed expression of rat GATA-1 and -2 (rGATA-1 and -2) in hippocampus. Figure 1a shows mRNA expression of rGATA-2. In contrast, rGATA-1 was not expressed at detectable levels in the hippocampus. Since the involvement of GATA-2 in cellular and behavioral abnormalities related to stress and depression remains an open question, we investigated the influence of acute and chronic stress on the expression levels of rGATA-2 mRNA in the hippocampus. Rats were exposed to acute restraint stress or chronic unpredictable stress (CUS), which results in anhedonic behavior that is reversed with antidepressant treatment, including the rapid acting agent ketamine [27]. While acute restraint had no effect, CUS exposure significantly increased levels of rGATA-2 mRNA in the hippocampus (Fig. 1b, c; $P<0.01$ compared with the nonstressed control). A single dose of ketamine (10 mg/kg) significantly decreased GATA-2 mRNA in acutely stressed rats, and completely reversed the effects of CUS (Fig. 1b, c; $P<0.05$).

Infection of cultured rat hippocampal neurons with AAV-hGATA1-eGFP or AAV-hGATA2-eGFP (Fig. 1a) induced an increase in the expression of hGATA-1 and hGATA-2 by RT-PCR, respectively, compared to control virus (vector only) as expected (Fig. 1b). Western blot analysis of nuclear extracts of the hippocampal neurons demonstrated that levels of hGATA-1 and hGATA-2 protein levels were also increased in response to AAV-hGATA1 and AAV-hGATA2 infection, respectively, compared to control virus (Fig. 1c). The majority of the cells transfected by AAV (with or without hGATA-1 and hGATA-2) differentiate into neurons as determined by the neuronal marker MAP2 (Fig. 1d, e). These experiments show that the hGATA proteins were produced in hippocampal neuronal cells. Infection of cells with AAV-hGATA1 or AAV-hGATA2 resulted in a similar total cell number compared to control virus (Fig. 1e), suggesting that cell survival was not affected by hGATA overexpression.

Dendritic length and spine density in rat hippocampal neurons

Viral expression of rat GATA1 significantly decreases the number of dendrite intersections in cultured rat cortical neurons, indicating decreased complexity (Kang et al., 2012). To investigate whether hGATA-1 and hGATA-2 can alter complexity of rat hippocampal neurons, we analyzed dendrite morphology by fixing and labeling neurons with a GFP-specific antibody (Fig. 2a), and

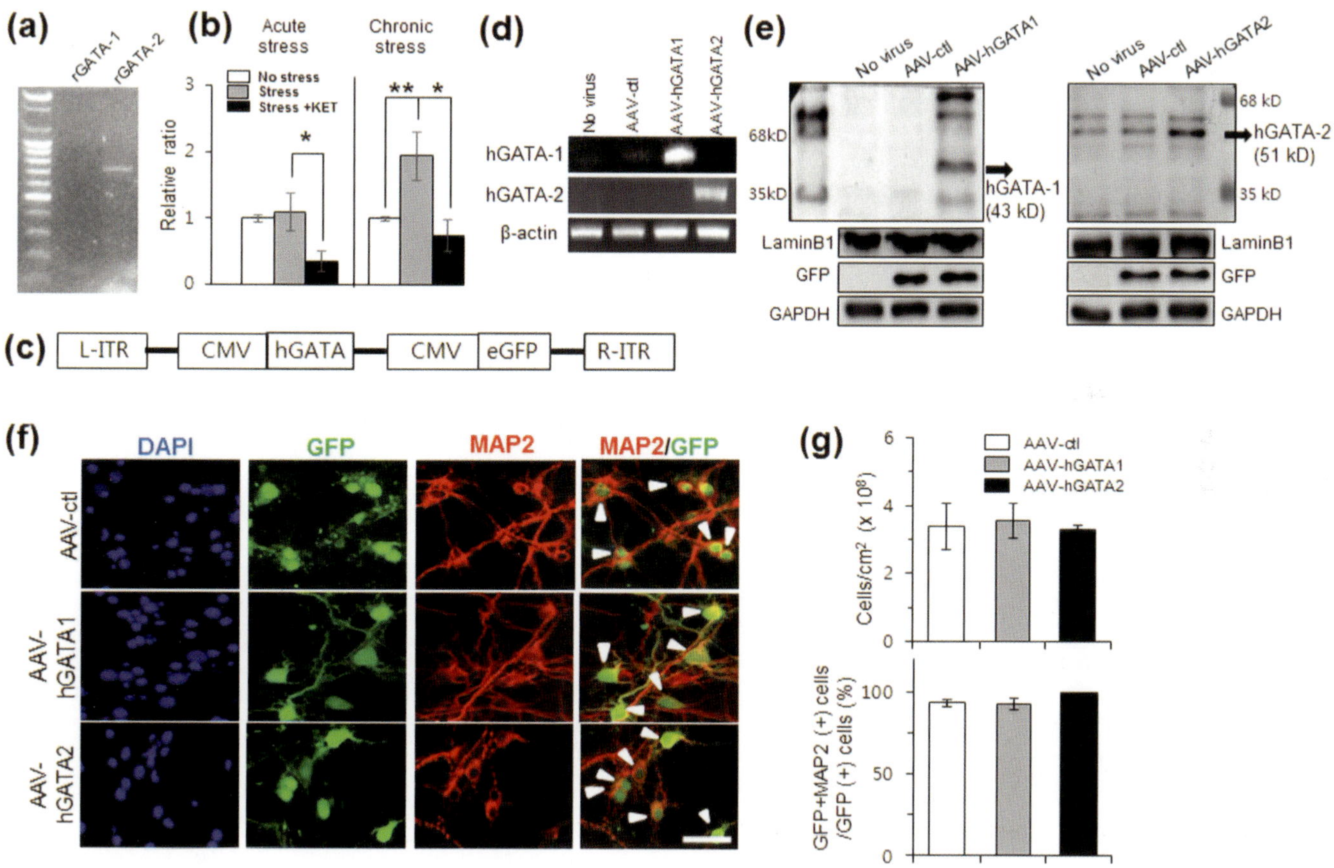

Figure 1. AAV-hGATA-enhanced GFP (eGFP) vector construction and expression in the hippocampal neurons. (a) RT-PCR analysis demonstrating expression of rGATA-2, but not r-GATA-1 in hippocampus. (b) Quantitative RT-PCR analysis of rGATA-2 in the rat hippocampus exposed to acute stress or CUS in the presence or absence of ketamine treatment. Rats were exposed to acute restraint stress for 2 h or CUS for 21 d and received either saline or ketamine (Stress+KET), and sections were subjected to quantitative RT-PCR. Results are expressed as a ratio of nonstressed controls and are the mean ± SEM, each analyzed in triplicate brain sections. rGATA-2 mRNA was increased in acute and CUS animals compared with nonstressed animals ($P<0.01$). CUS animals injected with KET showed a decrease in rGATA-2 mRNA compared with CUS animals ($P<0.05$; $n=6$ animals in each group). (c) L-ITR and R-ITR, left and right inverted terminal repeats, respectively; CMV, cytomegalovirus promoter. (d) RT-PCR of cDNA isolated from cultured hippocampal neurons transfected with AAV-hGATA1 and AAV-hGATA2. (e) Western blotting analysis was conducted to examine the expression of hGATA transcription factors, and representative blots were shown. The abundance of hGATA-1 (43 kD) and hGATA-2 (51 kD) protein in the nuclear extracts is increased in response to infection with AAV-hGATA1 or AAV-hGATA2. Nuclear extracts were determined by lamin B1, a nuclear marker. (f) Images of hippocampal neurons infected with AAV and stained with antibodies to GFP and MAP2. (g) The total number of cells was revealed by nuclear staining with DAPI. Transfection with AAV-hGATA1 or AAV-hGATA2 showed the same fraction of GFP(+) cells colabeled with MAP2 compared with transduction with AAV-ctl ($P>0.05$). The percentage of MAP2(+) cells among GFP(+) cells is shown as a fraction of the total GFP number of cells. Total MAP2(+) and GFP(+) cells (arrowheads) were counted with a microscope in 10 non-overlapping fields per well. Values represent mean ± s.e.m. from five independent experiments. Scale bar, 50 μm.

then measured the number of dendrite intersections using Sholl analysis [28]. Consistent with previous results in cortical neurons, viral expression of hGATA1 decreased the complexity of the dendritic arbor of hippocampal neurons (Fig. 2a). When dendritic length was plotted against the shell distances 10–100 μm, differences between AAV-ctl and AAV-hGATA1 were most marked for the middle 20–80 μm range (Fig. 2b; $P<0.05$). Decreased complexity in processes of GFP(+) cells that were infected with AAV-hGAT2 was greatest in the 20–50 μm range (Fig. 2b; $P<0.05$).

Since we observed a morphological change in the rat primary hippocampal neuronal cells that were transfected with AAV-hGATA1 and AAV-hGATA2, we then measured the spine density of those cells to further characterize the morphological changes. Spines protruding from second order dendrites were assessed separately for the proximal and distal dendrites, and results expressed as the number of spines per μm dendritic length (Fig. 2c, d). Infection of cells with AAV-hGATA1 significantly decreased spine density of proximal and distal dendrites compared to AAV-ctl (Fig. 2d; $P<0.001$). Spines of dendrites in cells transfected with AAV-hGATA2 also showed significant decreases in the proximal and distal segments (Fig. 2d; $P<0.01$). Alterations of spine-synapses are accompanied by regulation of postsynaptic proteins, including PSD-95 [27,29]. Consistent with this idea, the expression of PSD-95 was decreased in neurons transfected with AAV-hGAT1 and AAV-hGATA2 (Fig. 2e).

We then investigated protein levels of β-tubulin type III (Tuj1) and GAP-43, which are known to play an important role in

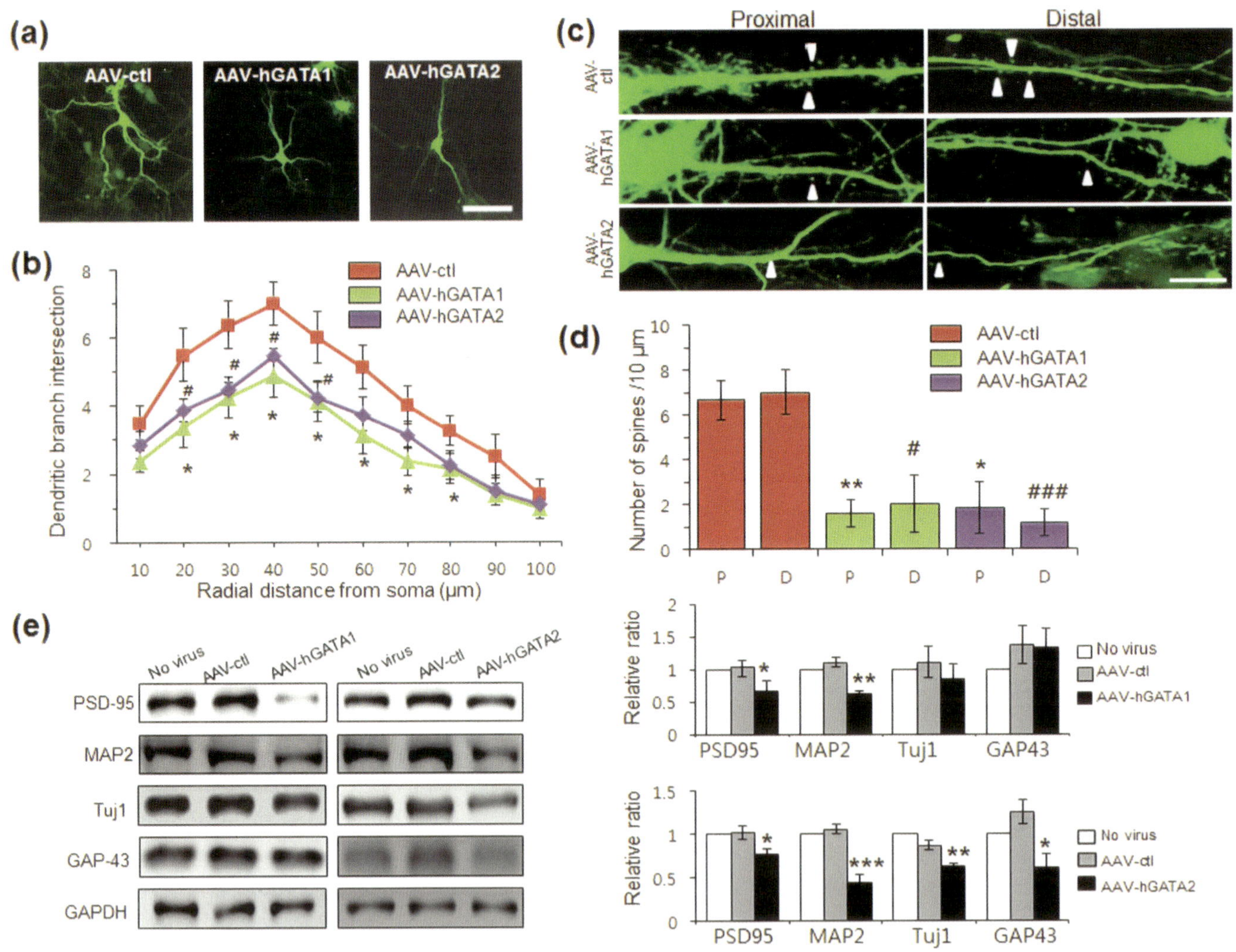

Figure 2. hGATA1 and hGATA-2 decreases dendritic arborization and spine density. Neuronal complexity in the hippocampal neurons transfected with AAV-hGATA1 or AAV-hGATA2 was analyzed based on three-dimensional projections of confocal stack images through complete neuritic extension of GFP(+) process. The neurons were transfected with AAV on 4 DIV and analyzed on 24 DIV. (a) An averaged image of multiple confocal planes across GFP(+) cells. (b) Sholl analysis of GFP(+) cells. Cells transfected with AAV-ctl presented neuritis with an increased ramification compared with cells transfected with AAV-hGAT1 and AAV-hGATA2 ($^{*}P<0.05$). (c) Representative images are shown of high-magnification Z-stack projections of dendrites of GFP(+) cells from AAV-ctl- and AAV-hGATA-transfected cells. A continuous stretch of dendritic processes was imaged. (d) The spine density (arrowheads) of proximal (P) and distal (D) segments was significantly decreased in AAV-hGATA-transfected cells compared to AAV-ctl-transfected rats ($^{*}P<0.05$, $^{**}P<0.01$ compared to proximal region of AAV-ctl; $^{\#}P<0.05$, $^{\#\#\#}P<0.001$ compared to distal region of AAV-ctl; $n=9$–12 neurons in each group). The data were expressed as the number of spines per 10 μm. (e) MAP2, PSD-95, Tuj1 and GAP-43 expression in the cells described in (a) determined by Western blot analysis. Expression levels are depicted relative to the level of cells that were not exposed to virus (: no virus) for comparison. ($n=3$–4 biological replicates per group). $^{*}P<0.05$, $^{**}P<0.01$, $^{***}P<0.001$ compared to control vector. Scale bars: *a*, 30 μm; *c*, 10 μm. Student's *t*-test.

neuronal differentiation, especially in neurite outgrowth [30]. Western blotting analyses showed a significant reduction in the protein levels of Tuj1 and GAP-43 in neurons transfected with AAV-hGATA2, but not AAV-hGATA1 (Fig. 2e). Protein levels of MAP2, which plays a role in neuronal maturation [23], were decreased by overexpression of hGATA1 or hGATA-2 (Fig. 2e).

hGATA-1 and hGATA-2 produces depressive behaviors

Given the negative effects of hGATA-1 and hGATA-2 on spine formation and dendritic arborization, we then examined the effects of hGATA-1 and hGATA-2 expression on behaviors in rat models of depression. The AAV vectors were bilaterally injected into the DG of adult rat hippocampus and behavioral testing was conducted 5 weeks after viral infusion (Fig. 3a). This resulted in widespread gene expression in the DG granule cell layer, as shown by viral expression of EGFP (Fig. 3b). Infusions of AAV-hGATA1 and AAV-hGATA2 into the hippocampus also increased levels of hGATA1 and hGATA2 mRNA, respectively, in microdissections of the infused DG area (Fig. 3c). Three models of depression/antidepressant response were tested, including the forced swim test (FST) and learned helplessness (LH), two behavioral despair models, and the sucrose preference test (SPT), a measure of anhedonia, a core symptom of depression [31]. These models are responsive to acute, subchronic, chronic antidepressants, respectively [31–33]. Both AAV-hGATA1 and AAV-hGATA2 infusions increased immobility in FST, a pro-depressive response during the initial period (300 sec) of testing (Fig. 3a; $P<0.05$, $P<0.001$, respectively). The depressant response was sustained in rats infused with AAV-hGATA2, but not AAV-hGATA1, during whole testing session (900 sec) ($P>0.1$, $P<0.05$, respectively). Spontaneous locomotor activity (LMA) was not different between these two groups, indicating that the effect observed in FST is not due to general ambulatory differences (Fig. 3e).

In the learned helplessness model, exposing animals to inescapable stress causes escape deficits. In the rats we studied here, infusion of both AAV-hGATA1 and AAV-hGATA2 increased the number of escape failures during the active avoidance testing, without exposure to an inescapable stressor (trials 1–30) (Fig. 3g, $P<0.05$). There were no significant differences in sucrose preference by AAV-hGATA-1 and AAV-hGATA2 compared to AAV-ctl groups (Fig. 3f, $P>0.05$). In addition, both AAV-hGATA1 and hGATA2 had no effect on the latency to feed NSFT, an animal model of anxiety that is responsive to chronic, but not acute antidepressant treatments [34] (Fig. 3h, $P>0.05$ compared to AAV-ctl). Home cage feeding and total fluid consumption were not different between the two groups (Fig. 3i, j). These results show that infusion of AAV-hGATA1 or AAV-hGATA2 produced depressive-like behaviors in two established rat models, the FST and LH.

hGATA-1 and hGATA-2 repress synapse-related genes

Previous chromatin immunoprecipitation studies have demonstrated that GATA-1 binds to the promoter elements of synapse-related genes, including Rab4b, indicating transcriptional control of these genes [10]. To investigate whether hGATA-1 and hGATA-2 could also regulate the expression of synapse-associated genes in hippocampus, mRNA levels were quantified by RT-PCR. Overexpression of hGATA1 or hGATA-2 in hippocampal DG results in down-regulation of Rab4b mRNA (Fig. 4a, b), a gene implicated in dendritic spine formation, consistent with previous results that elevated GATA-1 underlies the decreased transcription of Rab4b [10]. Given that AAV-hGATA1 and AAV-hGATA2 decrease levels of PSD-95 in cultured hippocampal neurons (Fig. 1a), we examined whether a similar effect is observed in DG transfected by AAV-hGATA1 and AAV-hGATA2. RT-PCR analysis demonstrated that PSD-95 and GAP-43 mRNA levels were decreased in response to AAV-hGATA1 or AAV-hGATA2 infusions into DG (Fig. 4). In addition, overexpression of hGATA-1 or hGATA-2 downregulated the levels of MAP2 mRNA, along with the glutamatergic neuronal marker vesicular glutamate transporter 1 (vGluT1) mRNA (Fig. 4d, e). However, overexpression of hGATA-1 or hGATA-2 had no effects on the differentiation of inhibitory neurons, as determined by quantitative RT-PCR analyzing glutamic acid decarboxylase 1 (GAD1) mRNA, the inhibitory neuronal marker (Fig. 4f). These results indicate that overexpressing hGATA might affect differentiation of glutamatergic neuron subpopulations, although it is possible that altered expression of vGluT1 is related to reduced spine formation. AAV-hGATA1 and AAV-hGATA2 infusion significantly decreased spine density by ~86% and ~50%, respectively (Fig. 4g, h, $P<0.001$, $P<0.05$, respectively, compared with the AAV-ctl group).

To directly test if synapse-related genes are regulated by GATA, we knocked down endogeneous GATA-2 with small hairpin RNAs (shRNAs) targeted against rat GATA-2 (shGATA-2) in hippocampal neuronal cultures; we did not examine knockdown of GATA-1 due to its low level of endogenous expression under baseline, non stress conditions [10], The transfection of shGATA-2 resulted in approximately 60% knockdown, as shown by real time RT-PCR and Western blot analysis (Fig. 5a, b). When compared to control neurons transfected with control vector alone, significant increases in the expression of Rab4b, PSD-95, GAP-43, MAP2 mRNAs were observed (Fig. 5c, d, e, f) in cells transfected with shGATA-2. The shGATA-2 incubation also significantly increased the spine density (Fig. 5g, h, $P<0.001$, compared with the control group). Regarding dendritic branch points in the MAP2(+) and GFP(+) neurons, we found that cultures differentiated with shGATA-2 contained neurons that had many more local secondary dendritic arborizations than the neurons in the control cultures (Fig. 5i, j, $P<0.001$ and $P<0.01$ compared to no transfection and control vectors, respectively). The shGATA-2 treatment significantly increased the length of spines (Figure S1 in File S1, $P<0.001$, compared with the control group). Together, these results suggest that hGATA-1 and hGATA-2 are involved in transcription of these synapse- and neurite-related genes, and in turn spine-synapse formation.

Discussion

Here we show that viral expression of hGATA-1 or hGATA-2 transcription factors suppress the expression of genes that are involved in spine formation and neurite outgrowth in the rat hippocampal cells. We also extend our previous studies and demonstrate that chronic stress exposure increases GATA-2 expression in the hippocampus and that this effect is reversed by the rapid acting antidepressant ketamine, supporting a role for GATA-2 in stress related behavioral alterations. Moreover, the results demonstrate that viral expression of hGATA-1 or hGAT-2 in the hippocampus of rat brain decrease in the expression of synapse related genes and cause depressive-like behaviors.

The results of behavioral testing indicate that expression of hGATA-1 and hGATA-2 increases vulnerability to developing 'depressive-like' behaviors. Notably, increased hGATA-1 and hGATA-2 levels in the hippocampal DG is sufficient to produce depressive-like effects in the FST and LH, models of behavioral despair and helplessness that are responsive to acute and subchronic antidepressant treatment, respectively. Expression of hGATA-1 or hGATA-2 had no effects on behavior in the SPT and NSFT, models of anhedonia and anxiety. The reasons for the

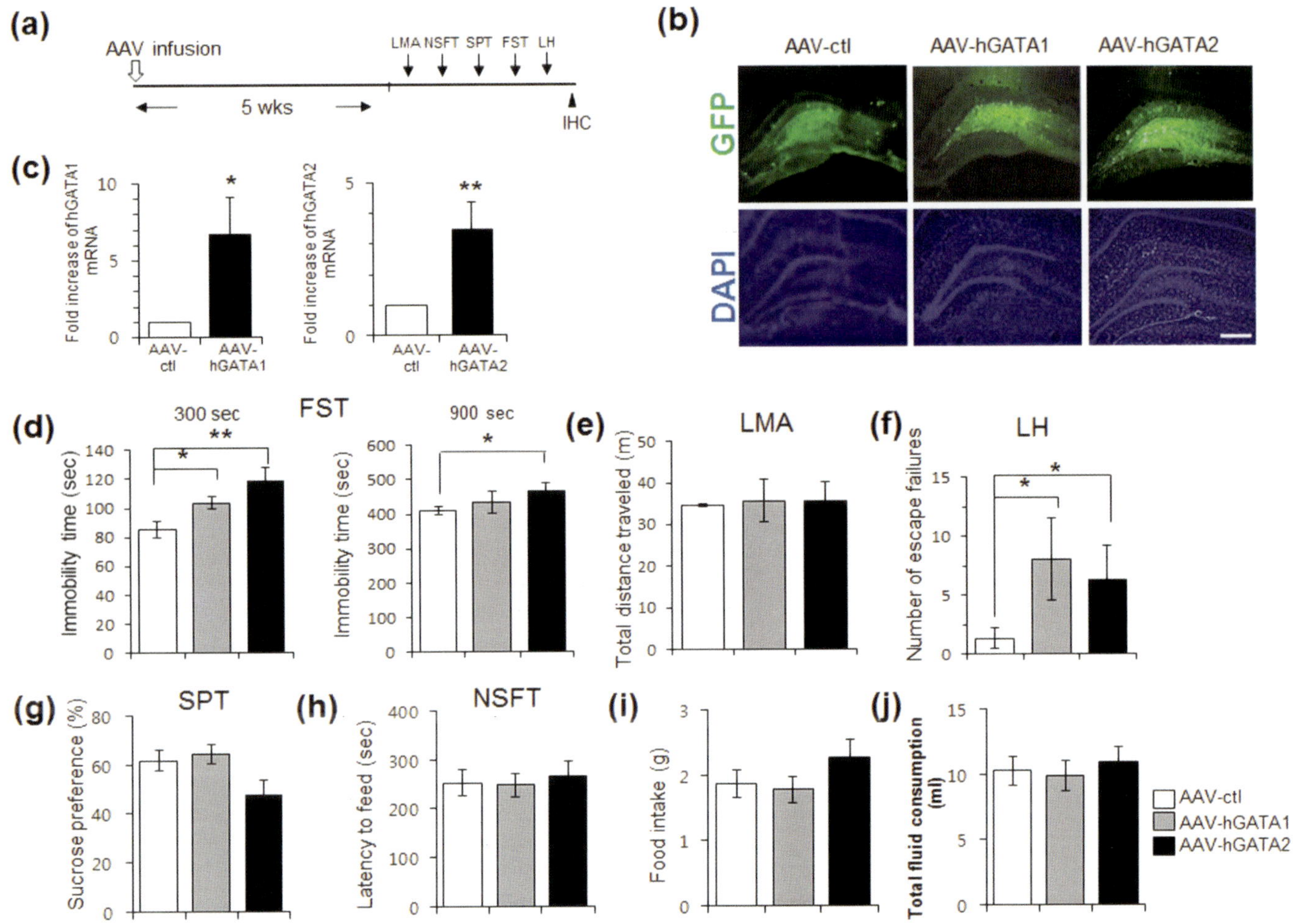

Figure 3. AAV-GATA infusions into hippocampus produce depression-like behavioral actions. (a) Experimental design. Animals were injected with AAV-ctl, AAV-hGATA1 or AAV-hGATA2 and 5 weeks later were tested in behavioral paradigms, and then hippocampal sections were harvested for and immunohistochemistry (IHC) and biochemistry. (b) Representative images of GFP(+) cells in DG from AAV-ctl-eGFP, AAV-hGATA1-eGFP and AAV-hGATA2-eGFP injected animals. (c) Quantitative RT-PCR analysis was conducted to examine the expression of hGATA1 and hGATA-2 mRNA ($^{**}P<0.01$). (d) FST. AAV-hGATA2 rats had a longer immobility score (time in seconds) than AAV-ctl-injected rats during the initial testing for 300 sec ($F_{1,12}=11.04$, $P=0.005$) and whole testing session for 900 sec ($F_{1,12}=5.12$, $P=0.042$). AAV-hGATA1 rats had a longer immobility score than AAV-ctl-injected rats during the initial testing for 300 sec ($F_{1,12}=5.79$, $P=0.034$; 900 sec: $F_{1,12}=0.52$, $P=0.48$). (e) Locomoter activity. The total distance moved in the box was similar between groups ($F_{1,10}=0.03$, $P=0.84$). (f) LH. AAV-hGATA1 or AAV-hGATA2 transduced rats had more escape failures than AAV-ctl animals (AAV-hGATA1: $F_{1,20}=7.09$, $P=0.028$; AAV-hGATA2: $F_{1,19}=5.85$, $P=0.038$). (g) SPT. Sucrose preference was not different both in AAV-hGATA1- or AAV-hGATA2-injected animals compared to AAV-ctl-injected animals (AAV-hGATA1: $F_{1,19}=0.08$, $P=0.67$; AAV-hGATA2: $F_{1,19}=0.19$, $P=0.78$). (h) NSFT. No differences in the latency to feed were shown between AAV-hGATA-injected animals and AAV-ctl-injected animals (AAV-hGATA1: $F_{1,19}=0.01$, $P=0.92$; AAV-hGATA2: $F_{1,19}=0.09$, $P=0.76$). (i-j) Home cage feeding and total fluid consumption. There was no difference in the home cage food intake (AAV-hGATA1: $F_{1,19}=0.08$, $P=0.76$; AAV-hGATA2: $F_{1,19}=0.79$, $P=0.38$) and total fluid consumption (AAV-hGATA1: $F_{1,19}=0.079$, $P=0.78$; AAV-hGATA2: $F_{1,19}=0.19$, $P=0.66$) between AAV-ctl-injected and AAV-hGATA-injected rats. Values represent mean ± s.e.m. from AAV-ctl ($n=10$), AAV-hGATA1 ($n=9$–11) and AAV-hGATA2 ($n=8$–11). Student's t-test (c). ANOVA test (d-j). $^{*}P<0.05$, $^{**}P<0.01$ compared to control vector. Scale bar: 200 μm.

lack of effects in SPT and NSFT are not clear but could be due to the responsiveness of these models to acute (FST), subchronic (LH), or chronic (SPT, NSFT) antidepressant treatments. Alternatively, the differential responses could be related to the role of hippocampus in these behaviors. It would be interesting in future studies to examine the influence of hGATA-1 and hGATA-2 expression in other brain regions, including the prefrontal cortex and amygdala on these behaviors. Nevertheless, the results demonstrate that hGATA-1 and hGATA-2 in the DG of hippocampus produces changes in neuronal morphology that contribute to the expression of depressive-like deficits in tests that assess despair and helplessness, but not anhedonia and anxiety.

Overexpression of GATA-1 in rat cortex has previously been shown to cause depressive behaviors that are associated with alterations of neuronal morphology [10]. Further evidence for a role of GATA1 in depression was provided by a recent genome microarray study of postmortem MDD subjects, which showed that levels of GATA1 mRNA were increased in the DG, but not CA1 subregion of the hippocampus [11]. Accordingly, we examined the influence of GATA transcription factors on the morphology of hippocampal neurons and depressive behaviors. This strategy allows analysis of the overall effects of these transcription factors on synapse related target genes that may occur via conserved GATA promoter sequences. An advantage of this approach is that we are examining the endogenous target

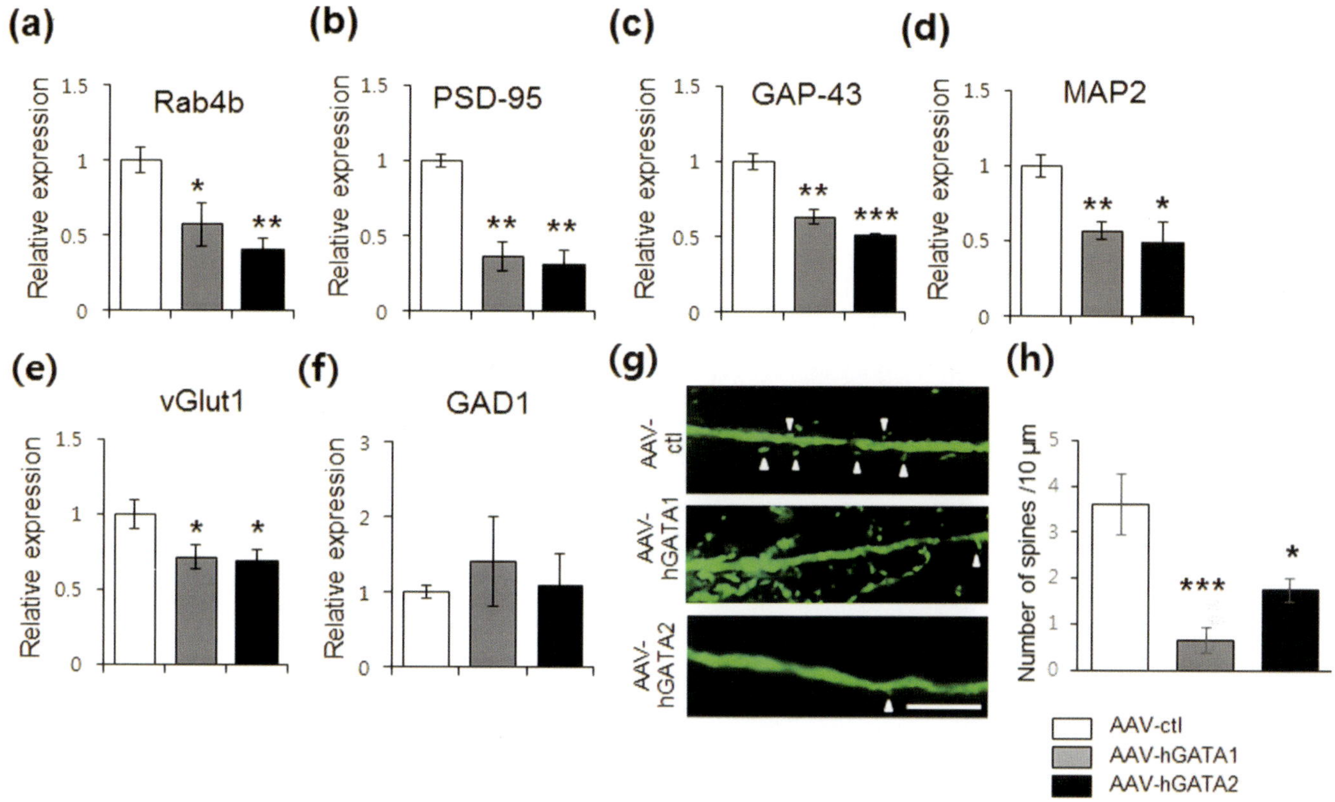

Figure 4. Transcriptional repression of synapse-related genes and a decrease in spine density by AAV-hGATA1 and AAV-hGATA2 in DG of the rat hippocampus. (a–d) Quantitative analysis of synapse-related genes in DG microdissected from rat hippocampus transfected with AAV-hGATA1 or AAV-hGATA2. Rab4b, AAV-hGATA1: $F_{1,4}=10.78$, $P=0.03$; AAV-hGATA2: $F_{1,4}=46.2$, $P=0.002$; PSD95, AAV-hGATA1: $F_{1,4}=31.73$, $P=0.004$; AAV-hGATA2: $F_{1,4}=42.8$, $P=0.002$; GAP43, AAV-hGATA1: $F_{1,4}=49.8$, $P=0.002$; AAV-hGATA2: $F_{1,4}=755.17$, $P=0.00001$; MAP2, AAV-hGATA1: $F_{1,4}=46.1$, $P=0.002$; AAV-hGATA2: $F_{1,4}=8.3$, $P=0.04$; vGlut1, AAV-hGATA1: $F_{1,4}=16.6$, $P=0.015$; AAV-hGATA2: $F_{1,4}=24.09$, $P=0.02$; GAD1, AAV-hGATA1: $F_{1,4}=0.004$, $P=0.95$; AAV-hGATA2: $F_{1,4}=1.59$, $P=0.27$. (g) Representative images are shown of high-magnification Z-stack projections of apical tuft segments of GFP(+) DG granule cells from AAV-ctl, AAV-hGATA1 and AAV-hGATA2-injected rats. (h) Density of dendritic spines (arrowheads) was significantly decreased in AAV-hGATA1- and AAV-hGATA2-injected rats compared with AAV-ctl-injected rats (a main effect of virus, $F_{2,13}=12.9$, $P<0.0001$; AAV-hGATA1: $F_{1,10}=21.15$, $P=0.0009$; AAV-hGATA2: $F_{1,7}=5.63$, $P=0.04$). The data were expressed as the number of spines per 10 µm. ANOVA test. $^{*}P<0.05$, $^{**}P<0.01$, $^{***}P<0.001$ compared to control vector. Values represent mean ± s.e.m. of 5–7 cells from three animals per group. Scale bar: 10 µm.

genes in their normal chromatin environment in rat hippocampal cells, which express GATA-2, and low levels of GATA-1 [14]. Based on low endogenous levels, viral expression of hGATA-1 may produce a distinct effect on the transactivation of genes. In contrast, because levels of endogenous GATA-2 are relatively high, viral expression of hGATA-2 may produce less physiological changes. However, hGATA-2 protein appears to exhibit a broader binding sequence specificity compared with that of mouse GATA-1 and hGATA-3 [35]. Thus even small changes in the level of hGATA-2 proteins might affect transactivation of GATA-2 responsive genes and in turn produces depressive-like deficits. Our results together with the previous finding [10] indicate that GATA1 induces depressive-like behaviors and a decrease in spine density when it is overexpressed either in the prefrontal cortex or hippocampus. Accordingly, hGATA-2, which produces similar depressive-like behaviors when expressed in hippocampal neurons, might have depressive effects on animal behaviors when it is overexpressed in the prefrontal cortex as well. Given that hGATA-1 and -2 control depressive-like behaviors in rats, one might assume there is a link between hGATA transcription factors and adult hippocampal neurogenesis, a form of neural plasticity that is increased by antidepressant treatments [36]. However, there have been no reports that GATA transcription factors regulate adult hippocampal neurogenesis, and further studies will be needed to address this question.

The results show that some of the synaptic plasticity-related genes normally expressed in neuronal cells respond to hGATA-1 and hGATA-2 transcription factor expression. Interestingly, besides previously known GATA-1 responding genes, PSD-95, GAP-43 and MAP2 showed a response to changes in levels of the hGATA-1/hGATA-2 *in vivo*. Our scans for canonical GATA sites throughout the locus based on aligned DNA sequences indicate that PSD-95, GAP-43 and MAP2 have potential GATA-1 and GATA-2 binding sites (http://www.cbrc.jp/research/db/TFSEARCH.html). Therefore, it appears that genes having conserved GATA sites showed a response to changes in levels of the GATA proteins. Indeed many genes have GATA promoter elements (conserved or not) because of the short recognition sequence (6 to 8 bp), which are frequently represented in genomic DNA (e.g. >50 sites in MAP2 gene) [35,37]. However, the functional regulation of GATA transcription factor binding *in vivo* is controlled by many different factors. The primary determinants of transcriptional outcome would be the context in which a potential binding site is embedded, local chromatin structure, and synergistic interactions with other transcription factors recognizing neighboring sites. Thus, the repressive effects of hGATA-1 and

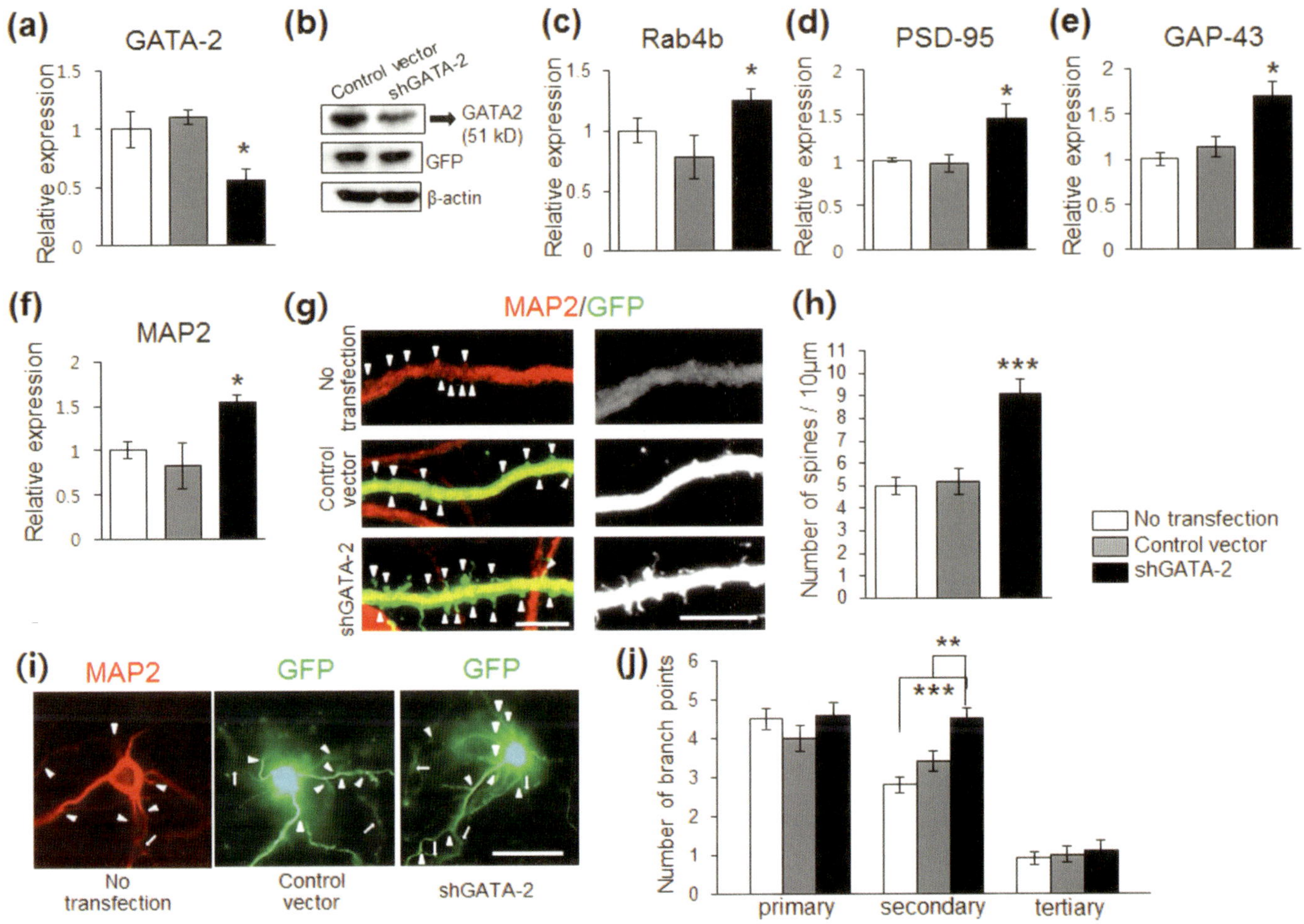

Figure 5. shGATA-2 increases synapse-related genes and spine density. (a–b) Transfection with shGATA-2 caused ~60% knockdown of GATA2 mRNA and protein expression in rat hippocampal cells. Western blotting analysis was conducted to examine the expression of endogeneous rat GATA-2, and representative blots were shown. The GATA-2 (51 kD) protein in the nuclear extracts is downregulated in response to transfection with shGATA-2 compared to control vector. (c–f) Quantitative analysis of synapse-related genes in rat hippocampal neurons transfected with shGATA-2. Rab4b, $P<0.05$; PSD95, $P<0.01$; GAP43, $P<0.05$; MAP2, $P<0.05$). (g) Representative images are shown of Z-stack projections of dendrites of MAP2(+) and GFP(+) cells from ctl- and shGATA2-transfected cells. A continuous stretch of dendritic processes was imaged. (right panel) high magnification. (h) Density of dendritic spines (arrowheads) was significantly increased in shGATA2-transfected cells compared with controls ($^{***}P<0.001$ compared to controls). The data were expressed as the number of spines per 10 μm. $n=5$–7 cells. (i) The number of dendritic branches exiting the soma (1′ dendrites), dendritic branches arborizing from 1′ dendrites (2′ dendrites, arrowheads) and dendritic branches arborizing from 2′ dendrites (3′ dendrites, arrows) were counted in neurons immunostained for MAP2 and GFP ($n=10$–15 cells per treatment). Student's *t* test. $^{*}P<0.05$, $^{**}P<0.01$, $^{***}P<0.001$ compared to control vector. Values represent mean ± s.e.m. Scale bar: 10 μm.

hGATA-2 on the synapse-related genes might not be solely due to the presence or number of DNA binding sites, but rather is related to the transcriptome environment of genes, which is also influenced by experiential and behavioral factors. Given the high degree of similarity of DNA binding zinc finger sequences between hGATA-1 and hGATA-2, hGATA-2 might be the primary repressor *in vivo* until hGATA-1 is induced by stimuli such as chronic stress. Further studies will be required to address how the mammalian GATA proteins regulate the transcription of synapse-related genes via different binding specificities at different sites *in vivo*.

Given that hGATA-1 and hGATA-2 may regulate spine morphology and synaptic function in hippocampal neurons and depressive behaviors in rats, further studies will be warranted to investigate whether hGATA-1 and hGATA-2 play distinct roles in neurons of the adult brain including hippocampus. Full evaluation of the expression and role of the hGATA-1 and hGATA-2 on the transcription of target genes in rodents, as well as the localization in different populations of neurons in human brain will further elucidate the molecular mechanisms that underlie the pathophysiology and eventually the treatment of stress related illnesses such as depression and related psychiatric disorders.

Supporting Information

File S1 Supporting Materials and Methods and Figure S1.

Author Contributions

Conceived and designed the experiments: HS. Performed the experiments: MC SEW SYK HJK SYC SHL YSK. Analyzed the data: HJK YSK HS. Contributed reagents/materials/analysis tools: RSD HS. Wrote the paper: RSD HS.

References

1. Gutierrez H, Davies AM (2011) Regulation of neural process growth, elaboration and structural plasticity by NF-kappaB. Trends Neurosci 34: 316–325.
2. Eyre H, Baune BT (2012) Neuroplastic changes in depression: a role for the immune system. Psychoneuroendocrinology 37: 1397–1416.
3. Kasai H, Matsuzaki M, Noguchi J, Yasumatsu N, Nakahara H (2003) Structure-stability-function relationships of dendritic spines. Trends Neurosci 26: 360–368.
4. Holtmaat A, Svoboda K (2009) Experience-dependent structural synaptic plasticity in the mammalian brain. Nat Rev Neurosci 10: 647–658.
5. Kasai H, Fukuda M, Watanabe S, Hayashi-Takagi A, Noguchi J (2010) Structural dynamics of dendritic spines in memory and cognition. Trends Neurosci 33: 121–129.
6. Glantz LA, Lewis DA (2000) Decreased dendritic spine density on prefrontal cortical pyramidal neurons in schizophrenia. Arch Gen Psychiatry 57: 65–73.
7. Pan X, Minegishi N, Harigae H, Yamagiwa H, Minegishi M, et al. (2000) Identification of human GATA-2 gene distal IS exon and its expression in hematopoietic stem cell fractions. J Biochem 127: 105–112.
8. Begley CG, Green AR (1999) The SCL gene: from case report to critical hematopoietic regulator. Blood 93: 2760–2770.
9. Shivdasani RA, Orkin SH (1996) The transcriptional control of hematopoiesis. Blood 87: 4025–4039.
10. Kang HJ, Voleti B, Hajszan T, Rajkowska G, Stockmeier CA, et al. (2012) Decreased expression of synapse-related genes and loss of synapses in major depressive disorder. Nat Med 18: 1413–1417.
11. Duric V, Banasr M, Licznerski P, Schmidt HD, Stockmeier CA, et al. (2010) A negative regulator of MAP kinase causes depressive behavior. Nat Med 16: 1328–1332.
12. Zhou Y, Yamamoto M, Engel JD (2000) GATA2 is required for the generation of V2 interneurons. Development 127: 3829–3838.
13. Craven SE, Lim KC, Ye W, Engel JD, de Sauvage F, et al. (2004) Gata2 specifies serotonergic neurons downstream of sonic hedgehog. Development 131: 1165–1173.
14. Wallach I, Zhang J, Hartmann A, van Landeghem FK, Ivanova A, et al. (2009) Erythropoietin-receptor gene regulation in neuronal cells. Pediatr Res 65: 619–624.
15. El Wakil A, Francius C, Wolff A, Pleau-Varet J, Nardelli J (2006) The GATA2 transcription factor negatively regulates the proliferation of neuronal progenitors. Development 133: 2155–2165.
16. Nardelli J, Thiesson D, Fujiwara Y, Tsai FY, Orkin SH (1999) Expression and genetic interaction of transcription factors GATA-2 and GATA-3 during development of the mouse central nervous system. Dev Biol 210: 305–321.
17. Morceau F, Schnekenburger M, Dicato M, Diederich M (2004) GATA-1: friends, brothers, and coworkers. Ann N Y Acad Sci 1030: 537–554.
18. Gong QH, Stern J, Dean A (1991) Transcriptional role of a conserved GATA-1 site in the human epsilon-globin gene promoter. Mol Cell Biol 11: 2558–2566.
19. Minegishi N, Ohta J, Suwabe N, Nakauchi H, Ishihara H, et al. (1998) Alternative promoters regulate transcription of the mouse GATA-2 gene. J Biol Chem 273: 3625–3634.
20. Kumari J, Bogwald J, Dalmo RA (2009) Transcription factor GATA-3 in Atlantic salmon (Salmo salar): molecular characterization, promoter activity and expression analysis. Mol Immunol 46: 3099–3107.
21. Son H, Banasr M, Choi M, Chae SY, Licznerski P, et al. (2012) Neuritin produces antidepressant actions and blocks the neuronal and behavioral deficits caused by chronic stress. Proc Natl Acad Sci U S A 109: 11378–11383.
22. Hommel JD, Sears RM, Georgescu D, Simmons DL, DiLeone RJ (2003) Local gene knockdown in the brain using viral-mediated RNA interference. Nat Med 9: 1539–1544.
23. Kim JS, Chang MY, Yu IT, Kim JH, Lee SH, et al. (2004) Lithium selectively increases neuronal differentiation of hippocampal neural progenitor cells both in vitro and in vivo. J Neurochem 89: 324–336.
24. Sholl DA (1953) Dendritic organization in the neurons of the visual and motor cortices of the cat. J Anat 87: 387–406.
25. Melia KR, Ryabinin AE, Schroeder R, Bloom FE, Wilson MC (1994) Induction and habituation of immediate early gene expression in rat brain by acute and repeated restraint stress. J Neurosci 14: 5929–5938.
26. Li N, Liu RJ, Dwyer JM, Banasr M, Lee B, et al. (2011) Glutamate N-methyl-D-aspartate receptor antagonists rapidly reverse behavioral and synaptic deficits caused by chronic stress exposure. Biol Psychiatry 69: 754–761.
27. Li N, Lee B, Liu RJ, Banasr M, Dwyer JM, et al. (2010) mTOR-dependent synapse formation underlies the rapid antidepressant effects of NMDA antagonists. Science 329: 959–964.
28. Beauquis J, Roig P, De Nicola AF, Saravia F (2010) Short-term environmental enrichment enhances adult neurogenesis, vascular network and dendritic complexity in the hippocampus of type 1 diabetic mice. PLoS One 5: e13993.
29. Keith D, El-Husseini A (2008) Excitation Control: Balancing PSD-95 Function at the Synapse. Front Mol Neurosci 1: 4.
30. Denny JB (2006) Molecular mechanisms, biological actions, and neuropharmacology of the growth-associated protein GAP-43. Curr Neuropharmacol 4: 293–304.
31. Banasr M, Duman RS (2008) Glial loss in the prefrontal cortex is sufficient to induce depressive-like behaviors. Biol Psychiatry 64: 863–870.
32. Hunsberger JG, Newton SS, Bennett AH, Duman CH, Russell DS, et al. (2007) Antidepressant actions of the exercise-regulated gene VGF. Nat Med 13: 1476–1482.
33. Banasr M, Chowdhury GM, Terwilliger R, Newton SS, Duman RS, et al. (2010) Glial pathology in an animal model of depression: reversal of stress-induced cellular, metabolic and behavioral deficits by the glutamate-modulating drug riluzole. Mol Psychiatry 15: 501–511.
34. Santarelli L, Gobbi G, Debs PC, Sibille ET, Blier P, et al. (2001) Genetic and pharmacological disruption of neurokinin 1 receptor function decreases anxiety-related behaviors and increases serotonergic function. Proc Natl Acad Sci U S A 98: 1912–1917.
35. Merika M, Orkin SH (1993) DNA-binding specificity of GATA family transcription factors. Mol Cell Biol 13: 3999–4010.
36. Malberg JE, Eisch AJ, Nestler EJ, Duman RS (2000) Chronic antidepressant treatment increases neurogenesis in adult rat hippocampus. J Neurosci 20: 9104–9110.
37. Gumina RJ, Kirschbaum NE, Piotrowski K, Newman PJ (1997) Characterization of the human platelet/endothelial cell adhesion molecule-1 promoter: identification of a GATA-2 binding element required for optimal transcriptional activity. Blood 89: 1260–1269.

Anxiety and Depression Mediate the Health-Related Quality of Life Differently in Patients with Cardiovascular Disease and Stroke–Preliminary Report of the Yilan Study: A Population-Based Community Health Survey

Nai-Wei Hsu[1,2,4], Hsuan-Ming Tsao[1,2], Hsi-Chung Chen[3], Pesus Chou[4]*

1 Division of Cardiology, Department of Internal Medicine, National Yang-Ming University Hospital, Yilan, Taiwan, **2** Department of Medicine, School of Medicine, National Yang-Ming University, Taipei, Taiwan, **3** Department of Psychiatry and Center of Sleep Disorders, National Taiwan University Hospital, Taipei, Taiwan, **4** Community Medicine Research Center & Institute of Public Health, National Yang-Ming University, Taipei, Taiwan

Abstract

Background: Cardiovascular disease and stroke have emerged as substantial and growing health challenges to populations around the world. Besides for the survival and medical prognosis, how to improve the health-related quality of life (HRQoL) might also become one of the goals of treatment programs. There are multiple factors that influence HRQol, including comorbidity, mental function and lifestyle. However, substantial research and investigation have still not clarified these underlying pathways, which merit further attention. The purpose of this study was to determine how psychological factors affect the link between cardiovascular disease and stroke with HRQoL.

Methods and Result: A total of 1,285 elder subjects at least 65 years of age (47.2% male) were enrolled. The mental function and HRQol of each patient was then measured using the Hospital Anxiety and Depression Scale and Short Form-12. After multiple regression analysis, anxiety, depression, cardiovascular disease, stroke, education level and age were shown to be associated with both mental component score (MCS) and physical component score (PCS). In the mediation analysis using the SPSS macro provided by Preacher and Hayes, cardiovascular disease and stroke affected HRQoL via anxiety and depression, respectively.

Conclusions: These results suggest that cardiovascular disease and stroke have negative impacts on patient MCS and PCS through different underlying pathways. Cardiovascular disease influences the HRQoL both directly and indirectly with the mediation of anxiety, and stroke influences the HRQoL by way of depression. These findings support the proposition that different combinations of both physical and psychological support are necessary to best manage these diseases.

Editor: Yong-hui Dang, Xi'an Jiaotong University School of Medicine, China

Funding: This study was funded by the Research Foundation of Cardiovascular Medicine (100-02-023) in Taiwan and HMT and NWH received the funding. However, the funder had no role in study design, data collection and analysis, decision to publish, or preparation of the manuscript.

Competing Interests: The authors have declared that no competing interests exist.

* Email: pschou@ym.edu.tw

Introduction

Cardiovascular disease and stroke have become potent and emerging threats to the world's health care systems. In 2008, cardiovascular disease and stroke caused more than 17 million deaths around the globe. [1] Furthermore, it has been projected that these diseases will become the two leading causes of death from 2020 to 2030. [2,3] However, most patients with cardiovascular disease and stroke can at best only be well-controlled and not cured. Therefore, many experts have suggested that maintaining and even improving the quality of life (QoL) for those patients, especially the elderly, might be one of the major goals of treatment [4–6].

Quality of life has been reported to be influenced by many factors with rather complex interactions. [5,7] Therefore, a conceptual model might be beneficial in explaining the relationships among such factors. [5] Wilson and Cleary have already suggested a 5-level model, including biological, physical and mental symptoms, functions, health satisfaction, age and environmental conditions, trying to classify and clarify the relationships between these variables. [8] By this model, Halvorsrud et al. demonstrated that QoL can be predicted by factors such as health satisfaction directly, and by environmental conditions through health satisfaction and depressive symptoms indirectly. [5] Therefore, health-related quality of life (HRQoL) seems to play an important role in influencing the QoL in people with cardiovascular disease and stroke.

Table 1. Univariate analysis of health-related quality of life among the elderly in Yilan from 2011–2012.

	Mental component score				Physical component score			
	n	mean	(SD)	P	n	mean	(SD)	P
Sex				**0.010**				0.644
Male	593	58.1	8.5		593	47.9	(11.1)	
Female	654	56.8	9.6		654	47.6	(10.0)	
Age				**0.001**				**<0.001**
65–<70 years	354	58.8	(7.7)		354	49.6	(8.9)	
70–<75 years	349	57.6	(9.3)		349	49.0	(8.8)	
75–<80 years	255	57.3	(8.5)		255	46.7	(11.6)	
80 years above	289	55.8	(10.6)		289	44.7	(12.5)	
BMI				0.209				**0.005**
<18.5	56	56.6	(8.3)		56	46.2	(12.8)	
18.5–<24	504	57.3	(8.6)		504	48.8	(9.8)	
24–<27	374	58.0	(9.0)		374	49.1	(9.3)	
≥27	267	58.5	(8.3)		267	46.7	(10.2)	
Education				**<0.001**				**<0.001**
Illiterate	204	55.8	(9.8)		204	45.3	(11.0)	
Primary school	461	56.8	(9.8)		461	47.3	(11.2)	
Secondary school	363	58.3	(8.2)		363	48.9	(9.6)	
College and above	207	59.3	(7.4)		207	49.1	(9.5)	
Living status				0.076				**0.010**
Solitary	127	56.1	(9.3)		127	49.8	(9.6)	
Not solitary	1,120	57.6	(9.1)		1,120	47.5	(10.6)	
Smoking				**0.010**				0.094
Never	969	57.5	(9.0)		969	48.0	(10.3)	
Current smoker	123	59.2	(7.9)		123	47.3	(10.4)	
Quitted	155	55.8	(10.2)		155	46.1	(12.2)	
Drinking				0.065				**0.001**
Never	1,009	57.3	(9.2)		1,009	47.3	(10.6)	
Current drinker	175	58.8	(7.3)		175	50.5	(9.0)	
Quitted	63	56.3	(10.8)		63	46.8	(12.9)	
Hyperlipidemia				0.541				0.310
No	964	57.5	(9.1)		964	47.9	(10.6)	
Yes	278	57.1	(9.2)		278	47.2	(10.1)	
Diabetes				0.514				**0.003**
No	979	57.5	(8.9)		979	48.2	(10.3)	
Yes	266	57.1	(9.7)		266	45.9	(11.2)	
Hypertension				0.655				**0.015**
No	602	57.6	(8.9)		602	48.5	(10.2)	
Yes	644	57.3	(9.3)		644	47.0	(10.8)	
Cardiovascular disease				**<0.001**				**0.001**
No	902	58.1	(8.7)		902	48.4	(10.1)	
Yes	336	55.9	(9.9)		336	46.0	(11.4)	
Stroke				**0.016**				**<0.001**
No	1,163	57.7	(8.7)		1,163	48.3	(10.0)	
Yes	79	53.9	(13.3)		79	39.4	(14.1)	
Hospital Anxiety and Depression Scale								
Anxiety subscore				**<0.001**				0.570
<3	781	59.8	(6.8)		781	47.9	(10.2)	
≥3	460	53.7	(10.8)		460	47.6	(11.0)	

Table 1. Cont.

	Mental component score				Physical component score			
	n	mean	(SD)	P	n	mean	(SD)	P
Depression subscore				**<0.001**				**<0.001**
<6	1,052	58.7	(8.0)		1,052	48.9	(9.8)	
≥6	189	51.1	(11.4)		189	41.4	(11.9)	
Short form 12 Health Survey								
Physical component score				**0.001**				
<50	584	58.4	(9.7)					
≥50	658	56.6	(8.5)					
Mental component score								**0.043**
<50					226	49.3	(13.5)	
≥50					1,021	47.4	(9.8)	

Health-related quality of life in patients with cardiovascular disease, stroke, and other chronic diseases has been studied extensively using different methods in recent years. [6,7,9–19] The results of these studies have suggested that the HRQoL might be associated with lifestyle, comorbidity and mental health. [6,7,9,10,12–15,17] Some studies disclosed that although chronic diseases usually exert a negative impact on quality of physical health, the status of mental health might be relatively unaffected. [7,12,20,21] Other studies also suggested that the major contribution of the chronic disease to the negative impact on HRQoL could be the symptoms and disabilities of the disease rather than the disease itself. [9,12,14,21] Besides, Spitzer et al. already proposed that both physical and mental disorders might have different effects on the components of HRQoL. [22] These seemingly controversial results raised the question that, even with similar outcomes, the underlying pathways for these disease to influence the HRQoL might be different, just as that proposed by Mayo et al., who used the Wilson and Cleary model to evaluate the HRQoL in people recovering from stroke. [23] Steca et al. also found a significant relationship of illness severity (predicted by left ventricular function) with health satisfaction and depression in cardiovascular disease patients, but these relationships were fully mediated by illness perception and self-efficacy beliefs (both were indicators of patients' psychological well-being). [24] Therefore, as mental disorders (such as anxiety and depression) are frequently comorbid with cardiovascular disease and stroke, [25–30] whether these two diseases influence the HRQoL directly or indirectly through some other mediators, such as psychological functions, requires further evaluation.

The purpose of this study is trying to determine how psychological factors affect the link between cardiovascular disease and stroke with the HRQoL. Additionally, the impacts of these diseases on the HRQoL will also be evaluated.

Method

1. Participants

This study is a part of the Yilan Study, which is a population-based community health survey conducted by the Community Medicine Research Center at the National Yang-Ming University and the National Yang-Ming University Hospital in Taiwan. Since 2012, with the help of the Community Angels (social volunteers) and the Yang-Ming Crusade (student volunteers of the National Yang-Ming University), all people at least 65 years of age living in the 7 most populated villages of Yilan City, a city located in the northeastern part of Taiwan, have been visited at their homes by well-trained project assistants. In addition to recording the body weight and height, the demographic data, lifestyles and a self-reported medical history, including education level, living status, smoking and drinking habits, hypertenion, diabetes, cardiovascular disease (including coronary heart disease, heart failure and valvular heart disease), stroke, and hyperlipidemia were collected. Then, measurement of anxiety and depression tendency and the HRQoL were also performed. All the questionnaires have been completed by trained project assistants through face to face interview. Those people who did not agree to join the project, could not provide past medical history, had never visited a physician to confirm a medical diagnosis, or could not complete the questionnaires were excluded. All participants provided written informed consent and the Institutional Review Board of the National Yang-Ming University Hospital approved this study (IRB No. 2011A016).

2. Measurement of anxiety and depression symptoms

Measurement of anxiety and depression in study participants was performed by use of the Hospital Anxiety and Depression Scale (HADS). The HADS is a short, simple and reliable method for measuring both clinical and subclinical anxiety and depression symptoms in a general clinical setting and general population. [31,32] The scale is composed of 14 items designed to obtain the participant's feelings in the past one week, with 7 items rating anxiety and 7 rating depression. Each item is scored from 0 to 3 and the total range of both anxiety and depression subscores are 0–21, with higher scores indicating more anxious and depressive tendency. The Chinese translation of the HADS has been proven valid with the optimal cut-off points of 3 for the anxiety subscore and 6 for the depression subscore [33,34].

3. Measurement of HRQoL

We used the Short Form 12 Health Survey Version 2 (SF-12v2) to evaluate the HRQoL of study participants. Twelve items derived from the Short Form 36 Health Survey Version 2 (SF-36v2) are used to constitute the mental component summary (MCS) and physical component summary (PCS) for measuring the participant's mental and physical function status in the past four weeks. [35,36] The SF-36 is one of the most widely used

Table 2. Multiple regression analysis for factors associated with health-related quality of life among the elderly in Yilan from 2011–2012.

	Mental component score				Physical component score		
	Beta	***P***	**Cumulative R^2**		**Beta**	***P***	**Cumulative R^2**
Final stepwise model				**Final stepwise model**			
(Constant)	86.877	<0.001		(Constant)	100.546	<0.001	
Anxiety	−0.832	**<0.001**	0.173	Depression	−1.422	**<0.001**	0.103
Physical component score	−0.366	**<0.001**	0.244	Mental component score	−0.536	**<0.001**	0.250
Depression	−1.068	**<0.001**	0.355	Age	−0.231	**<0.001**	0.277
Age	−0.144	**<0.001**	0.373	Stroke	−5.489	**<0.001**	0.292
Education	0.748	**0.001**	0.378	Cardiovascular disease	−2.100	**<0.001**	0.303
Cardiovascular disease	−1.567	**0.001**	0.383	Anxiety	−0.297	**<0.001**	0.311
Stroke	−2.848	**0.002**	0.388	Diabetes	−2.007	**0.001**	0.319
Body mass index	0.123	**0.029**	0.390	Education	0.710	**0.006**	0.323
Forced-enter full model			0.395	Forced-enter full model			0.329
Controlling Variables: sex, living status, smoking~current, smoking~quit, drinking~current, drinking~quit, diabetes, hypertension, and hyperlipidemia.				Controlling Variables: sex, body mass index, living status, smoking~current, smoking~quit, drinking~current, drinking~quit, hypertension, and hyperlipidemia.			

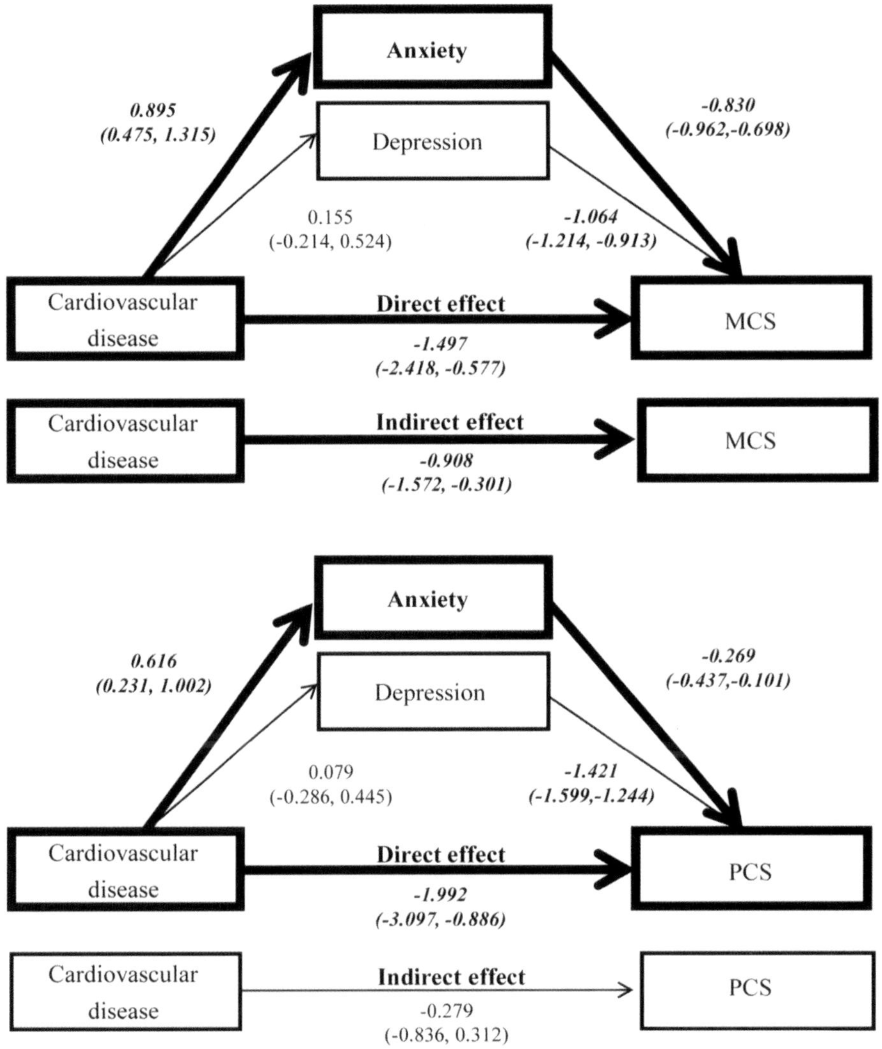

Figure 1. The estimation of the direct and indirect effect of cardiovascular disease on MCS & PCS (Bootstrap resamples: 5000). Footnote: Controlling covariates: Age, sex, body mass index, education, living status, smoking, drinking, diabetes, hypertension, hyperlipidemia, stroke, and PCS (or MCS). MCS: mental component score, PCS: physical component score, (): bias-corrected and accelerated 95% confidence interval. Bolded lines indicate significant direct and indirect effects.

measurements of the HRQoL of people in the world, and the SF-12 has been shown to closely mirror the results. [37,38] The translation of SF-36 and SF-12 Health Survey from English into Chinese has been carefully developed and proven to be valid. [39–41] Besides, because the mean of the norm during standardization was 50, we also divided the results of the MCS and the PCS with the cutoff points of 50 for purposes of additional comparisons. [42] For further validation of the HRQoL, two more questions have been asked: "How do you rate your happiness?" and "How do you rate your health status?" Each item score ranges from 0 to 100. A higher score indicates a greater level of happiness or a healthier life.

4. Statistical analysis

The IBM SPSS Statistics version 21 has been used to analyze all data. In the univariate analysis, the independent *t*-test and the one-way analysis of variance (ANOVA) were utilized. The Pearson Correlation coefficient was used to measure the correlations between MCS vs happiness rating, and PCS vs health status rating. Those variables found to be associated with significantly different results of HRQoL by literature review and by univariate analysis were included in the multiple regression analysis. Then, for statiscal efficiency, we choose stepwise multiple regression method to analyze the relationships between HRQoL (MCS & PCS) and major factors of lifestyle and comorbidity in order to find out those variables playing the major roles in the association. The dichotomous values of the HADS, MCS and PCS were used for univariate analysis, and the row scores of them for multivariate and mediation analysis. All reported p values are two-tailed and are considered significant if $p \leq 0.05$.

We used the SPSS macro provided by Preacher and Hayes in the assessment of the direct and indirect effects of cardiovascular disease and stroke affecting the HRQoL. [43] This macro utilizes a bootstrapping strategy to test the validity of the indirect effects and is able to partial out the effects of covariates without the assumption of multivariate normal distribution. [44] In the present study, each test would be resampled 5,000 times to estimate the bias-corrected and accelerated 95% confidence interval (BCa 95%

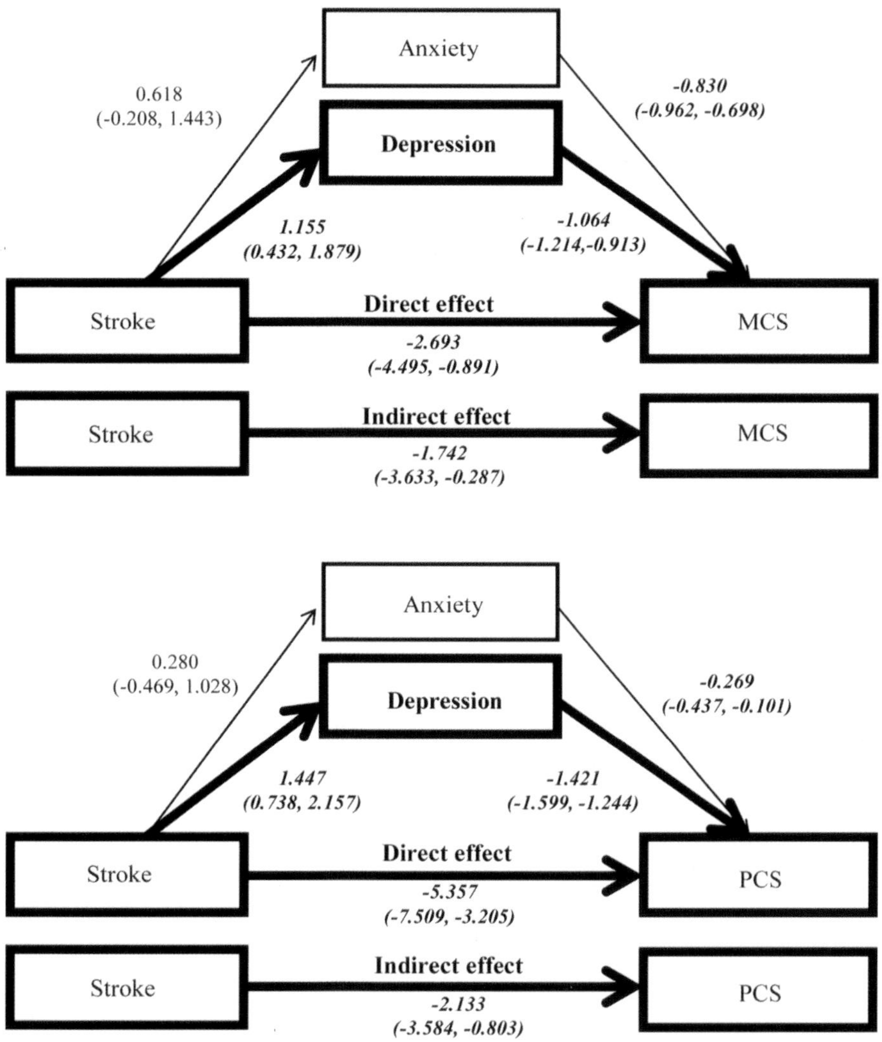

Figure 2. The estimation of the direct and indirect effect of stroke on MCS & PCS (Bootstrap resamples: 5000). Footnote: Controlling covariates: Age, sex, body mass index, education, living status, smoking, drinking, diabetes, hypertension, cardiovascular disease, hyperlipidemia, and PCS (or MCS). MCS: mental component score, PCS: physical component score, (): bias-corrected and accelerated 95% confidence interval. Bolded lines indicate significant direct and indirect effects.

CI). In the multiple mediation model, depression and anxiety were hypothesized to be intervening variables between medical illness and HRQoL. The SPSS macro estimated the direct effect that medical illness confers on HRQoL and provided the estimated indirect effects that were mediated by all intervening variables. All the effects of other factors have also been controlled by this Macro during the analysis (as showing in the figure legends).

Results

There was a total of 1,285 elderly study participants (≥65 years) with 606 male participants comprising 47.2% of that group. The mean age was 74.6±6.9 years with 56.1% of the participants between 65–75 years of age. The prevalences of the reported medical conditions of these participants were hypertension (51.3%), cardiovascular disease (27.1%), hyperlipidemia (22.4%), diabetes (21.4%), and stroke (7.0%). The mean anxiety subscore, depression subscore, MCS and PCS were 2.5±3.2, 2.7±3.0, 57.5±9.1 and 47.7±10.5, respectively. All the relevant data are shown in Supporting Information S1 and Supporting Information S2.

The MCS and PCS were different in elderly subjects with different lifestyles and comorbidities. Table 1 summarized the results of univariate analysis of HRQoL and showed that male and younger participants with higher education level had higher MCS scores. On the contrary, those who had quit smoking and drinking had lower MCS score. Regarding PCS, people with younger age, normal or slightly higher BMI, higher education level, solitary living status, and status of current drinker obtained a higher measurement of physical health quality. Those people with cardiovascular disease, stroke, and depression had both poorer MCS and PCS measurements. Besides, those participants with anxiety and PCS over 50 typically had lower MCS scores, and those with diabetes, hypertension, and MCS over 50 showed poorer PCS. Significant positive correlations between MCS vs happiness, and PCS vs health status were also noted (MCS/happiness rating: $r = 0.336$, $p < 0.001$, PCS/health status rating: $r = 0.365$, $p < 0.001$).

Table 2 showed the results of multiple regression analysis of HRQoL with different lifestyles and comorbidities. After controlling for possible confounding effects, anxiety, depression, age, education level, cardiovascular disease and stroke were shown to be significantly correlated with both MCS and PCS. We also found that BMI and quit smoking status were correlated with MCS and diabetes with PCS. Besides, the MCS and PCS were negatively correlated with each other. The R square of the final selected model was 0.390 in MCS and 0.323 in PCS, as compared to 0.395 of the full model in MCS and 0.329 in PCS.

Another interesting finding was that anxiety entered the model earlier than depression in the regression analysis of MCS, but vice versa in that of PCS. Besides, cardiovascular disease also entered the model earlier than the stroke in MCS analysis, but with reversed sequence in PCS analysis. The different sequences meant various impacts of these variables on the MCS and PCS. Therefore, it would be reasonable to assume that psychological factors might influence the link of cardiovascular disease and stroke with HRQoL by different pathways. Figure 1 and 2 shows the results of the estimation of the pathways that cardiovascular disease and stroke affect HRQoL. These figures suggested that in addition to the direct effect, cardiovascular disease exerted its impact on the HRQoL (both MCS & PCS) indirectly through anxiety. On the contrary, stroke affected the MCS and PCS both directly and indirectly through depression.

Discussion

In this study, we found that cardiovascular disease and stroke are both negatively associated with health related quality of life through different pathways. The cardiovascular disease influences the MCS and PCS both directly and indirectly through anxiety. On the other hand, with a direct effect on both kinds of HRQoL, stroke also has an impact on MCS and PCS mediated by depression indirectly. These results provide an evidence to clarify the possible underlying mechanisms between HRQoL and cardiovascular disease and stroke. Depression and anxiety are common comorbidities in patients with cardiovascular disease and stroke. [25–30,45–50]. There are several assumptions for such high prvalence. First, both depression and anxiety have been proposed to be the risk factors or preictors of cardiovascular disease and stroke. [25,27,29,45] Second, cardiovascular disease and stroke may also precipitate the development of depression and anxiety through biological and behavioral mechanisms. From biological aspects, Hare et al. have summaried the possible mechanisms of post-cardiovascular disease depression, which included alterations in the autonomic nervous system, platelet receptors and function, coagulopathic factors (such as plasminogen activator inhibitor-1 and fibrinogen), pro-inflammatory cytokines, endothelial function, neurohormonal factors, and genetic linkages. [29] Feng C. also reviewed the possible neurobiological pathogenesis for post-stroke depression, which included neuroanatomical factors (lesion location, infarction size, vascular depression hypothesis), neuronal biochemical factors (neurotransmitter, immune dysfunction, hypothalamic-pituitary-adrenal axis activation), and neurogenesis hypothesis. [51] Hellmann-Regen J at al. even proposed that stroke might share many pathophysiological features and risk factors with cardiovascular disease in the association with depression. [45] Besides, though there were relatively less researches about whether cardiovascular disease and stroke might precipitate the development of anxiety, Hare and Knutson have still suggested that both diseases might lead the development of anxiety through at least partially similar pathogenesis as those of the development of depression. [29,52] From behavior aspects, Hare at al. have summarized that cardiovascular disease might be associated with perceived loss (such as health, functional capacity, employmernt, and independence) and social isolation, which might lead to depression and anxiety. [29] Afanasiev et al. also suggested that physical disability, stroke severity, and cognitive decline were so far the main predictors of depressive symptoms. [53] Besides, there were also studies suggested that the anxious symptoms induced by fears (such as the recurrent attacks of disease, falling and returning to work) after disease attacks might influence the daily life. [27] Both depression an anxiety have been proposed to be negatively associated with HRQoL. [17,22,27,29,30,46,48,50,54–56] Our study results show similar results, however, that the mediators of the effects of both diseases on the HRQoL are different. We believe the neuroanatomic factors (such as the lesion location and infarction size) of stroke and neurogenesis post stroke, both involving the neurological pathways mediating the emotional responses and being different from those possible mechanisms of post-cardiovascular depression, might be two of the possible reasons for such difference. [51] However, more further detailed investigations to valide the porposal are necessary. Besides, we also believe that the reversibility of the symptoms of these two diseases might also play an important role. For example, most of the symptoms (such as dyspnea, angina, etc.) of the cardiovascular disease are reversible, therefore making those patients prone to worry about when and how to return the work and thus precipitated them to anxiety. On the other hand, those stroke patients usually got irreversible physical disability, which has been one of the predictors of depression. Our results also support Mayo et al.'s hypothesis that with similar outcomes of HRQoL across various health conditions, the pathways to these outcomes might be different. [23] Besides, the various pathways may also have important clinical implications. For example, in those people with cardiovascular disease, management of disease progression alone may not be enough. Adequate education to promote good illness perception with resultant positive self-efficacy belief, as proposed by Steca et al., should also be included to relieve the possible anxiety of these people. [24] On the other hand, for those people with stroke, because of the high prevalence of depression after stroke, [30] the goal of treatment should focus on both functional recovery and psychological support, as proposed by Mayo et al., who has suggested that interventions should not only focus on functional recovery during the first 3 months post-stroke. [23] However, this assumption of different pathways still needs further evaluation and validation.

Though both anxiety and depression are negatively associatd with HRQoL, the early entrance into the regression model with higher R square suggests that anxiety might have a greater correlation with MCS than depression, and depression is correlated with PCS more closely than that of anxiety. The findings suggest that various emotional responses to these diseases might influence the HRQoL components differently. The explanation of this result might be partially attributed to the various underlying mechanisms precipitating the development of these emotional responses. These different patterns also give support to Spitzer's presumption. [22] Besides, the results further suggest that responsible management of mental functions in patients with cardiovascular disease and stroke may become one of the crucial issues.

After controlling for lifestyles, mental functions, and other medical conditions, our results show that cardiovascular disease and stroke are still negatively correlated with HRQoL, which are compatible with those results from the EUROASPIRE III, IQOLA, etc. [6,12,20] Previous studies have suggested that diseases which are more symptomatic and disabling have increased negative impacts on the HRQoL. [12,21] In our study, we believe those patients with cardiovascular disease and stroke would suffer from morefunctional deteriorations, such as angina, dyspnea on exertion, lower leg edema, and paralysis, than those of patients with other kind of diseases. These functional deteriorations, without the mediation of the negative emotional responses, would also directly decrease the HRQoL. However, the underlying mechanisms and whether other kinds of chronic disease might have such similar effects still need further evaluation.

Our study results also show that both MCS and PCS are significantly but negatively associated with each other. Taft et al. have suggested that because of the construction of the summaries, there might be reciprocal effects of subscale scores on PCS and MCS, especially in those cases with extremely unbalanced profiles. [57,58] Thus, high MCS may represent either good mental health or poor physical status, and vice versa. Therefore, clinical interpretation of MCS and PCS scores should be in conjunction with the assessment of patient well-being and functioning. [57] The positive correlations between MCS/happiness and PCS/health status in our study suggest that the results of SF-12V2 have faithfully reflected the real status of the participants, and the negative association between MCS and PCS might have been resulted from their positive mental satisfaction.

There are still some limitations in this study. First, although we aggressively attempted to visit all the elderly adults dwelling in this area, nearly 30% of the registered inhabitants refused to join this study. Though the age and sex distribution were similar between the participants and all registered inhabitants, those who did not agree to join the study could be those suffering from more physical or mental disabilities. This could lead to an underestimate of the correlation between diseases and HRQoL. Second, some of the participants might have diseases but they have not previously requested any medical help, so the prevalence of diseases might also be underestimated. Third, as proposed by Tseng et al., there might be some cultural influences upon illness attribution and perception in the measurement of HRQoL. Therefore our results should be interpreted taking these concerns into consideration. [40] Finally, though there are some overlapping of the pathophysiological features between cardiovascular disease and stroke, there are still some differences among these diseases. [29,45] Therefore further analysis of the interrelationship between HRQoL with each individual disease are indicated. However, the results of the present study still suggest that different diseases might have different effects on the HRQoL, and even with different pathways. These findings also provide the basis for further analysis.

In conclusion, after controlling for possible confounders, our study results have suggested that cardiovascular disease and stroke have negative impacts on both the mental and physical part of HRQoL through different pathways. Separate and apart from the direct effect, cardiovascular disease affects the HRQoL indirectly with the mediation of anxiety while stroke with depression. These findings support the proposition that different combinations of physical and psychological support in the managements of these diseases are necessary.

Supporting Information

Supporting Information S1 Dataset.

Supporting Information S2 Meta file.

Acknowledgments

We are grateful for the tremendous help from Mr. De-Wei Lin and Miss Yu-Huei Lin, who are the professional project assistants and visited all the participants and recorded the data. We also thank Yu-Chun Chen, M. D., Ph. D., for his knowledgeable suggestions during the preparation of this article.

Author Contributions

Conceived and designed the experiments: NWH HCC PC. Performed the experiments: NWH HMT PC. Analyzed the data: NWH HMT HCC. Contributed reagents/materials/analysis tools: NWH HMT HCC. Contributed to the writing of the manuscript: NWH HMT HCC PC.

References

1. World Health Organization (2011) Global status report on noncommunicable diseases 2010. Italy: World Health Organization.
2. Murray CJ, Lopez AD (1997) Alternative projections of mortality and disability by cause 1990–2020: Global Burden of Disease Study. Lancet 349: 1498–1504.
3. Mathers CD, Loncar D (2006) Projections of global mortality and burden of disease from 2002 to 2030. PLoS Med 3: e442.
4. Oldridge N, Saner H, McGee HM (2005) The Euro Cardio-QoL Project. An international study to develop a core heart disease health-related quality of life questionnaire, the HeartQoL. Eur J Cardiovasc Prev Rehabil 12: 87–94.
5. Halvorsrud L, Kirkevold M, Diseth A, Kalfoss M (2010) Quality of life model: predictors of quality of life among sick older adults. Res Theory Nurs Pract 24: 241–259.
6. De Smedt D, Clays E, Annemans L, Doyle F, Kotseva K, et al. (2013) Health related quality of life in coronary patients and its association with their cardiovascular risk profile: results from the EUROASPIRE III survey. Int J Cardiol 168: 898–903.
7. Wikman A, Wardle J, Steptoe A (2011) Quality of life and affective well-being in middle-aged and older people with chronic medical illnesses: a cross-sectional population based study. PLoS One 6: e18952.
8. Wilson IB, Cleary PD (1995) Linking clinical variables with health-related quality of life. A conceptual model of patient outcomes. JAMA 273: 59–65.
9. Stewart AL, Greenfield S, Hays RD, Wells K, Rogers WH, et al. (1989) Functional status and well-being of patients with chronic conditions. Results from the Medical Outcomes Study. JAMA 262: 907–913.
10. Lyons RA, Lo SV, Littlepage BN (1994) Comparative health status of patients with 11 common illnesses in Wales. J Epidemiol Community Health 48: 388–390.
11. Spertus JA, Jones P, McDonell M, Fan V, Fihn SD (2002) Health status predicts long-term outcome in outpatients with coronary disease. Circulation 106: 43–49.
12. Alonso J, Ferrer M, Gandek B, Ware JE Jr, Aaronson NK, et al. (2004) Health-related quality of life associated with chronic conditions in eight countries: results from the International Quality of Life Assessment (IQOLA) Project. Qual Life Res 13: 283–298.
13. Singh JA, Borowsky SJ, Nugent S, Murdoch M, Zhao Y, et al. (2005) Health-related quality of life, functional impairment, and healthcare utilization by veterans: Veterans' Quality of Life Study. J Am Geriatr Soc 53: 108–113.
14. Netuveli G, Wiggins RD, Hildon Z, Montgomery SM, Blane D (2006) Quality of life at older ages: evidence from the English longitudinal study of aging (wave 1). J Epidemiol Community Health 60: 357–363.
15. Landman GW, van Hateren KJ, Kleefstra N, Groenier KH, Gans RO, et al. (2010) Health-related quality of life and mortality in a general and elderly population of patients with type 2 diabetes (ZODIAC-18). Diabetes Care 33: 2378–2382.
16. Maatouk I, Wild B, Wesche D, Herzog W, Raum E, et al. (2012) Temporal predictors of health-related quality of life in elderly people with diabetes: results of a German cohort study. PLoS One 7: e31088.
17. Lim L, Jin AZ, Ng TP (2012) Anxiety and depression, chronic physical conditions, and quality of life in an urban population sample study. Soc Psychiatry Psychiatr Epidemiol 47: 1047–1053.
18. Grool AM, van der Graaf Y, Visseren FL, de Borst GJ, Algra A, et al. (2012) Self-rated health status as a risk factor for future vascular events and mortality in patients with symptomatic and asymptomatic atherosclerotic disease: the SMART study. J Intern Med 272: 277–286.
19. van Mierlo ML, Schroder C, van Heugten CM, Post MW, de Kort PL, et al. (2014) The influence of psychological factors on health-related quality of life after stroke: a systematic review. Int J Stroke 9: 341–348.
20. Hopman WM, Harrison MB, Coo H, Friedberg E, Buchanan M, et al. (2009) Associations between chronic disease, age and physical and mental health status. Chronic Dis Can 29: 108–116.
21. Singer MA, Hopman WM, MacKenzie TA (1999) Physical functioning and mental health in patients with chronic medical conditions. Qual Life Res 8: 687–691.

22. Spitzer RL, Kroenke K, Linzer M, Hahn SR, Williams JB, et al. (1995) Health-related quality of life in primary care patients with mental disorders. Results from the PRIME-MD 1000 Study. JAMA 274: 1511–1517.
23. Mayo NE, Scott SC, Bayley M, Cheung A, Garland J, et al. (2013) Modeling health-related quality of life in people recovering from stroke. Qual Life Res.
24. Steca P, Greco A, Monzani D, Politi A, Gestra R, et al. (2013) How does illness severity influence depression, health satisfaction and life satisfaction in patients with cardiovascular disease? The mediating role of illness perception and self-efficacy beliefs. Psychol Health 28: 765–783.
25. Tully PJ, Cosh SM, Baune BT (2013) A review of the affects of worry and generalized anxiety disorder upon cardiovascular health and coronary heart disease. Psychol Health Med 18: 627–644.
26. Goodwin RD, Davidson KW, Keyes K (2009) Mental disorders and cardiovascular disease among adults in the United States. J Psychiatr Res 43: 239–246.
27. Campbell Burton CA, Murray J, Holmes J, Astin F, Greenwood D, et al. (2013) Frequency of anxiety after stroke: a systematic review and meta-analysis of observational studies. Int J Stroke 8: 545–559.
28. Musselman DL, Evans DL, Nemeroff CB (1998) The relationship of depression to cardiovascular disease: epidemiology, biology, and treatment. Arch Gen Psychiatry 55: 580–592.
29. Hare DL, Toukhsati SR, Johansson P, Jaarsma T (2013) Depression and cardiovascular disease: a clinical review. Eur Heart J.
30. Hackett ML, Yapa C, Parag V, Anderson CS (2005) Frequency of depression after stroke: a systematic review of observational studies. Stroke 36: 1330–1340.
31. Zigmond AS, Snaith RP (1983) The Hospital Anxiety and Depression Scale. Acta Psychiatr Scand 67: 361–370.
32. Bjelland I, Dahl AA, Haug TT, Neckelmann D (2002) The validity of the Hospital Anxiety and Depression Scale. An updated literature review. J Psychosom Res 52: 69–77.
33. Leung CM, Ho S, Kan CS, Hung CH, Chen CN (1993) Evaluation of the Chinese version of the Hospital Anxiety and Depression Scale. A cross-cultural perspective. Int J Psychosom 40: 29–34.
34. Lam CL, Pan PC, Chan AW, Chan SY, Munro C (1995) Can the Hospital Anxiety and Depression (HAD) Scale be used on Chinese elderly in general practice? Fam Pract 12: 149–154.
35. Maruish ME, Turner-Bowker DM (2009) A guide to the development of certified modes of Short Form survey administration.; Lincoln R, editor: QualityMetric Incorporated.
36. Maruish ME, DeRosa MA (2009) A guide to the integration of certified Short Form survey scoring and data quality evaluation capabilities.; Lincoln R, editor: QualityMetric Incorporated.
37. Ware JE Jr, Kosinski M, Bayliss MS, McHorney CA, Rogers WH, et al. (1995) Comparison of methods for the scoring and statistical analysis of SF-36 health profile and summary measures: summary of results from the Medical Outcomes Study. Med Care 33: As264–279.
38. Ware J Jr, Kosinski M, Keller SD (1996) A 12-Item Short-Form Health Survey: construction of scales and preliminary tests of reliability and validity. Med Care 34: 220–233.
39. Bullinger M, Alonso J, Apolone G, Leplege A, Sullivan M, et al. (1998) Translating health status questionnaires and evaluating their quality: the IQOLA Project approach. International Quality of Life Assessment. J Clin Epidemiol 51: 913–923.
40. Tseng HM, Lu JF, Gandek B (2003) Cultural issues in using the SF-36 Health Survey in Asia: results from Taiwan. Health Qual Life Outcomes 1: 72.
41. Tseng HM, Lu JF, Tsai YJ (2003) Assessment of health-related quality of life in Taiwan (II): norming and validation of SF-36 Taiwan version. Taiwan J Public Health 22: 512–518.
42. Maruish ME, Kosinski M (2009) A guide to the development of certified Short Form interpretation and reporting capabilities.; Lincoln R, editor: QualityMetric Incorporated.
43. Preacher KJ, Hayes AF (2004) SPSS and SAS procedures for estimating indirect effects in simple mediation models. Behav Res Methods Instrum Comput 36: 717–731.
44. Hayes AF (2009) Beyond Baron and Kenny: Statistical Mediation Analysis in the New Millennium. Communication Monographs 76: 4: 408–420.
45. Hellmann-Regen J, Piber D, Hinkelmann K, Gold SM, Heesen C, et al. (2013) Depressive syndromes in neurological disorders. Eur Arch Psychiatry Clin Neurosci 263 Suppl 2: S123–136.
46. Ayerbe L, Ayis S, Wolfe CD, Rudd AG (2013) Natural history, predictors and outcomes of depression after stroke: systematic review and meta-analysis. Br J Psychiatry 202: 14–21.
47. Hackett ML, Kohler S, O'Brien JT, Mead GE (2014) Neuropsychiatric outcomes of stroke. Lancet Neurol 13: 525–534.
48. Huang CY, Hsu MC, Hsu SP, Cheng PC, Lin SF, et al. (2010) Mediating roles of social support on poststroke depression and quality of life in patients with ischemic stroke. J Clin Nurs 19: 2752–2762.
49. D'Aniello GE, Scarpina F, Mauro A, Mori I, Castelnuovo G, et al. (2014) Characteristics of anxiety and psychological well-being in chronic post-stroke patients. J Neurol Sci 338: 191–196.
50. Ayerbe L, Ayis SA, Crichton S, Wolfe CD, Rudd AG (2013) Natural history, predictors and associated outcomes of anxiety up to 10 years after stroke: the South London Stroke Register. Age Ageing.
51. Feng C, Fang M, Liu XY (2014) The neurobiological pathogenesis of poststroke depression. ScientificWorldJournal 2014: 521349.
52. Knutson KM, Rakowsky ST, Solomon J, Krueger F, Raymont V, et al. (2013) Injured brain regions associated with anxiety in Vietnam veterans. Neuropsychologia 51: 686–694.
53. Afanasiev S, Aharon-Peretz J, Granot M (2013) Personality type as a predictor for depressive symptoms and reduction in quality of life among stroke survivals. Am J Geriatr Psychiatry 21: 832–839.
54. Benyamini Y, Roziner I, Goldbourt U, Drory Y, Gerber Y (2013) Depression and anxiety following myocardial infarction and their inverse associations with future health behaviors and quality of life. Ann Behav Med 46: 310–321.
55. Tang WK, Lau CG, Mok V, Ungvari GS, Wong KS (2013) Impact of anxiety on health-related quality of life after stroke: a cross-sectional study. Arch Phys Med Rehabil 94: 2535–2541.
56. Creed F, Morgan R, Fiddler M, Marshall S, Guthrie E, et al. (2002) Depression and anxiety impair health-related quality of life and are associated with increased costs in general medical inpatients. Psychosomatics 43: 302–309.
57. Taft C, Karlsson J, Sullivan M (2001) Do SF-36 summary component scores accurately summarize subscale scores? Qual Life Res 10: 395–404.
58. Schroder A, Oernboel E, Licht RW, Sharpe M, Fink P (2012) Outcome measurement in functional somatic syndromes: SF-36 summary scores and some scales were not valid. J Clin Epidemiol 65: 30–41.

Drinking Pattern, Abstention and Problem Drinking as Risk Factors for Depressive Symptoms: Evidence from Three Urban Eastern European Populations

Steven Bell[1]*, Annie Britton[1], Ruzena Kubinova[2], Sofia Malyutina[3,4], Andrzej Pajak[5], Yuri Nikitin[3], Martin Bobak[1]

1 Research Department of Epidemiology and Public Health, University College London, London, United Kingdom, **2** National Institute of Public Health, Prague, Czech Republic, **3** Institute of Internal and Preventive Medicine, Novosibirsk, Russia, **4** Novosibirsk State Medical University, Novosibirsk, Russia, **5** Institute of Public Health, Jagiellonian University, Krakow, Poland

Abstract

Purpose: To examine whether the frequency and amount of alcohol consumed in binge drinking sessions, total annual volume of alcohol consumed, problem drinking and abstaining from alcohol are associated with depressive symptoms in Eastern Europe.

Subjects and Methods: Cross-sectional data from a total of 24,381 participants from general population samples of the Czech Republic (N = 7,601), Russia (N = 6,908) and Poland (N = 9,872) aged 45–69 years in 2002–2005. Depressive symptoms were defined as ≥16 points on the Centre for Epidemiological Studies – Depression (CES-D) scale. Several alcohol related measures were derived using responses from the graduated frequency questionnaire. Binge drinking was defined at several sex-specific thresholds (ranging from 60+ to 140+ g of ethanol) and two frequencies (at least monthly or weekly). Total annual alcohol intake in grams was also extracted. Problem drinking was defined as ≥2 positive answers on the CAGE questionnaire.

Results: Problem drinking was consistently associated with approximately a 2-fold increase in odds of depressive symptoms across all countries and in both sexes. Abstaining from alcohol was typically associated with increased odds of depressive symptoms. Analyses separating lifelong abstainers and former drinkers in the Russian cohort revealed that this increased odds was driven by former drinkers. Amongst men, heavy frequent binge drinking was associated with increased odds of depressive symptoms in the Czech Republic and Poland. In women, heavy infrequent binge drinking was associated with increased odds of depressive symptoms in Russia and Poland. Only in Polish men was higher annual volume of alcohol intake associated with increased odds of depressive symptoms.

Conclusion: Abstaining from alcohol and problem drinking were associated with increased odds of depressive symptoms in these Eastern European populations. Annual volume of alcohol intake as well as frequency and amount of alcohol consumed in a binge drinking session were less consistently associated with depressive symptoms.

Editor: Antonio Verdejo García, University of Granada, Spain

Funding: SB was supported by a UK Economic and Social Research Council PhD Studentship. Both SB and AB are currently funded by the European Research Council (309337, PI: Britton, http://www.ucl.ac.uk/alcohol-lifecourse). The HAPIEE study was supported by grants from the Wellcome Trust (064947/Z, 081081/Z), the US National Institute of Aging (1R01 AG23522) and the MacArthur Foundation. The funders had no role in study design, data collection and analysis, decision to publish, or preparation of the manuscript.

Competing Interests: The authors have declared that no competing interests exist.

* Email: steven.bell@ucl.ac.uk

Introduction

Depression [1–3] and alcohol consumption [4] are widely acknowledged as important public health problems and there is ample evidence that the two are related [5,6]. The majority of research on the topic has focussed on the relationship between clinical disorders [7–9] with less attention drawn to the association between alcohol intake and depressive symptoms in the general (non-clinical) population [10,11]. Studies that have looked at the relationship between alcohol intake and depressive symptoms have produced conflicting findings [10–14].

Both the prevalence of depression [15,16] and alcohol consumption [4] are high in Eastern Europe compared to other regions. Little is known about the extent to which drinking patterns in this region, marked by heavy alcohol consumption and binge drinking [4,17], are linked with the high prevalence of depression. Examining the association between drinking pattern and depressive symptoms in populations with both high overall volume of alcohol intake combined with a pattern of heavy episodic drinking would allow for comparisons to be made to other drinking cultures whereby overall drinking volume is similar but drinking pattern is different (for example, Southern Europe [4]) or where drinking pattern is similar but overall volume of intake is lower (e.g. the Nordic regions [4]) to determine the extent to which drinking pattern plays a role in the development of depressive symptoms or whether it is mostly due to overall volume consumed.

Differentiating between different patterns of heavy drinking has been particularly encouraged in the context of Eastern Europe where a high prevalence of episodic heavy drinking exists [18–20]. Yet little research has specifically focussed on the effect of increasing dose of alcohol consumed per occasion *and* frequency of consuming these different doses of alcohol as risk factors for depression. It is probable that the biological effect of alcohol on the brain/body depends on cumulative dose, therefore examining the effect of different doses of consumption as well as the frequency of drinking makes intuitive sense. Others have, however, argued that it is problem drinking which is harmful to psychological health [21], but surprisingly few studies have examined the relationship between problem drinking and depression in Eastern Europe [22,23]. On the other spectrum of drinking, the extent to which non-drinking is associated with depression is also underexplored. The main uncertainty here relates to the degree to which the supposed beneficial psychological effects of moderate consumption [24,25] may be confounded by including former drinkers alongside lifelong abstainers in the non-drinking group [26,27].

Given the paucity of research on these important public health issues, the purpose of this study was to determine the extent to which binge drinking at different intensities (i.e. doses) and frequencies (e.g. on a monthly or weekly basis), annual drinking volume, problem drinking and abstention from alcohol are related to depressive symptoms in Eastern Europe.

Materials and Methods

Ethical statement

The University College London Hospital Research Ethics Committee Alpha approved the HAPIEE study. Ethical approval was also obtained from local research ethics committees at each HAPIEE site: National Institute of Public Health Ethics Committee (Prague, the Czech Republic), Jagellonian University Medical College Bioethics Committee (Krakow, Poland), and Institute of Internal and Preventive Medicine Ethics Committee (Novosibirsk, Russia). Participants provided written, informed consent.

The HAPIEE Study

Cross-sectional data from the baseline wave (2003–2005) of the Health, Alcohol and Psychosocial factors in Eastern Europe (HAPIEE) study [28] were used to explore the relationship between drinking pattern, problem drinking and abstaining from alcohol as risk factors for depressive symptoms. The study randomly recruited individuals aged between 45 to 69 years from electoral lists in Novosibirsk (Russia), and population registers in Krakow (Poland), Havirov/Karvina, Hradec Kralove, Jihlava, Kromeriz, Liberec and Usti nad Labem (Czech Republic). Questionnaires were identical across study sites and were translated to each language and back-translated to English to ensure comparability. The only difference between centres was the fact that the Polish questionnaire also included a filter question allowing those who reported not drinking in the previous 12 months to skip the other questions in the alcohol section. A total of 28,947 subjects (overall response rate of 59%) were recruited. The analytic sample consisted of 24, 381 individuals after those with missing information on depressive symptom status (N = 3,274), alcohol consumption (N = 376) and covariates (N = 509) were excluded (categories not mutually exclusive). A multivariable logistic regression model revealed that those with missing data were more likely to have lower educational attainment and belong to the high deprivation group.

Assessment of dose and frequency of binge drinking

Data on drinking patterns come from the graduated frequency questionnaire [29,30]. The graduated frequency questionnaire asks participants how often in the previous 12 months they consumed more than X amount of alcohol with separate doses, equivalent to: ≥10 g, ≥40 g, ≥60 g, ≥100 g, ≥140 g and ≥ 180 g of pure ethanol (based on original local units defined as 0.5 litre of beer, 0.2 litre of wine and 0.05 litre of spirits, ranging from "10 and above" to "less than one" - 100 ml of beer, wine and spirit was assumed to contain 4 g, 10 g, or 36 g of ethanol, respectively). There were nine frequency responses, spanning from never to daily.

Given gender differences in alcohol consumption and metabolism [31], combined with low cell counts for certain response categories in women, separate binge drinking variables were derived for men and women. In men it was coded as follows: (1, reference category) always consuming between 1–59 g of alcohol per single drinking occasion, (2) consuming 60+ g on an occasional basis (defined as less than monthly), (3) 60–99 g in a single sitting at least monthly, (4) 100–139 g in a single sitting at least monthly, (5) 140+g in a single sitting at least monthly, (6) 60–99 g in a single sitting at least weekly, (7) 100–139 g in a single sitting at least weekly, (8) 140+g in a single sitting at least weekly and (9) past-year abstainers (those who reported no alcohol consumption in the previous 12 months on the graduated frequency questionnaire). For women, categories 4 and 5, and 7 and 8 were combined to form 100+g on an at least monthly or weekly basis respectively. We used frequency to determine the category drinkers belonged to in cases whereby participants reported exceeding one threshold on a monthly basis and another on a weekly basis (e.g. if a participant consumed 140+ g on a monthly basis and 60–99 g on a weekly basis then they would be classified as belonging to the 60–99 g on a weekly basis group). The rationale behind this decision is that frequency better reflects usual drinking habits than overall amount alone. Approximately 18 and 11% of men categorised as belonging to the 60–99 g in a single sitting on a weekly basis category drank 100 g or 140 g in a single occasion on a monthly basis, respectively. Around 19% of men belonging to the 100–139 g on a weekly basis category drank 140+ g in a single drinking episode on a monthly basis. Almost 13% of women belonging to the category of 60–99 g in a single sitting on a weekly basis drank 100+ g on one occasion monthly.

The purpose of deriving this variable was to compare each dose/frequency category (as well as abstention) with a non-binge drinking reference group always consuming between 1 and <59 g of alcohol per occasion; not simply, for example, looking at those who drank ≥100 grams in a single sitting on a monthly basis compared to those who did not consume this amount (a category which would then also include participants who were themselves binge drinkers albeit at a lower threshold). However, for the sake of completeness, we also estimated models examining the relationship between frequency of consuming 60+, 100+ and 140+g and depressive symptoms separately. For each dose of alcohol, frequency responses were as follows: (1) never, (2) 1–11 times per year, (3) 1–3 times per month, (4) weekly, and (5) past year abstainers. At doses of 100+ and 140+ g per occasion the category of never was divided into those always consuming between 1–59 g of alcohol per single drinking occasion (referent) and those who drank above 60 g but always less than X g per occasion. The estimates from these models can be found in *Information S1*.

Drinking volume

From the graduated frequency we also derived a measure of total volume of alcohol consumed in the previous year. We categorised consumption levels above 240 g (a threshold reflecting less than one drink per month) into sex-specific tertiles of consumption derived from the entire sample. These were 260–1740 g, 1750–6020 g and >6400 g for men, and 260–420 g, 430–1200 g and >1210 g for women. The final variable used in analyses consisted of the following categories: (1) abstainers, (2) ≤ 240 g per annum, (3) first tertile of consumption, (4) second tertile of consumption (reference category), and (5) third tertile of consumption.

Problem drinking

Problem drinking was assessed using the CAGE questionnaire [32,33]. CAGE is an acronym of the first four letters of the key words in each question: 1) "Have you ever felt you should Cut down on your drinking?", 2) "Have people ever Annoyed you by criticising your drinking?", 3) "Have you ever felt bad or Guilty about your drinking?", and 4) "Have you ever had a drink first thing in the morning to steady your nerves or get rid of a hangover (as an "Eye opener")?". Positive responses to two or more of the questions are commonly used as an indicator of problem drinking [34].

Former drinkers and lifelong abstainers

In the Russian cohort those who reported having not consumed alcohol in the past 12 months were asked whether they had previously consumed alcohol. These questions were used to stratify the abstainer group into former drinkers and life-long abstainers.

Assessment of depressive symptoms

Depressive symptoms were assessed using the 20-item Center for Epidemiologic Studies Depression (CES-D) scale [35]. The CES-D is a self-report questionnaire aimed to measure the presence of depressive symptoms in the past week (e.g. "I felt depressed" or "I was bothered by things that usually don't bother me"). Items are scored on a 4-point Likert scale, with response options relating to how frequent the participant experienced each of the 20 symptoms: (0) rarely or none of the time (less than 1 day); (1) some or a little of the time (1–2 days); (2) occasionally or a moderate amount of time (3–4 days); and (3) most or all of the time (5–7 days). Scores were combined to form an aggregate depression score on a scale of 0 to 60 and those with scores of 16 or above were considered to have depressive symptoms [36,37]. This threshold has been demonstrated to have acceptable specificity and sensitivity in comparison to clinical interview based measures of depressive disorder [38,39].

Covariates

The following covariates were used in analyses: age, marital status (married/cohabiting [reference category], single, divorced/separated and widowed) [40,41], educational attainment (university, secondary/vocational [reference category], primary or less) [42,43], material deprivation level score [44,45] which was based on three questions concerning how often the participants' household did not have enough money to buy food or clothes, or to pay bills such as housing, heating and electricity, with the possible answers "never", "rarely", "sometimes", "often" or "all the time", coded as 0–4. These items were summed and then categorised into three groups: low (reference category; scores of 0–1), intermediate (scores of 2–8) and high (scores of 9–12). Smoking status (never smoked [reference category], current smoker, ex-smoker) was also controlled for [40,46].

Statistical Analysis

Logistic regression was used to estimate odds ratios (ORs) and associated 95% confidence intervals (CIs) for depressive symptoms by binge drinking dose/frequency, annual volume of alcohol intake as well as problem drinking. Separate models were fitted for each drinking measure as including all drinking components in the same model would likely represent over-adjustment [47] and therefore bias the effect estimates (estimates from models including all drinking variables simultaneously are made available for interested readers in *Information S2*).

To compare the consistency of associations across countries, we tested for interactions between drinking variables and cohort; we found p-values <0.01 in all interaction tests. Models were further stratified by gender (frequency/dose variables differed by sex). Within all centres, we present two models: model 1 was adjusted for age only, and model 2 was adjusted for all covariates.

All models were fitted using Stata 13.1 [48]. An alpha level of 0.05 was considered statistically significant for all analyses.

Results

Sample composition

Table 1 outlines descriptive statistics by country and gender. Briefly, among men, problem drinking was more common in Russia followed by Poland and the Czech Republic. Binge drinking in general was also more common in Russian men with almost 30% of respondents reporting binge drinking on a weekly basis compared to approximately 18% of Czech Republic men and 7% of Polish men. Men from the Czech Republic and Russia consumed a higher volume of alcohol annually than those from Poland. A greater proportion of Polish men abstained from alcohol in the previous year, followed by Russia and the Czech Republic. Depressive symptoms were also more common in Polish men.

Among women, abstaining rates were high in Poland doubling the rate of both Russia and the Czech Republic. Problem drinking was highest for women from the Czech Republic followed by those from Russia and Poland. A greater proportion of those from the Czech Republic and Russia engaged in binge drinking on a monthly or weekly basis, although the behaviour was not common in any country (especially heavy binge drinking). Women from the Czech Republic had a higher annual intake of alcohol than women from Russia and Poland. Depressive symptoms were more common amongst women; almost a quarter of women from the Czech Republic and, 34 and 33% of women from Russia and Poland were identified as having depressive symptoms.

Regression estimates

For men (Table 2), in the Czech Republic significant increased odds of depressive symptoms were observed for those drinking 140+g on a weekly basis (OR 1.92, CI 1.16–3.17) in comparison to those always drinking <60 g in a single sitting. In Poland, binge drinking on a weekly basis was associated with increased odds of depressive symptoms irrespective of the amount consumed in a single session (however upon adjustment for confounding factors the effects were attenuated). Russian men who consumed between 100 to 139 g of ethanol in a single sitting on a monthly basis had lower odds of depressive symptoms (OR 0.53, CI 0.31–0.89) than those who always drank <60 g in a single sitting and this reduced odds was maintained after adjustment for confounding factors (OR 0.47, CI 0.28–0.81). Men who abstained from alcohol in the previous 12 months also had higher odds of depressive symptoms

Table 1. Descriptive information by country and sex.

	Czech				Russia				Poland			
	Men		Women		Men		Women		Men		Women	
	N	%	N	%	N	%	N	%	N	%	N	%
Depressive symptoms												
No	3052	86.2	3092	76.2	2636	85.0	2526	66.4	3789	79.3	3412	67.0
Yes	489	13.8	968	23.8	465	15.0	1281	33.6	988	20.7	1683	33.0
Drinking session dose/frequency												
Abstainer	227	6.4	738	18.2	418	13.5	620	16.3	1090	22.8	2439	47.9
Always <60 g in a single sitting	887	25.1	2091	51.5	444	14.3	2451	64.4	1511	31.6	2069	40.6
60+g occasionally	1091	30.8	837	20.6	579	18.7	464	12.2	1215	25.4	443	8.7
60–99 g monthly	450	12.7	226	5.6	358	11.5	173	4.5	361	7.6	87	1.7
100–139 g† monthly	159	4.5	78	1.9	205	6.6	32	0.8	131	2.7	26	0.5
140+g monthly	107	3.0	—	—	170	5.5	—	—	152	3.2	—	—
60–99 g weekly	399	11.3	56	1.4	462	14.9	53	1.4	186	3.9	23	0.5
100–139 g† weekly	121	3.4	34	0.8	259	8.4	14	0.4	62	1.3	8	0.2
140+g weekly	100	2.8	—	—	206	6.6	—	—	69	1.4	—	—
Annual drinking volume												
Abstainer	227	6.4	738	18.2	418	13.5	620	16.3	1090	22.8	2439	47.9
<=240 g	389	11.0	1165	28.7	137	4.4	1274	33.5	565	11.8	1185	23.3
1st tertile	753	21.3	388	9.6	757	24.4	933	24.5	1315	27.5	423	8.3
2nd tertile	888	25.1	669	16.5	820	26.4	581	15.3	1140	23.9	589	11.6
3rd tertile	1284	36.3	1100	27.1	969	31.3	399	10.5	667	14.0	458	9.00
CAGE score												
<2	2940	90.0	3193	97.3	2066	77.0	3126	98.1	3198	88.2	2556	98.3
2+	326	10.0	88	2.7	617	23.0	61	1.9	430	11.8	45	1.7
Age (mean, SD)	3541	58.4 (7.2)	4060	57.7 (7.1)	3101	58.1 (7.0)	3807	57.9 (7.1)	4777	57.9 (7.0)	5095	57.5 (7.0)
Marital status												
Married/cohabiting	2976	84.0	2776	68.4	2743	88.5	2308	60.6	4139	86.6	3399	66.7
Single	105	3.0	98	2.4	70	2.3	172	4.5	197	4.1	357	7.0
Divorced/separated	347	9.8	615	15.1	166	5.4	549	14.4	261	5.5	465	9.1
Widowed	113	3.2	571	14.1	122	3.9	778	20.4	180	3.8	874	17.2
Educational attainment												
Primary or less	205	5.8	725	17.9	182	5.9	227	6.0	464	9.7	718	14.1
Secondary/vocational	2667	75.3	2900	71.4	1870	60.3	2524	66.3	2920	61.1	3025	59.4
University	669	18.9	435	10.7	1049	33.8	1056	27.7	1393	29.2	1352	26.5
Smoking status												

Table 1. Cont.

	Czech				Russia				Poland			
	Men		Women		Men		Women		Men		Women	
	N	%	N	%	N	%	N	%	N	%	N	%
Never	1121	31.7	2214	54.5	759	24.5	3225	84.7	1325	27.7	2602	51.1
Current	1055	29.8	962	23.7	1505	48.5	392	10.3	1717	35.9	1442	28.3
Former	1365	38.6	884	21.8	837	27.0	190	5.0	1735	36.3	1051	20.6
Material deprivation												
Low	2247	66.3	2396	59.0	1462	47.2	961	25.2	2854	59.7	2544	49.9
Intermediate	1140	32.2	1580	38.9	1493	48.2	2498	65.6	1680	35.2	2203	43.2
High	54	1.5	84	2.1	146	4.7	348	9.1	243	5.09	348	6.8

†The figures presented for the category of 100–139 g in a single sitting for women also contain those drinking 140+ g; see methods section.
Some percentage totals may exceed 100 due to rounding.

in the Czech Republic (adjusted OR 1.55, CI 1.05–2.28) as well as Poland (adjusted OR 1.59, CI 1.31–1.94). In terms of annual volume of alcohol consumed, those who abstained from alcohol had consistently higher odds of depressive symptoms than those in the second tertile of consumption (after full adjustment this effect was attenuated and became non-significant in the Czech Republic but the overall OR continued to indicate increased odds). In Russia and Poland, those drinking ≤240 g of alcohol annually had increased odds of depressive symptoms when compared to those in the second tertile of consumption, as did those belonging to the first tertile of consumption in Russia (adjusted OR 1.39, CI 1.04, 1.87). Only in Poland was there an increased risk in the third tertile of annual alcohol consumption (adjusted OR 1.42, CI 1.11, 1.81)

For women (Table 3), those who abstained from alcohol in the previous 12 months had increased odds of depressive symptoms when compared to those always drinking <60 g in a single sitting in the Czech Republic (adjusted OR 1.30, CI 1.07–1.59) and Poland (adjusted OR 1.35, CI 1.18, 1.54). In the Czech Republic, women consuming 100 g+ on a weekly basis had increased odds of depressive symptoms (OR 2.45, CI 1.23–4.90) however this was attenuated after controlling for confounding factors (OR 1.93, CI 0.94–3.96). In both Russia (adjusted OR 3.31, CI 1.52–6.55) and Poland (adjusted OR 2.84, CI 1.26–6.41) women consuming 100+ g on a monthly basis had increased odds of depressive symptoms in comparison to those who always drank <60 g in a single sitting. When looking at differences in the odds of depressive symptoms by total volume of alcohol consumed in the previous year, abstainers in all countries had higher odds than those in the second tertile of alcohol intake. In Russia, those with an intake of ≤240 g had higher odds of depressive symptoms (adjusted OR 1.31, CI 1.05–1.64).

Problem drinking was consistently associated with increased odds of depressive symptoms across all countries in both men (Table 2) and women (Table 3).

When stratifying the abstainer group into former drinkers and life-long abstainers (Table 4) in the Russian cohort, neither abstainer category had increased odds of depressive symptoms compared to those always drinking <60 g in a single sitting for men, while for women, former drinkers had increased odds (adjusted OR 1.37, CI 1.09–1.72) but not lifelong abstainers. Former drinkers had higher odds of depressive symptoms in all models relating to annual alcohol intake in comparison to those in the second tertile of consumption (adjusted ORs of 1.55, CI 1.10, 2.17 and 1.64, CI 1.23, 2.17 for men and women respectively).

Discussion

Summary of findings

In this large population based study in Eastern Europe, we found that problem drinking was consistently associated with an increased prevalence of depressive symptoms in all populations and both sexes. With binge drinking, the results were slightly less consistent. In men, frequent heavy binge drinking (140+ g in a sitting at least once a week) was associated with increased odds of depressive symptoms in the Czech Republic and Poland. Interestingly, Russian men who drank 100–139 g of alcohol in a single sitting on a monthly basis had lower odds of depressive symptoms than those always drinking less than 60 g in a single sitting. Among women, there was a tendency for those who engaged in heavy binge drinking (100+g in a single sitting) to have higher odds of depressive symptoms but the odds ratios were not statistically significant in the case of at least weekly binge drinking.

Table 2. Odds ratios (95% confidence intervals) for depressive symptoms by binge drinking dose/frequency, annual drinking volume and problem drinking by country in men.

	Czech (N = 3541)		Russia (N = 3101)		Poland (N = 4777)	
	Age adjusted	**Fully adjusted‡**	**Age adjusted**	**Fully adjusted**	**Age adjusted**	**Fully adjusted**
Binge drinking dose/frequency						
Abstainer	1.73** [1.19,2.51]	1.55* [1.05,2.28]	1.12 [0.79,1.59]	1.03 [0.71,1.48]	1.67*** [1.38,2.01]	1.59*** [1.31,1.94]
Always <60 g in a single sitting	1.00 (ref.)	1.00 (ref.)	1.00 (ref.)	1.00 (ref.)	1.00 (ref.)	1.00 (ref.)
60+g occasionally	0.88 [0.68,1.16]	0.98 [0.74,1.28]	0.77 [0.55,1.08]	0.77 [0.55,1.10]	0.88 [0.72,1.08]	0.88 [0.72,1.08]
60–99 g monthly	0.92 [0.66,1.30]	1.01 [0.71,1.44]	0.86 [0.59,1.25]	0.81 [0.55,1.21]	0.98 [0.73,1.31]	0.92 [0.68,1.25]
100–139 g monthly	0.91 [0.55,1.51]	1.01 [0.60,1.69]	0.53* [0.31,0.89]	0.47** [0.28,0.81]	1.06 [0.68,1.67]	0.97 [0.61,1.55]
140+g monthly	1.30 [0.76,2.23]	1.18 [0.68,2.05]	1.18 [0.75,1.87]	1.02 [0.63,1.66]	0.78 [0.50,1.24]	0.67 [0.42,1.07]
60–99 g weekly	0.84 [0.59,1.21]	0.83 [0.57,1.21]	0.66* [0.45,0.97]	0.68 [0.46,1.00]	1.44* [1.01,2.06]	1.38 [0.95,2.01]
100–139 g weekly	0.92 [0.52,1.62]	0.89 [0.50,1.59]	0.78 [0.51,1.21]	0.77 [0.49,1.21]	2.36** [1.38,4.04]	1.71 [0.96,3.04]
140+g weekly	1.92* [1.16,3.17]	1.67 [1.00,2.81]	0.98 [0.62,1.53]	0.83 [0.52,1.32]	1.93* [1.14,3.26]	1.53 [0.88,2.65]
Annual drinking volume						
Abstainer	1.72** [1.18,2.50]	1.43 [0.97,2.11]	1.64** [1.18,2.26]	1.55** [1.11,2.17]	1.89*** [1.53,2.32]	1.88*** [1.52,2.34]
≤240 g	1.08 [0.76,1.52]	0.99 [0.70,1.41]	1.68* [1.05,2.69]	1.61 [0.99,2.63]	1.25 [0.96,1.62]	1.32* [1.01,1.72]
1st tertile	0.97 [0.73,1.28]	0.97 [0.73,1.30]	1.36* [1.02,1.81]	1.39* [1.04,1.87]	1.04 [0.84,1.28]	1.08 [0.87,1.34]
2nd tertile	1.00 (ref.)	1.00 (ref.)	1.00 (ref.)	1.00 (ref.)	1.00 (ref.)	1.00 (ref.)
3rd tertile	0.87 [0.68,1.12]	0.83 [0.64,1.07]	1.18 [0.90,1.56]	1.17 [0.88,1.55]	1.48** [1.17,1.88]	1.42** [1.11,1.81]
Problem drinking†						
No	1.00 (ref.)	1.00 (ref.)	1.00 (ref.)	1.00 (ref.)	1.00 (ref.)	1.00 (ref.)
Yes	2.18*** [1.65,2.89]	2.09*** [1.56,2.78]	1.82*** [1.44,2.31]	1.66*** [1.29,2.13]	3.17*** [2.55,3.94]	2.76*** [2.20,3.48]

*** $p<0.001$;
** $p<0.01$;
* $p<0.05$.
†Models concerning problem drinking (CAGE score 2+) are restricted to those who consumed alcohol in the previous 12 months (Czech N = 3266, Russia N = 2683, Poland N = 3828).
‡Full adjustment = age, marital status, educational attainment, material deprivation level and smoking status.

Abstaining from alcohol was also associated with increased odds of depressive symptoms in comparison to moderate drinking except in Russia; however, compared to the second tertile of annual alcohol consumption, abstainers had consistently higher odds of depressive symptoms. Analyses attempting to disentangle lifelong non-drinkers from former drinkers typically revealed significantly increased odds of depressive symptoms in former drinkers.

Interpretation and comparison to other work

These findings corroborate previous studies in Central and Eastern Europe which have found binge drinking to be associated with increased rates of depressive symptoms [22], including earlier analyses of the HAPIEE data [15]. However, the models used previously [15] differ substantially from those used here. The previous analyses used a relatively low dose of alcohol (<20 g, including abstainers) as the reference category (in comparison to the referent group used in this study, i.e. always consuming <60 g in a single sitting and excluding abstainers) and they used the mean dose of alcohol in a single drinking session as the main exposure (using a maximum dose of ≥80 g). While the previous analyses found increased odds of depressive symptoms in binge drinkers, the previous definition did not take into account the frequency of binge drinking or the graded increase in the amount of alcohol consumed in a binge drinking session (i.e. different doses above 60 g). When the intensity and frequency of binge drinking are accounted for, as in our analyses, it appears that both elements are important in terms of the association with depressive symptoms.

An unexpected finding was that Russian men who consumed 100–139 g in a single sitting at least monthly had lower odds of depressive symptoms than those who always consumed less than 60 g in a drinking occasion. A possible explanation for this finding is that those who drank heavily did so with friends and therefore social participation served as a protective factor against depression, whilst also increasing the opportunity to drink at hazardous levels [49,50]. However, given that this result was not replicated in the Czech Republic or Polish cohorts (or in women) appropriate caution should be applied in the interpretation this this finding.

To our knowledge only one other study has examined abstaining from alcohol as a risk factor for poor mental health in Eastern Europe, focussing on Russian men [51]. Our findings are generally consistent with that study in that we found abstaining was not associated with greater odds of depressive symptoms in Russia when looking at drinking pattern (effect estimates indicated poorer mental health for abstaining Russians in both studies but these effects did not reach statistical significance) but in analyses of the association between annual drinking volume and depressive symptoms, Russians who abstained from alcohol actually had significantly increased odds of depression.

Table 3. Odds ratios (95% confidence intervals) for depressive symptoms by binge drinking dose/frequency, annual drinking volume and problem drinking by country in women.

	Czech (N = 4060)		Russia (N = 3807)		Poland (N = 5095)	
	Age adjusted	**Fully adjusted‡**	**Age adjusted**	**Fully adjusted**	**Age adjusted**	**Fully adjusted**
Binge drinking dose/frequency						
Abstainer	1.48*** [1.22,1.79]	1.30** [1.07,1.59]	1.19 [0.99,1.44]	1.14 [0.94,1.37]	1.43*** [1.25,1.62]	1.35*** [1.18,1.54]
Always <60 g in a single sitting	1.00 (ref.)	1.00 (ref.)	1.00 (ref.)	1.00 (ref.)	1.00 (ref.)	1.00 (ref.)
60+g occasionally	1.06 [0.88,1.29]	1.10 [0.90,1.35]	0.91 [0.73,1.13]	0.85 [0.68,1.07]	1.24 [1.00,1.55]	1.17 [0.93,1.47]
60–99 g monthly	0.80 [0.56,1.14]	0.81 [0.57,1.17]	1.02 [0.73,1.43]	1.01 [0.72,1.41]	0.99 [0.62,1.59]	0.90 [0.54,1.48]
100+g monthly	1.46 [0.89,2.41]	1.38 [0.82,2.32]	3.31** [1.62,6.77]	3.16** [1.52,6.55]	2.85** [1.31,6.19]	2.84* [1.26,6.41]
60–99 g weekly	1.06 [0.56,1.99]	1.09 [0.57,2.08]	1.22 [0.69,2.16]	1.26 [0.71,2.25]	0.86 [0.34,2.20]	0.81 [0.31,2.13]
100+g weekly	2.45* [1.23,4.90]	1.93 [0.94,3.96]	1.30 [0.43,3.90]	0.96 [0.31,2.97]	1.47 [0.35,6.17]	1.53 [0.34,6.86]
Annual drinking volume						
Abstainer	1.52*** [1.19,1.95]	1.32* [1.02,1.70]	1.39** [1.09,1.78]	1.37* [1.06,1.76]	1.56*** [1.28,1.91]	1.48*** [1.19,1.83]
≤240 g annually	1.14 [0.90,1.43]	1.11 [0.88,1.41]	1.31* [1.06,1.63]	1.31* [1.05,1.64]	1.22 [0.98,1.52]	1.18 [0.94,1.49]
1st tertile	1.05 [0.78,1.42]	0.97 [0.71,1.32]	1.04 [0.83,1.30]	1.10 [0.87,1.38]	1.01 [0.76,1.34]	1.00 [0.74,1.33]
2nd tertile	1.00 (ref.)	1.00 (ref.)	1.00 (ref.)	1.00 (ref.)	1.00 (ref.)	1.00 (ref.)
3rd tertile	0.98 [0.78,1.24]	1.00 [0.79,1.27]	1.25 [0.95,1.64]	1.28 [0.96,1.69]	1.29 [0.99,1.68]	1.30 [0.99,1.72]
Problem drinking†						
No	1.00 (ref.)	1.00 (ref.)	1.00 (ref.)	1.00 (ref.)	1.00 (ref.)	1.00 (ref.)
Yes	2.36*** [1.52,3.66]	2.28*** [1.45,3.59]	2.51*** [1.51,4.18]	2.38** [1.41,4.03]	3.89*** [2.12,7.16]	3.37*** [1.77,6.42]

*** $p<0.001$;
** $p<0.01$;
* $p<0.05$.
†Models concerning problem drinking (CAGE score 2+) are restricted to those who consumed alcohol in the previous 12 months (Czech N = 3541, Russia N = 3101, Poland N = 4777).
‡Full adjustment = age, marital status, educational attainment, material deprivation level and smoking status.

In our data, problem drinkers had consistently increased odds of depressive symptoms. This finding is in line with previous findings on the topic of depression and alcohol consumption in Eastern Europe [22,23]. In studies elsewhere, problem drinking has been demonstrated to increase the risk of prevalent [9,22,52–56] and incident [6–8,57] depression independent of the amount of alcohol a person consumes or the manner in which that they consume it [21,58].

Table 4. Odds ratios (95% confidence intervals) for former drinkers and lifelong abstainers on depressive symptoms in the Russian HAPIEE cohort.

	Men			Women		
	N	**Age adjusted**	**Fully adjusted‡**	**N**	**Age adjusted**	**Fully adjusted**
Binge drinking dose/frequency						
Always <60 g in a single sitting	—	1.00 [1.00,1.00]	1.00 [1.00,1.00]	—	1.00 [1.00,1.00]	1.00 [1.00,1.00]
Former drinker	388	1.12 [0.78,1.59]	1.02 [0.71,1.48]	369	1.41** [1.13,1.77]	1.37** [1.09,1.72]
Lifelong abstainer	30	1.17 [0.46,2.98]	1.07 [0.41,2.80]	251	0.92 [0.70,1.22]	0.86 [0.65,1.14]
Annual drinking volume						
2nd tertile	—	1.00 [1.00,1.00]	1.00 [1.00,1.00]	—	1.00 [1.00,1.00]	1.00 [1.00,1.00]
Former drinker	388	1.63** [1.17, 2.27]	1.55** [1.10, 2.17]	369	1.65*** [1.25, 2.18]	1.64*** [1.23, 2.17]
Lifelong abstainer	30	1.72 [0.69, 4.33]	1.63 [0.63, 4.23]	251	1.07 [0.78, 1.48]	1.03 [0.74, 1.43]

*** $p<0.001$;
** $p<0.01$;
* $p<0.05$.
‡Full adjustment = age, marital status, educational attainment, material deprivation level and smoking status.

Strengths and weaknesses

Specific strengths of this analysis include the large sample size of each country – providing relatively good statistical power (with certain exceptions outlined below). Furthermore, standardised internationally validated tools were used to collect information on individual drinking episodes and depressive symptoms. Data from the graduated frequency questionnaire were then used to create a variable which took into account both dose and frequency of binge drinking and derive total annual alcohol intake.

There are, however, also several shortcomings. First, these analyses are based on cross-sectional data. It is plausible that the relationship would differ over time and examining the association over multiple occasions may provide additional aetiological insights into the possibly bi-directional relationship between alcohol consumption and depressive symptoms [5,59,60] (that is, depressive symptoms may cause people to drink in binges, and drinking in binges may exacerbate depressive symptoms). Therefore further work using longitudinal data is warranted.

Another limitation is that in some of our statistical models, abstainers had to be grouped into a single aggregate category of past year non-drinkers, although the reasons for present/recent non-drinking are likely to be heterogeneous. Many other investigators have pointed out the weaknesses of using an aggregate group of abstainers [26,27,61] as a comparison group for moderate (and other) drinkers. There are valid concerns that moderate drinking may inadvertently be attributed as having beneficial effects compared to non-drinking when the reality may be that this difference is due to residual confounding [62] or failure to distinguish former drinkers and occasional drinkers from the lifelong abstaining group [27,63]. In our study we were able to stratify the abstainer group into former drinkers and lifelong abstainers in Russia (Table 4). We found that there were increased odds of depressive symptoms amongst former drinkers, supporting the argument that the increased odds of depressive symptoms among abstainers may largely be driven by former drinkers as previously reported elsewhere [64].

A third limitation is that the frequency of consuming <60 g in a single sitting was not taken into account. The reference group used in these analyses may therefore contain a number of occasional or, conversely, frequent drinkers which may bias the relationship observed [27]. However, additional analyses did not detect a significant association between depressive symptoms and drinking frequency in this group (with the exception of Russian women, where those drinking very infrequently (only 1–5 times per year) had increased odds of depression; data not presented). It is also possible that the reference group contains some individuals who have reduced their alcohol consumption over time due to ill-health [65,66]. There was no information available to account for this possibility at baseline, and interpretation of the above findings should be made with this in mind.

Fourth, there may also be concerns about the small number of female binge drinkers identified in the study, especially categories relating to heavy and frequent binge drinking. The odds ratios for female drinkers have wide confidence intervals and should be interpreted with appropriate caution.

A fifth limitation relates to both alcohol and depressive symptom measures being based on self-reported data. Self-report measures of alcohol consumption have been consistently demonstrated to provide inaccurate estimates of consumption [67,68] and self-report measures of depressive symptoms are not (necessarily) equivalent to clinical diagnoses [69].

Sixth, participants were aged between 45 and 69 years of age. It is plausible that the same relationship might not be present in younger or older populations. Studies examining the relationship between alcohol use disorders and major depression earlier in the life-course also find a consistent relationship between problematic drinking and depression [7] suggesting that the association between these two measures might be consistent across the life-course. However, drinking pattern is known to fluctuate over time [70] and hazardous drinking declines with age [71] – this may explain why we do not see a consistent picture with respect to the association between binge drinking or annual volume of alcohol consumed and depressive symptoms in our sample. Analyses focussed on life-course patterns of alcohol intake in relation to depressive symptomology may provide important additional information, such as whether there are periods in the life-course whereby binge drinking is most commonly linked with depressive symptoms or if the relationship between drinking pattern and depressive symptoms is best explained by accumulated exposure of life-time drinking. Such hypotheses strengthen the argument that longitudinal work on this topic is warranted.

Finally, the rates of abstention in Poland were higher than in other populations in HAPIEE and than what we would expect from population level surveys [4]. Almost 35% of the Polish sample reported being non-drinkers at baseline. The reason for such a high rate is believed to be related to the Polish questionnaire containing a filter question which allowed for participants to skip the alcohol related questions if they indicated being non-drinkers in the last 12 months. However, the associations of abstention with depressive symptoms in Polish subjects were similar to Czech participants, as would be expected from the geographical and cultural closeness of these two populations. This suggests that the filter questions did not introduce a major bias.

Conclusions

Our findings indicate that dose of alcohol consumed in a binge drinking session and the frequency of doing so may contribute to the burden of depression in Eastern Europe but problem drinking was the alcohol variable consistently associated with increased odds of depressive symptoms in all countries, indicating that it is likely to be a useful predictor of depression in Eastern Europe. It is possible that the increased odds of depressive symptoms observed amongst non-drinkers is driven by former drinkers. Future work will however need to investigate whether this relationship holds when predicting depressive symptoms prospectively using a longitudinal design.

Supporting Information

Information S1 Estimates from models relating the frequency of drinking >60, 100 and 140 g in the past year to depressive symptoms.

Information S2 Estimates from models whereby binge drinking dose/frequency, annual drinking volume and problem drinking are simultaneously included in the same model.

Acknowledgments

We would like to thank all individuals participating in the HAPIEE study as well as all members of the HAPIEE study team.

Author Contributions

Conceived and designed the experiments: SB AB MB RK SM AP YN. Performed the experiments: SB AB MB RK SM AP YN. Analyzed the data: SB. Wrote the paper: SB. Revised the manuscript critically for important intellectual content and approved the final draft: AB RK SM AP YN MB.

References

1. Becker AE, Kleinman A (2013) Mental Health and the Global Agenda. N Engl J Med 369: 66–73. doi:10.1056/NEJMra1110827
2. Mathers CD, Loncar D (2006) Projections of Global Mortality and Burden of Disease from 2002 to 2030. PLoS Med 3: e442. doi:10.1371/journal.pmed.0030442
3. Patel V, Jenkins R, Lund C, the PLoS Medicine Editors (2012) Putting Evidence into Practice: The PLoS Medicine Series on Global Mental Health Practice. PLoS Med 9: e1001226. doi:10.1371/journal.pmed.1001226
4. World Health Organisation (2012) Alcohol in the European Union. Consumption, harm and policy approaches. Copenhagen, Denmark: World Health Organisation Regional Office for Europe. Available: http://www.euro.who.int/__data/assets/pdf_file/0003/160680/e96457.pdf. Accessed 25 April 2012.
5. Mueser KT, Drake RE, Wallach MA (1998) Dual diagnosis: A review of etiological theories. Addict Behav 23: 717–734. doi:10.1016/S0306-4603(98)00073-2
6. Boden JM, Fergusson DM (2011) Alcohol and depression. Addiction 106: 906–914. doi:10.1111/j.1360-0443.2010.03351.x
7. Fergusson DM, Boden JM, Horwood LJ (2009) Tests of Causal Links Between Alcohol Abuse or Dependence and Major Depression. Arch Gen Psychiatry 66: 260–266. doi:10.1001/archgenpsychiatry.2008.543
8. Boschloo L, van den Brink W, Penninx BWJH, Wall MM, Hasin DS (2012) Alcohol-use disorder severity predicts first-incidence of depressive disorders. Psychol Med 42: 695–703. doi:10.1017/S0033291711001681
9. Grant BF, Harford TC (1995) Comorbidity between DSM-IV alcohol use disorders and major depression: results of a national survey. Drug Alcohol Depend 39: 197–206. doi:10.1016/0376-8716(95)01160-4
10. Haynes JC, Farrell M, Singleton N, Meltzer H, Araya R, et al. (2005) Alcohol consumption as a risk factor for anxiety and depression: Results from the longitudinal follow-up of the National Psychiatric Morbidity Survey. Br J Psychiatry 187: 544–551. doi:10.1192/bjp.187.6.544
11. Paljärvi T, Koskenvuo M, Poikolainen K, Kauhanen J, Sillanmäki L, et al. (2009) Binge drinking and depressive symptoms: a 5-year population-based cohort study. Addiction 104: 1168–1178. doi:10.1111/j.1360-0443.2009.02577.x
12. Wang J, Patten SB (2001) Alcohol consumption and major depression: findings from a follow-up study. Can J Psychiatry 46: 632–638.
13. Wang J, Patten SB (2002) Prospective study of frequent heavy alcohol use and the risk of major depression in the Canadian general population. Depress Anxiety 15: 42–45. doi:10.1002/da.1084
14. Graham K, Massak A, Demers A, Rehm J (2007) Does the Association Between Alcohol Consumption and Depression Depend on How They Are Measured? Alcohol Clin Exp Res 31: 78–88. doi:10.1111/j.1530-0277.2006.00274.x
15. Bobak M, Pikhart H, Pajak A, Kubinova R, Malyutina S, et al. (2006) Depressive symptoms in urban population samples in Russia, Poland and the Czech Republic. Br J Psychiatry 188: 359–365. doi:10.1192/bjp.188.4.359
16. Ferrari AJ, Charlson FJ, Norman RE, Patten SB, Freedman G, et al. (2013) Burden of Depressive Disorders by Country, Sex, Age, and Year: Findings from the Global Burden of Disease Study 2010. PLoS Med 10: e1001547. doi:10.1371/journal.pmed.1001547
17. Popova S, Rehm J, Patra J, Zatonski W (2007) Comparing alcohol consumption in central and eastern Europe to other European countries. Alcohol Alcohol 42: 465–473. doi:10.1093/alcalc/agl124
18. Room R (2005) Commentary: Pattern of drinking and the Russian heart. Int J Epidemiol 34: 788–790. doi:10.1093/ije/dyi117
19. Bobak M, Room R, Pikhart H, Kubinova R, Malyutina S, et al. (2004) Contribution of drinking patterns to differences in rates of alcohol related problems between three urban populations. J Epidemiol Community Health 58: 238–242. doi:10.1136/jech.2003.011825
20. Leon DA, Shkolnikov VM, McKee M (2009) Alcohol and Russian mortality: a continuing crisis. Addiction 104: 1630–1636. doi:10.1111/j.1360-0443.2009.02655.x
21. Bulloch A, Lavorato D, Williams J, Patten S (2012) Alcohol Consumption and Major Depression In The General Population: The Critical Importance of Dependence. Depress Anxiety 29: 1058–1064. doi:10.1002/da.22001
22. Zhan W, Shaboltas A, Skochilov R, Kozlov A, Krasnoselskikh T (2012) Gender Differences in the Relationship between Alcohol Use and Depressive Symptoms in St. Petersburg, Russia. J Addict Res Ther 3. doi:10.4172/2155-6105.1000124
23. Averina M, Nilssen O, Brenn T, Brox J, Arkhipovsky V, et al. (2005) Social and lifestyle determinants of depression, anxiety, sleeping disorders and self-evaluated quality of life in Russia. Soc Psychiatry Psychiatr Epidemiol 40: 511–518. doi:10.1007/s00127-005-0918-x
24. Peele S, Brodsky A (2000) Exploring psychological benefits associated with moderate alcohol use: a necessary corrective to assessments of drinking outcomes? Drug Alcohol Depend 60: 221–247. doi:10.1016/S0376-8716(00)00112-5
25. Baum-Baicker C (1985) The psychological benefits of moderate alcohol consumption: A review of the literature. Drug Alcohol Depend 15: 305–322. doi:10.1016/0376-8716(85)90008-0
26. Fillmore KM, Stockwell T, Chikritzhs T, Bostrom A, Kerr W (2007) Moderate Alcohol Use and Reduced Mortality Risk: Systematic Error in Prospective Studies and New Hypotheses. Ann Epidemiol 17: S16–S23.
27. Stockwell T, Greer A, Fillmore K, Chikritzhs T, Zeisser C (2012) How good is the science? BMJ 344: e2276.
28. Peasey A, Bobak M, Kubinova R, Malyutina S, Pajak A, et al. (2006) Determinants of cardiovascular disease and other non-communicable diseases in Central and Eastern Europe: Rationale and design of the HAPIEE study. BMC Public Health 6: 255. doi:10.1186/1471-2458-6-255
29. Rehm J (1998) Measuring Quantity, Frequency, and Volume of Drinking. Alcohol Clin Exp Res 22: 4s–14s. doi:10.1111/j.1530-0277.1998.tb04368.x
30. Greenfield TK (2000) Ways of measuring drinking patterns and the difference they make: experience with graduated frequencies. J Subst Abuse 12: 33–49. doi:10.1016/S0899-3289(00)00039-0
31. Bell S, Britton A (2011) Alcohol and men's health. Trends Urol Mens Health 2: 9–12. doi:10.1002/tre.206
32. Mayfield D, McLeod G, Hall P (1974) The CAGE questionnaire: validation of a new alcoholism screening instrument. Am J Psychiatry 131: 1121–1123.
33. Ewing JA (1984) Detecting Alcoholism: The CAGE Questionnaire. JAMA J Am Med Assoc 252: 1905–1907. doi:10.1001/jama.1984.03350140051025
34. Fiellin DA, Reid MC, O'Connor PG (2000) Screening for alcohol problems in primary care: a systematic review. Arch Intern Med 160: 1977–1989. doi:10.1001/archinte.160.13.1977
35. Radloff LS (1977) The CES-D Scale. Appl Psychol Meas 1: 385–401. doi:10.1177/014662167700100306
36. Beekman ATF, Deeg DJ., van Tilburg T, Smit JH, Hooijer C, et al. (1995) Major and minor depression in later life: a study of prevalence and risk factors. J Affect Disord 36: 65–75. doi:10.1016/0165-0327(95)00061-5
37. Ferketich AK, Schwartzbaum JA, Frid DJ, Moeschberger ML (2000) Depression as an Antecedent to Heart Disease Among Women and Men in the NHANES I Study. Arch Intern Med 160: 1261–1268. doi:10.1001/archinte.160.9.1261
38. Breslau N (1985) Depressive symptoms, major depression, and generalized anxiety: A comparison of self-reports on CES-D and results from diagnostic interviews. Psychiatry Res 15: 219–229. doi:10.1016/0165-1781(85)90079-4
39. Beekman AT, Deeg D, Van Limbeek J, Braam A, De Vries M, et al. (1997) Criterion validity of the Center for Epidemiologic Studies Depression scale (CES-D): results from a community-based sample of older subjects in The Netherlands. Psychol Med 27: 231–236.
40. Merrick EL, Horgan CM, Hodgkin D, Garnick DW, Houghton SF, et al. (2008) Unhealthy Drinking Patterns in Older Adults: Prevalence and Associated Characteristics. J Am Geriatr Soc 56: 214–223. doi:10.1111/j.1532-5415.2007.01539.x
41. Van de Velde S, Bracke P, Levecque K (2010) Gender differences in depression in 23 European countries. Cross-national variation in the gender gap in depression. Soc Sci Med 71: 305–313. doi:10.1016/j.socscimed.2010.03.035
42. Bjelland I, Krokstad S, Mykletun A, Dahl AA, Tell GS, et al. (2008) Does a higher educational level protect against anxiety and depression? The HUNT study. Soc Sci Med 66: 1334–1345. doi:10.1016/j.socscimed.2007.12.019
43. Grittner U, Kuntsche S, Gmel G, Bloomfield K (2013) Alcohol consumption and social inequality at the individual and country levels—results from an international study. Eur J Public Health 23: 332–339. doi:10.1093/eurpub/cks044
44. Bobak M, Mckee M, Rose R, Marmot M (1999) Alcohol consumption in a national sample of the Russian population. Addiction 94: 857–866. doi:10.1046/j.1360-0443.1999.9468579.x
45. Pikhartova J, Chandola T, Kubinova R, Bobak M, Nicholson A, et al. (2009) Neighbourhood socioeconomic indicators and depressive symptoms in the Czech Republic: a population based study. Int J Public Health 54: 283–293. doi:10.1007/s00038-009-8029-1
46. Boden JM, Fergusson DM, Horwood LJ (2010) Cigarette smoking and depression: tests of causal linkages using a longitudinal birth cohort. Br J Psychiatry 196: 440–446. doi:10.1192/bjp.bp.109.065912
47. Schisterman EF, Cole SR, Platt RW (2009) Overadjustment Bias and Unnecessary Adjustment in Epidemiologic Studies. Epidemiology 20: 488–495. doi:10.1097/EDE.0b013e3181a819a1
48. StataCorp (2013) Stata Statistical Software: Release 13. College Station, TX: StataCorp LP.
49. Bobrova N, West R, Malyutina D, Malyutina S, Bobak M (2010) Gender Differences in Drinking Practices in Middle Aged and Older Russians. Alcohol Alcohol 45: 573–580. doi:10.1093/alcalc/agq069
50. Peirce RS, Frone MR, Russell M, Cooper ML, Mudar P (2000) A longitudinal model of social contact, social support, depression, and alcohol use. Health Psychol 19: 28–38. doi:10.1037/0278-6133.19.1.28
51. Dissing AS, Gil A, Keenan K, McCambridge J, McKee M, et al. (2013) Alcohol consumption and self-reported (SF12) physical and mental health among working-aged men in a typical Russian city: a cross-sectional study. Addiction 108: 1905–1914. doi:10.1111/add.12257
52. Swendsen JD, Merikangas KR, Canino GJ, Kessler RC, Rubio-Stipec M, et al. (1998) The comorbidity of alcoholism with anxiety and depressive disorders in four geographic communities. Compr Psychiatry 39: 176–184. doi:10.1016/S0010-440X(98)90058-X
53. Burns L, Teesson M (2002) Alcohol use disorders comorbid with anxiety, depression and drug use disorders: Findings from the Australian National Survey

of Mental Health and Well Being. Drug Alcohol Depend 68: 299–307. doi:10.1016/S0376-8716(02)00220-X
54. Smith GW, Shevlin M (2008) Patterns of Alcohol Consumption and Related Behaviour in Great Britain: A Latent Class Analysis of the Alcohol Use Disorder Identification Test (AUDIT). Alcohol Alcohol 43: 590–594. doi:10.1093/alcalc/agn041
55. Bolton JM, Robinson J, Sareen J (2009) Self-medication of mood disorders with alcohol and drugs in the National Epidemiologic Survey on Alcohol and Related Conditions. J Affect Disord 115: 367–375. doi:10.1016/j.jad.2008.10.003
56. Boschloo L, Vogelzangs N, van den Brink W, Smit JH, Veltman DJ, et al. (2012) Alcohol use disorders and the course of depressive and anxiety disorders. Br J Psychiatry 200: 476–484. doi:10.1192/bjp.bp.111.097550
57. Flensborg-Madsen T, Mortensen EL, Knop J, Becker U, Sher L, et al. (2009) Comorbidity and temporal ordering of alcohol use disorders and other psychiatric disorders: results from a Danish register-based study. Compr Psychiatry 50: 307–314. doi:10.1016/j.comppsych.2008.09.003
58. Boschloo L, Vogelzangs N, van den Brink W, Smit JH, Veltman DJ, et al. (2012) Authors' reply. Br J Psychiatry 201: 326–327. doi:10.1192/bjp.201.4.326a
59. Meyer RE (1986) Psychopathology and addictive disorders. New York, USA: Guildford Press. 362 p.
60. Bell S, Britton A (2014) An exploration of the dynamic longitudinal relationship between mental health and alcohol consumption: a prospective cohort study. BMC Med 12: 91. doi:10.1186/1741-7015-12-91
61. Kerr WC, Ye Y (2010) Relationship of Life-Course Drinking Patterns to Diabetes, Heart Problems, and Hypertension Among Those 40 and Older in the 2005 U.S. National Alcohol Survey. J Stud Alcohol Drugs 71: 515–525.
62. Naimi TS, Brown DW, Brewer RD, Giles WH, Mensah G, et al. (2005) Cardiovascular risk factors and confounders among nondrinking and moderate-drinking U.S. adults. Am J Prev Med 28: 369–373. doi:10.1016/j.amepre.2005.01.011
63. Caldwell TM, Rodgers B, Power C, Clark C, Gamble SA (2006) Drinking histories of self-identified lifetime abstainers and occasional drinkers: findings from the 1958 British Birth cohort study. Alcohol Alcohol 41: 650–654. doi:10.1093/alcalc/agl088
64. Lucas N, Windsor TD, Caldwell TM, Rodgers B (2010) Psychological Distress in Non-Drinkers: Associations with Previous Heavy Drinking and Current Social Relationships. Alcohol Alcohol 45: 95–102. doi:10.1093/alcalc/agp080
65. Shaper AG, Wannamethee G, Walker M (1988) Alcohol and mortality in British men: explaining the U-shaped curve. The Lancet 332: 1267–1273.
66. Hu Y, Pikhart H, Malyutina S, Pajak A, Kubinova R, et al. (2014) Alcohol consumption and physical functioning among middle-aged and older adults in Central and Eastern Europe: Results from the HAPIEE study. Age Ageing: Advance Access. doi:10.1093/ageing/afu083
67. Chikirzhs T, Fillmore K, Stockwell T (2009) A healthy dose of scepticism: Four good reasons to think again about protective effects of alcohol on coronary heart disease. Drug Alcohol Rev 28: 441–444. doi:10.1111/j.1465-3362.2009.00052.x
68. Laatikainen T, Alho H, Vartiainen E, Jousilahti P, Sillanaukee P, et al. (2002) Self-reported alcohol consumption and association to carbohydrate-deficient transferrin and gamma-glutamyltransferase in a random sample of the general population in the Republic of Karelia, Russia and in North Karelia, Finland. Alcohol Alcohol 37: 282–288. doi:10.1093/alcalc/37.3.282
69. Myers JK, Weissman MM (1980) Use of a self-report symptom scale to detect depression in a community sample. Am J Psychiatry 137: 1081–1084.
70. Fillmore KM (1987) Prevalence, Incidence and Chronicity of Drinking Patterns and Problems Among Men as a Function of Age: a longitudinal and cohort analysis. Br J Addict 82: 77–83. doi:10.1111/j.1360-0443.1987.tb01440.x
71. O'Malley PM (2004) Maturing out of problematic alcohol use. Alcohol Res Health 28: 202–204.

Permissions

All chapters in this book were first published in PLOS ONE, by The Public Library of Science; hereby published with permission under the Creative Commons Attribution License or equivalent. Every chapter published in this book has been scrutinized by our experts. Their significance has been extensively debated. The topics covered herein carry significant findings which will fuel the growth of the discipline. They may even be implemented as practical applications or may be referred to as a beginning point for another development.

The contributors of this book come from diverse backgrounds, making this book a truly international effort. This book will bring forth new frontiers with its revolutionizing research information and detailed analysis of the nascent developments around the world.

We would like to thank all the contributing authors for lending their expertise to make the book truly unique. They have played a crucial role in the development of this book. Without their invaluable contributions this book wouldn't have been possible. They have made vital efforts to compile up to date information on the varied aspects of this subject to make this book a valuable addition to the collection of many professionals and students.

This book was conceptualized with the vision of imparting up-to-date information and advanced data in this field. To ensure the same, a matchless editorial board was set up. Every individual on the board went through rigorous rounds of assessment to prove their worth. After which they invested a large part of their time researching and compiling the most relevant data for our readers.

The editorial board has been involved in producing this book since its inception. They have spent rigorous hours researching and exploring the diverse topics which have resulted in the successful publishing of this book. They have passed on their knowledge of decades through this book. To expedite this challenging task, the publisher supported the team at every step. A small team of assistant editors was also appointed to further simplify the editing procedure and attain best results for the readers.

Apart from the editorial board, the designing team has also invested a significant amount of their time in understanding the subject and creating the most relevant covers. They scrutinized every image to scout for the most suitable representation of the subject and create an appropriate cover for the book.

The publishing team has been an ardent support to the editorial, designing and production team. Their endless efforts to recruit the best for this project,\has resulted in the accomplishment of this book. They are a veteran in the field of academics and their pool of knowledge is as vast as their experience in printing. Their expertise and guidance has proved useful at every step. Their uncompromising quality standards have made this book an exceptional effort. Their encouragement from time to time has been an inspiration for everyone.

The publisher and the editorial board hope that this book will prove to be a valuable piece of knowledge for researchers, students, practitioners and scholars across the globe.

List of Contributors

Brian Oldenburg
School of Population and Global Health, University of Melbourne, Melbourne, Australia

Fiona Cocker
School of Population and Global Health, University of Melbourne, Melbourne, Australia
Menzies Research Institute Tasmania, University of Tasmania, Hobart, Australia

Jan M. Nicholson
Judith Lumley Centre, La Trobe University, Melbourne, Australia

Nicholas Graves
School of Public Health, Queensland University of Technology, Queensland, Australia

Alison Venn, Kristy Sanderson and Andrew J. Palmer
Menzies Research Institute Tasmania, University of Tasmania, Hobart, Australia

Angela Martin
Tasmanian School of Business and Economics, University of Tasmania, Hobart, Australia

Jenn Scott
School of Psychology, University of Tasmania, Hobart, Tasmania, Australia

Eric W. de Heer
TopClinical Center for Body, Mind, and Health, GGz Breburg Tilburg, Tilburg, The Netherlands
Tilburg School of Behavioral and Social Sciences, Tranzo Department, University of Tilburg, Tilburg, The Netherlands

Christina M. van der Feltz-Cornelis
TopClinical Center for Body, Mind, and Health, GGz Breburg Tilburg, Tilburg, The Netherlands
Tilburg School of Behavioral and Social Sciences, Tranzo Department, University of Tilburg, Tilburg, The Netherlands
Trimbos Institute, Utrecht, the Netherlands

Brenda W. J. H. Penninx and Marloes M. J. G. Gerrits
Department of Psychiatry, EMGO Institute for Health and Care research, VU University Medical Centre, Amsterdam, The Netherlands

Aartjan T. F. Beekman
Department of Psychiatry, EMGO Institute for Health and Care research, VU University Medical Centre, Amsterdam, The Netherlands
GGZ inGeest, Mental Health Institute, Amsterdam, The Netherlands

Jack Dekker
Arkin, Mental Health Institute, Amsterdam, The Netherlands
Department of Clinical Psychology, VU University, Amsterdam, The Netherlands

Harm W. J. van Marwijk
Department of General Practice, EMGO Institute for Health and Care Research, VU University Medical Centre, Amsterdam, The Netherlands

Margot W. M. de Waal
Department of Public Health and Primary Care, Leiden university Medical Centre, Leiden, The Netherlands

Philip Spinhoven
Institute of Psychology, Leiden University, Leiden, The Netherlands
Department of Psychiatry, Leiden University Medical Centre, Leiden, The Netherlands

Anna Radkovsky
Department of Clinical Psychology and Psychotherapy, University of Marburg, Marburg, Hesse, Germany

Carolin M. Wirtz
Department of Clinical Psychology and Psychotherapy, University of Marburg, Marburg, Hesse, Germany, Department of Clinical Psychology and Psychotherapy, University of Erlangen- Nuremberg, Erlangen, Baveria, Germany

David D. Ebert
Department of Clinical Psychology and Psychotherapy, University of Marburg, Marburg, Hesse, Germany
Division for Clinical Psychology and Psychotherapy, Department for Psychology, Leuphana University Lueneburg, Lueneburg, Lower Saxony, Germany

Matthias Berking
Department of Clinical Psychology and Psychotherapy, University of Erlangen- Nuremberg, Erlangen, Baveria, Germany

Jiu Chen and Zhijun Zhang
Neurologic Department of Affiliated ZhongDa Hospital, Neuropsychiatric Institute and Medical School of Southeast University, Nanjing, Jiangsu Province, China
Wentao Ma, Yan Zhang, Xingqu Wu, Dunhong Wei, Guangxiong Liu, Zihe Deng and Laiqi Yang

Center for Mental Disease Control and Prevention, Third Hospital of the People's Liberation Army, Baoji, Shaanxi Province, China

Tsukasa Kato
Toyo University, Department of Social Psychology, Bunkyo-ku, Tokyo, Japan

Mohd Fareed and Mohammad Afzal
Human Genetics and Toxicology Laboratory, Section of Genetics, Department of Zoology, Faculty of Life Sciences, Aligarh Muslim University, Aligarh, Uttar Pradesh, India

Carmen K. M. Wong, Dicken C. C. Chan, Samuel Y. S. Wong and Martin C. S. Wong
Division of Family Medicine and Primary Health Care, JC School of Public Health and Primary Care, The Chinese University of Hong Kong, 4/F, School of Public Health building, Prince of Wales Hospital, Shatin, New Territories, Hong Kong SAR

Jun Liang, Man L. Chan, Yin H. Chan, Laam Chan, Kwong Y. Wan and Ming S. Ng
The Hong Kong Primary Care Research Network, F2029A, Special Block, Tuen Mun Hospital, New Territories, Hong Kong SAR

Chih-Chao Hsu and Ti Lu
Department of Psychiatry, Kaohsiung Veterans General Hospital, Kaohsiung, Taiwan

Wan-Shan Lin
Department of Psychiatry, Kaohsiung Veterans General Hospital, Kaohsiung, Taiwan

Li-Yu Hu
Department of Psychiatry, Kaohsiung Veterans General Hospital, Kaohsiung, Taiwan
Institute of Public Health, National Yang-Ming University, Taipei, Taiwan
School of Medicine, National Yang-Ming University, Taipei, Taiwan

Chia-Jen Liu
Institute of Public Health, National Yang-Ming University, Taipei, Taiwan
School of Medicine, National Yang-Ming University, Taipei, Taiwan
Division of Hematology and Oncology, Department of Medicine, Taipei Veterans General Hospital, Taipei, Taiwan

Yen-Po Wang
School of Medicine, National Yang-Ming University, Taipei, Taiwan
Endoscopy Center of Diagnosis and Treatment, Taipei Veterans General Hospital, Taipei, Taiwan
Division of Gastroenterology, Department of Medicine, Taipei Veterans General Hospital, Taipei, Taiwan

Yu-Wen Hu
School of Medicine, National Yang-Ming University, Taipei, Taiwan
Cancer Center, Taipei Veterans General Hospital, Taipei, Taiwan

Chia-Fen Tsai and Tung-Ping Su
School of Medicine, National Yang-Ming University, Taipei, Taiwan
Department of Psychiatry, Taipei Veterans General Hospital, Taipei, Taiwan

Tzeng-Ji Chen
School of Medicine, National Yang-Ming University, Taipei, Taiwan
Department of Family Medicine, Taipei Veterans General Hospital, Taipei, Taiwan

Cheng-Che Shen
Department of Psychiatry, Chiayi Branch, Taichung Veterans General Hospital, Taipei, Taiwan

Chiu-Mei Yeh
Department of Family Medicine, Taipei Veterans General Hospital, Taipei, Taiwan

Pan-Ming Chen
Department of Psychiatry, Su-Ao and Yuanshan Branch, Taipei Veterans General Hospital, Taipei, Taiwan

Masatoshi Suzuki, Michio Takahashi, Katsumasa Muneoka, Koichi Sato and Yukihiko Shirayama
Department of Psychiatry, Teikyo University Chiba Medical Center, Ichihara, Japan

Kenji Hashimoto
Division of Clinical Neuroscience, Chiba University Center for Forensic Mental Health, Chiba, Japan

Matthew S. Stratton, Michelle Staros, Brian T. Searcy, Connor Nash and Chad Eitel
Department of Biomedical Sciences, Colorado State University, Fort Collins, Colorado, United States of America

Stuart A. Tobet
Department of Biomedical Sciences, Colorado State University, Fort Collins, Colorado, United States of America
School of Biomedical Engineering, Colorado State University, Fort Collins, Colorado, United States of America

Gregor Majdic and Tomaz Budefeld
Center for Animal Genomics, Veterinary Faculty, University of Ljubljana, Ljubljana, Slovenia

David Carbone and Robert J. Handa
Department of Basic Medical Sciences, University of Arizona College of Medicine, Phoenix, Arizona, United States of America

Bart P. de Kwaasteniet and Guido A. van Wingen
Department of Psychiatry, Academic Medical Center, Amsterdam, the Netherlands
Brain Imaging Center, Academic Medical Center, Amsterdam, the Netherlands

Damiaan Denys
Department of Psychiatry, Academic Medical Center, Amsterdam, the Netherlands
Brain Imaging Center, Academic Medical Center, Amsterdam, the Netherlands
The Institute for Neuroscience, an institute of the Royal Netherlands Academy of Arts and Sciences, Amsterdam, the Netherlands

Eric H. G. Ruhe´
Department of Psychiatry, Academic Medical Center, Amsterdam, the Netherlands
Brain Imaging Center, Academic Medical Center, Amsterdam, the Netherlands
University of Groningen, University Medical Center Groningen, Mood and Anxiety Disorders, Department of Psychiatry, Groningen, the Netherlands

Jan Booij
Brain Imaging Center, Academic Medical Center, Amsterdam, the Netherlands
Department of Nuclear Medicine, Academic Medical Center, Amsterdam, the Netherlands

Chedwa Pinto
Department of Psychiatry, MC groep, Lelystad, the Netherlands

Peter A. Coventry Linda Gask
Collaboration for Leadership in Applied Health Research and Care, Centre for Primary Care and Manchester Academic Health Science Centre, University of Manchester, Manchester, United Kingdom

Joanna L. Hudson
Health Psychology Section, Psychology Department, Institute of Psychiatry, King's College London, London, United Kingdom

Evangelos Kontopantelis and Peter Bower
NIHR School for Primary Care Research, Centre for Primary Care and Manchester Academic Health Science Centre, University of Manchester, Manchester, United Kingdom

Karina Lovell and Janine Archer
School of Nursing, Midwifery and Social Work, University of Manchester, Manchester, United Kingdom

Chris Dickens and David A. Richards
Institute of Health Service Research, University of Exeter Medical School, University of Exeter, Exeter, United Kingdom

Simon Gilbody
Mental Health Research Group, Department of Health Sciences and Hull York Medical School, University of York, York, United Kingdom

Waquas Waheed
Lancashire Care NHS Foundation Trust, Preston, United Kingdom

Faith Martin and Steve Russell
School of International Development (DEV), University of East Anglia, Norwich, United Kingdom

Janet Seeley
London School of Hygiene and Tropical Medicine, London, United Kingdom
Uganda Research Unit on AIDS, Medical Research Council/Uganda Virus Research Institute, Entebbe, Uganda

Sarah A. Sullivan, Nicola Wiles, Daphne Kounali, Jon Heron and Liam Mahedy
Centre for Academic Mental Health, School of Social and Community Medicine, University of Bristol, Bristol, United Kingdom

Stan Zammit
Centre for Academic Mental Health, School of Social and Community Medicine, University of Bristol, Bristol, United Kingdom
Institute of Psychological Medicine and Clinical Neurosciences, University of Cardiff, Cardiff, United Kingdom

Glyn Lewis
Division of Psychiatry, University College London, London, United Kingdom

Mary Cannon
Department of Psychiatry, Royal College of Surgeons in Ireland, Dublin, Ireland

Peter B. Jones and Jan Stochl
Department of Psychiatry, Cambridge Neuroscience, University of Cambridge, Cambridge, United Kingdom

Lin-Chien Lee
Institute of Brain Science, National Yang-Ming University, Taipei, Taiwan
Department of Physical Medicine and Rehabilitation, Cheng Hsin General Hospital, Taipei, Taiwan
Integrated Brain Research Unit, Division of Clinical Research, Department of Medical Research, Taipei Veterans General Hospital, Taipei, Taiwan

Li-Fen Chen and Jen-Chuen Hsieh
Institute of Brain Science, National Yang-Ming University, Taipei, Taiwan
Integrated Brain Research Unit, Division of Clinical Research, Department of Medical Research, Taipei Veterans General Hospital, Taipei, Taiwan

Cheng-Hao Tu
Institute of Brain Science, National Yang-Ming University, Taipei, Taiwan
Integrated Brain Research Unit, Division of Clinical Research, Department of Medical Research, Taipei Veterans General Hospital, Taipei, Taiwan
Department of Education and Research, Taipei City Hospital, Taipei, Taiwan

Horng-Der Shen
Division of Basic Research, Department of Medical Research, Taipei Veterans General Hospital, Taipei, Taiwan

Ming-Wei Lin
Division of Basic Research, Department of Medical Research, Taipei Veterans General Hospital, Taipei, Taiwan
Institute of Public Health, National Yang-Ming University, Taipei, Taiwan

Hsiang-Tai Chao
Department of Obstetrics and Gynecology, Taipei Veterans General Hospital, Taipei, Taiwan
Department of Obstetrics and Gynecology, Faculty of Medicine, School of Medicine, National Yang-Ming University, Taipei, Taiwan

John A. Naslund
The Dartmouth Institute for Health Policy and Clinical Practice, Dartmouth College, Hanover, New Hampshire, United States of America

Glyn Elwyn
The Dartmouth Institute for Health Policy and Clinical Practice, Dartmouth College, Hanover, New Hampshire, United States of America
The Dartmouth Center for Health Care Delivery Science, Dartmouth College, Hanover, New Hampshire, United States of America

Kelly A. Aschbrenner
The Dartmouth Institute for Health Policy and Clinical Practice, Dartmouth College, Hanover, New Hampshire, United States of America
Department of Psychiatry, Geisel School of Medicine at Dartmouth, Hanover, New Hampshire, United States of America

Stuart W. Grande
The Dartmouth Center for Health Care Delivery Science, Dartmouth College, Hanover, New Hampshire, United States of America

Kadir Özdel, Seher Olga Guriz, Riza Gö kcer Tulaci and Erkan Kuru
Diskapi Yildirim Beyazit Teaching and Research Hospital, Department of Psychiatry, Ankara, Turkey

Ibrahim Taymur
Sevket Yilmaz Teaching and Research Hospital, Department of Psychiatry, Bursa, Turkey

Mehmet Hakan Turkcapar
Hasan Kalyoncu University, Department of Psychology, Istanbul, Turkey

Martine M. Veehof and Ernst T. Bohlmeijer
University of Twente, Department of Psychology, Health and Technology, Enschede, the Netherlands

Wendy T. M. Pots
University of Twente, Department of Psychology, Health and Technology, Enschede, the Netherlands
Dimence, Community Mental Health Center, Almelo, the Netherlands

Peter A. M. Meulenbeek
University of Twente, Department of Psychology, Health and Technology, Enschede, the Netherlands
GGNET, Community Mental Health Center, Warnsveld, the Netherlands

Jorinde Klungers
GGNET, Community Mental Health Center, Warnsveld, the Netherlands

Cheng-Ho Chang and Li-Yu Hu
Department of Psychiatry, Kaohsiung Veterans General Hospital, Kaohsiung, Taiwan
Shu-Li Wang
Department of Dental Laboratory Technology, Central Taiwan University of Science and Technology, Taichung, Taiwan

Shih-Jen Tsai
Department of Psychiatry, Taipei Veterans General Hospital, Taipei, Taiwan
School of Medicine, National Yang-Ming University, Taipei, Taiwan

Albert C. Yang
Department of Psychiatry, Taipei Veterans General Hospital, Taipei, Taiwan
School of Medicine, National Yang-Ming University, Taipei, Taiwan
Center for Dynamical Biomarkers and Translational Medicine, National Central University, Chungli, Taiwan

Zi-Hong You
Division of Nephrology, Department of Internal Medicine, Taichung Veterans General Hospital, Chia-Yi Branch, Chia-Yi, Taiwan
Institute of Medicine, Chung Shan Medical University, Taichung, Taiwan

Miyeon Choi
Department of Biochemistry and Molecular Biology, College of Medicine, Hanyang University, Seoul, Korea

Yong-Seok Kim and Hyeon Son
Department of Biochemistry and Molecular Biology, College of Medicine, Hanyang University, Seoul, Korea
Graduate School of Biomedical Science and Engineering, Hanyang University, Seoul, Korea

Sung Eun Wang, Seung Yeon Ko, Seung Yeun Chae and Seung Hoon Lee
Graduate School of Biomedical Science and Engineering, Hanyang University, Seoul, Korea

Hyo Jung Kang
Department of Life Science, Chung-Ang University, Seoul, Korea

Ronald S. Duman
Laboratory of Molecular Psychiatry, Center for Genes and Behavior, Departments of Psychiatry, Neurobiology, and Laboratory Medicine, Yale University School of Medicine, New Haven, Connecticut, United States of America

Hsuan-Ming Tsao
Division of Cardiology, Department of Internal Medicine, National Yang-Ming University Hospital, Yilan, Taiwan
Department of Medicine, School of Medicine, National Yang-Ming University, Taipei, Taiwan

Nai-Wei Hsu
Division of Cardiology, Department of Internal Medicine, National Yang-Ming University Hospital, Yilan, Taiwan
Department of Medicine, School of Medicine, National Yang-Ming University, Taipei, Taiwan
Community Medicine Research Center and Institute of Public Health, National Yang-Ming University, Taipei, Taiwan

Hsi-Chung Chen
Department of Psychiatry and Center of Sleep Disorders, National Taiwan University Hospital, Taipei, Taiwan

Pesus Chou
Community Medicine Research Center and Institute of Public Health, National Yang-Ming University, Taipei, Taiwan

Steven Bell, Annie Britton and Martin Bobak
Research Department of Epidemiology and Public Health, University College London, London, United Kingdom

Ruzena Kubinova
National Institute of Public Health, Prague, Czech Republic

Yuri Nikitin
Institute of Internal and Preventive Medicine, Novosibirsk, Russia

Sofia Malyutina
Institute of Internal and Preventive Medicine, Novosibirsk, Russia
Novosibirsk State Medical University, Novosibirsk, Russia

Andrzej Pajak
Institute of Public Health, Jagiellonian University, Krakow, Poland

Index

R

S

T

W